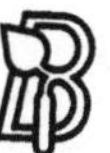

Series Editor

Michael J. Parnham
PLIVA
Research Institute
Prilaz baruna Filipovica 25
1000 Zagreb
Croatia

T Cells in Arthritis

Pierre Miossec
Wim B. van den Berg
Gary S. Firestein

Editors

Springer Basel AG

Editors

Prof. Pierre Miossec
University Claude Bernard
Departments of Immunology and Rheumatology
Hôpital Edouard Herriot
F-69437 Lyon Cedex 03
France

Prof. Dr. Wim B. van den Berg
Department of Rheumatology
University Hospital Nijmegen
Geert Grooteplein 8
NL-6525 Nijmegen
The Netherlands

Prof. Gary S. Firestein
Division of Rheumatology
UCSD School of Medicine
9500 Gilman Drive
San Diego, CA 92093-0656
USA

A CIP catalogue record for this book is available from the Library of Congress, Washington D.C., USA

Deutsche Bibliothek Cataloging-in-Publication Data
T cells in arthritis / ed. by Pierre Miossec ... - Basel ; Boston ;
Berlin : Birkhäuser, 1998
(Progress in inflammation research)
ISBN 978-3-0348-9787-7 ISBN 978-3-0348-8823-3 (eBook)
DOI 10.1007/978-3-0348-8823-3

Cover illustration: Immunostaining of a T cell producing IL-17 in the rheumatoid synovium. (From J.M. Durand and P. Miossec)

The publisher and editor can give no guarantee for the information on drug dosage and administration contained in this publication. The respective user must check its accuracy by consulting other sources of reference in each individual case.

Originally published by Birkhäuser Verlag in 1998
Softcover reprint of the hardcover 1st edition 1998

Printed on acid-free paper produced from chlorine-free pulp. TCF ∞
Cover design: Markus Etterich, Basel
ISBN 978-3-0348-9787-7

9 8 7 6 5 4 3 2 1

Contents

List of contributors vii

Preface ix

Katherine H.Y. Nguyen and Gary S. Firestein
T cells as secondary players in rheumatoid arthritis 1

David A. Fox and Nora G. Singer
T cell receptor rearrangements in arthritis 19

Juliane K. Franz, Thomas Pap, Ulf Müller-Ladner, Renate E. Gay, Gerd R. Burmester and Steffen Gay
T cell-independent joint destruction 55

Wim B. van den Berg
Role of T cells in arthritis: Lessons from animal models 75

Pierre Miossec
The Th1/Th2 cytokine balance in arthritis 93

Danielle Burger and Jean-Michel Dayer
Interactions between T cell plasma membranes and monocytes 111

Nancy Oppenheimer-Marks and Peter E. Lipsky
Adhesion molecules in arthritis: Control of T cell migration into the synovium 129

Marc Bonneville, Emmanuel Scotet, Marie-Alix Peyrat, Annick Lim, Jacques David-Ameline and Elisabeth Houssaint
T cell reactivity to Epstein-Barr virus in rheumatoid arthritis 149

Joachim Sieper and Jürgen Braun
T cell responses in reactive and Lyme arthritis 169

Ferdinand C. Breedveld
T cell directed therapies and biologics 189

Michael T. Falta and Brian L. Kotzin
T cells as primary players in rheumatoid arthritis 201

Index 233

List of contributors

Marc Bonneville, INSERM U463, Institut de Biologie, 9 quai Moncousu, F-44035 Nantes Cedex 01, France; e-mail: bonnevil@nantes.inserm.fr

Jürgen Braun, Department of Medicine, Division of Nephrology and Rheumatology, Klinikum Benjamin Franklin, Free University, Hindenburgdamm 30, D-12200 Berlin, Germany; e-mail: jbraun@zedat.fu-berlin.de

Ferdinand C. Breedveld, Leiden University Medical Center, Department of Rheumatology, C4-R, P.O.Box 9600, NL-2300 RC Leiden, The Netherlands; e-mail: F.C.Breedveld@Rheumatology.MedFac.LeidenUniv.nl

Danielle Burger, Division of Immunology and Allergy, Hans Wilsdorf Laboratory, University Hospital, 24 rue Micheli-du-Crest, CH-1211 Geneva 14, Switzerland; e-mail: danielle.burger@hcuge.ch

Gerd R. Burmester, Department of Rheumatology and Clinical Immunology, Charité University Hospital, Humboldt University of Berlin, Department of Rheumatology and Clinical Immunology, Schumannstr. 20-21, D-10117 Berlin, Germany

Jacques David-Ameline, INSERM U463, Institut de Biologie, 9 quai Moncousu, F-44035 Nantes Cedex 01, France

Jean-Michel Dayer, Division of Immunology and Allergy, Hans Wilsdorf Laboratory, University Hospital, 24 rue Micheli-du-Crest, CH-1211 Geneva 14, Switzerland; e-mail: jmda@diogenes.hcuge.ch

Gary S. Firestein, Division of Rheumatology, #0656, UCSD School of Medicine, 9500 Gilman Drive, La Jolla, CA 92093-0656, USA; e-mail: gfirestein@ucsd.edu

Michael T. Falta, Division of Basic Sciences, National Jewish Medical and Research Center, 1400 Jackson Street, Denver, CO 80206, USA; e-mail: faltam@njc.org

David A. Fox, Division of Rheumatology, Specialized Center of Research in Rheumatoid Arthritis and Multipurpose Arthritis and Musculoskeletal Diseases Center, University of Michigan, 3918 Taubman Center, Ann Arbor, MI 48109-0358, USA; e-mail: dfox@umich.edu

Juliane K. Franz, Center of Experimental Rheumatology, Department of Rheumatology, University Hospital Zürich, Gloriastr. 25, CH-8091 Zürich, Switzerland; and Department of Rheumatology and Clinical Immunology, Charité University Hospital, Humboldt University of Berlin, Schumannstr. 20–21, D-10117 Berlin, Germany

Renate E. Gay, Center of Experimental Rheumatology, Department of Rheumatology, University Hospital Zürich, Gloriastr. 25, CH-8091 Zürich, Switzerland; e-mail: ruzgar@ruz.unizh.ch

Steffen Gay, Center of Experimental Rheumatology, Department of Rheumatology, University Hospital Zürich, Gloriastr. 25, CH-8091 Zürich, Switzerland; e-mail: ruzgay@ruz.unizh.ch

Elisabeth Houssaint, INSERM U463, Institut de Biologie, 9 quai Moncousu, F-44035 Nantes Cedex 01, France

Brian L. Kotzin, Division of Basic Sciences, National Jewish Medical and Research Center, 1400 Jackson Street, Denver, CO 80206; and Departments of Medicine and Immunology, University of Colorado Health Sciences Center, 4200 East Ninth Avenue, Denver, CO 80262, USA; e-mail: Kotzinb@njc.org

Annick Lim, INSERM U277, Institut Pasteur, 25, rue du Dr. Roux, F-75724 Paris, France

Peter E. Lipsky, Rheumatic Diseases Division of The Depatment of Internal Medicine, The University of Texas Southwestern Medical School, 5323 Harry Hines Blvd., Dallas, TX 75235-3577, USA; e-mail: PLipsky@mednet.swmed.edu

Pierre Miossec, Clinical Immunology Unit, Departments of Immunology and Rheumatology, Hôpital Edouard Herriot, F-69437 Lyon Cedex 03, France; e-mail: miossec@cimac-res.univ-lyon1.fr

Ulf Müller-Ladner, Center of Experimental Rheumatology, Department of Rheumatology, University Hospital, Zürich, Gloriastr. 25, CH-8091 Zürich, Switzerland; and Department of Internal Medicine, Division of Rheumatology and Clinical Immunology, University of Regensburg, Franz-Josef-Strauss-Allee 11, D-93042 Regensburg, Germany

Nancy Oppenheimer-Marks, Rheumatic Diseases Division of The Depatment of Internal Medicine, The University of Texas Southwestern Medical School, 5323 Harry Hines Blvd., Dallas, TX 75235-3577, USA;
e-mail: PLipsky@mednet.swmed.edu

Katherine H.Y. Nguyen, Division of Rheumatology, #0656, UCSD School of Medicine, 9500 Gilman Drive, La Jolla, CA 92093-0656, USA;
e-mail: knguyen@ucsd.edu

Thomas Pap, Center of Experimental Rheumatology, Department of Rheumatology, University Hospital Zürich, Gloriastr. 25, CH-8091 Zürich, Switzerland;
e-mail: ruzpat@unizh.ch

Marie-Alix Peyrat, INSERM U463, Institut de Biologie, 9 quai Moncousu, F-44035 Nantes Cedex 01, France

Emmanuel Scotet, INSERM U463, Institut de Biologie, 9 quai Moncousu, F-44035 Nantes Cedex 01, France

Joachim Sieper, Department of Medicine, Division of Nephrology and Rheumatology, Klinikum Benjamin Franklin, Free University, Hindenburgdamm 30, D-12200 Berlin, Germany; e-mail: hjsieper@zedat.fu-berlin.de

Nora G. Singer, Department of Internal Medicine Division of Rheumatic Diseases, Case Western Reserve University Medical School, 11100 Rainbow Babies & Childrens Hospital, Cleveland, OH 44106, USA

Wim B. van den Berg, Dept. of Rheumatology, University Hospital Nijmegen, Geert Grooteplein 8, NL-6500 HB Nijmegen, The Netherlands;
e-mail: w.vandenberg@reuma.azn.nl

Preface

The pathogenesis of rheumatoid arthritis (RA) has been the subject of intense scrutiny for several decades. The prevailing hypotheses have changed over the years, and have attempted to incorporate the most recent data. The first major clue to an immune-mediated process was the discovery that an autoantibody, i.e. rheumatoid factor, was associated with the disease. This led to the simple assumption that antibody responses to a defined antigen were responsible for articular inflammation.

However, the complexity of RA soon led to alternative paradigms, and the "immune complex" model, which invoked intra-articular activation of complement by rheumatoid factor-containing complexes, reconciled some of these problems.

The 1980's ushered in the era of the T cell. The molecular events involved with antigen recognition, T cell response, cytokine production, and chronic inflammation led to the hypothesis that cell-mediated (rather than antigen-mediated) processes orchestrated synovial immune responses. Once again, this attractive model represented an over-simplification of the incredibly complex interactions between cells in the rheumatoid synovium.

Recent data on cytokine profiles, the role of macrophages, and partial transformation of fibroblast-like synoviocytes have raised some questions about this model. Nevertheless, compelling evidence supports at least some (and perhaps most) of the key conclusions.

The goal of this book is to outline the major arguments and data suggesting that T cells may, or may not, be central players in the pathogenesis of chronic RA. While each of the editors has his own bias (as will be clear by reading the respective chapters), our hope is that the readers will enjoy a complete and balanced view of the critical questions and experiments. This is not just an intellectual exercise; a great deal is at stake when considering these important questions. Most significant, the direction of future therapeutic interventions depends heavily on how one interprets the pathogenesis of RA.

Considerable time and resources need to be devoted to these interventions. Should they be focused on eliminating articular T cells, or enhancing T cell function (especially Th2 cells)? Should T cell approaches be abandoned in order to focus on the cytokine-producing macrophages or the metalloproteinase-producing fibroblasts? If synoviocytes are partially transformed, will this depend on T cell-dependent processes? Are synoviocytes truly transformed aggressors, passively responders, or a combination of both?

These questions will not be fully answered in this book. However, the reader will have the opportunity to arrive at his or her own conclusions and devote their time and effort towards that particular end.

We would like to thank all the contributors for their invaluable input. Such response to be on time is for us a sign of friendship which we are most grateful for. This extends to Katrin Serries, Janine Kern and others at Birkhäuser Publishing.

Pierre Miossec
Wim van den Berg
Gary S. Firestein

T cells as secondary players in rheumatoid arthritis

Katherine H.Y. Nguyen and Gary S. Firestein

Division of Rheumatology, UCSD School of Medicine, 9500 Gilman Drive, La Jolla, CA 92093, USA

Rheumatoid arthritis (RA) is a chronic inflammatory disease that affects about 1% of the general population worldwide [1]. The pathogenesis of RA remains a subject of debate, and many paradigms have been proposed and disputed over the years. The concept of autoimmunity in RA appeared in the 1940's when it was first appreciated that self-reacting antibodies (rheumatoid factors) are present in the blood of most patients with RA [2]. Subsequently, advances in immunological techniques established the framework for the "extravascular immune complex" hypothesis in the early 1970's [3–5]. This theory speculated that the inflammatory response in RA is initiated by the local production of rheumatoid factors and/or antibody directed against an undefined antigen. This, in turn, leads to complement fixation and generation of chemotactic molecules that attract polymorphonuclear leukocytes into joints. Hydrolytic enzymes contained within lysozomal granules are then released during phagocytosis of immune complexes and mediate the destructive process in the RA joint [6]. However, many questions remain unanswered by this model, especially mechanisms of synoviocyte invasion into articular cartilage.

T cells were subsequently recognized as critical players in the initiation and perpetuation of RA in part because: (1) histopathology of RA resembles a local immune response with an exuberant T cell infiltrate; and (2) RA is exquisitely associated with critical amino acid sequences in the human leukocyte antigen-D (HLA-D) locus (see Tab. 1). These observations formed the basis of the "T cell" hypothesis and provided the rationale for many experimental studies and therapeutic trials during the past two decades. Initial success in open trials using anti-T cell antibodies lent further credence to this model. However, evidence accumulated during the last 10 years raised some questions about the putative role of T cells in established RA. This review will focus on some of these controversial issues and explore alternative hypotheses that explain the perpetuation of RA.

It has generally been assumed that T lymphocytes are a crucial component of the early rheumatoid response. Histopathological studies of RA reveal an abundance of T cells, which comprise about 30–50% of synovial tissue cells. The predominant T cell subset in the sublining of RA patients is the $CD4^+$ helper/inducer lymphocyte

T Cells in Arthritis, edited by P. Miossec, W.B. van den Berg and G.S. Firestein

Table 1 – The role of T cells in rheumatoid arthritis (RA)

Evidence supporting the central role of T cells in chronic RA
• Histopathology of RA synovium reveals abundance of T cells
• Majority of T cells display markers of prior activation
• Strong linkage with specific class II MHC molecules
• Many experimental animal models of arthritis are T cell-dependent
• Modest efficacy of anti-T cell therapy

Evidence that does not support a central role of T cells in chronic RA
• Incomplete response to anti-T cell therapy despite marked immunosuppression
• Synovial T cells are already hyporesponsive
• Relative deficiency of T cell lymphokines in the joint
• No specific etiologic antigen identified
• Disease can progress despite co-existent AIDS
• Independent inflammatory and destructive processes

and the CD4/CD8 ratio ranges from 4:1 to 14:1. The T cell infiltrate is generally organized in two patterns. The first pattern consists of aggregates of lymphocytes which contain up to several hundred T cells in the sublining, especially near blood vessels. The number of aggregates varies widely among patients and ranges from a few scattered aggregates to the complete replacement of sublining areas by many organized lymphoid collections. A second pattern is characterized by diffuse T cell infiltration immediately below the synovial lining without obvious organization. In some patients, the sublining has a sparse lymphocytic infiltrate in a fibrotic extracellular matrix.

The majority of sublining lymphocytes display markers of prior activation, including CD45RO, CD27, VLA-4, VLA-1, VLA-5, and HLA class II molecules [7–9]. However, it is not at all certain whether these cells are activated *in situ* or arrive at the joint and are subsequently stimulated. Immunohistochemistry studies to look for evidence of cell division using cell-cycle specific, nuclear antigens Ki67 and proliferating cell nuclear antigen (PCNA) suggest only a low rate of cell division [10, 11]. Only rare cells incorporate tritiated thymidine and these are generally of the $CD8^+$ subset [12]. More likely, the synovial lymphocyte infiltration results from increased recruitment from the blood in combination with decreased apoptosis. The phenotype observed for synovial resident T cells matches that of cells which are preferentially recruited from peripheral blood by the activated endothelium of RA synovium and does not necessarily reflect local activation [13]. Furthermore, high expression of bcl-2 in T cells blocks cell death and probably contributes to local lymphocyte accumulation [14]. It is important to remember, however, that only a small percentage of activated or proliferating T cells might be required to orchestrate a synovial immune response.

Perhaps the most compelling evidence for the importance of antigen-specific responses is the association of RA with specific HLA-DR molecules, which are known to participate in antigen recognition and processing. In 1978, Stastny provided evidence that RA was associated with an antigen of the HLA-D locus, specifically the HLA-Dw4 allele [15]. Since then, a large number of population studies in diverse ethnic groups have documented the association of DR4 and Dw4 with classic and definite RA [16]. The disease-associated DRB1 allelic variants share a conserved sequence homology (QKRAA) that has been mapped to position 67–74 in the third hypervariable region (HVR) of the HLA-DRB1 gene [17]. This observation forms the basis for the "shared-epitope" hypothesis in which cross reactivity between the QKRAA motif and an arthritogenic antigen could lead to an antigen specific T cell response directed towards HLA-DR molecules.

Despite the simple elegance of this antigen-specific model, there are a number of caveats that should be recognized. First, unique peptides that are displayed selectively by RA-associated DRB1 molecules have not been identified by isolating and sequencing a repertoire of peptides displayed by each major histocompatibility complex (MHC) allele. This contrasts with other autoimmune diseases such as autoimmune thyroiditis or diabetes where pathogenic autoantigens appear to have been identified [18, 19]. Second, the specific amino acids 67–74 border the antigen binding groove of HLA-DR and are theoretically responsible for antigen binding specificity. Hence, individuals with this haplotype might efficiently present an arthritogenic epitope and be more susceptible to RA. A recent study by Penzotti and colleagues suggests that this is not necessarily the case [20]. Using molecular model building techniques, they found direct interactions via hydrogen bonds between β-chain residues Q70 and R71 and T cell receptor (TCR) CDR3bQ97 of the T cell clone EM025. This leads to recognition of DRB1*0404 itself and suggests that the interaction is peptide-independent. Therefore, the QKRAA amino acids, which are mainly directed away from the binding cleft, can regulate T cell responses without the involvement of an arthritogenic peptide.

In addition, some data support the role of DR4-positive RA-associated alleles as a severity rather than a susceptibility gene. If HLA-DR linkage of disease susceptibility is a function of recognition of an arthritogenic peptide, possession of a single copy of the disease-associated HLA-DR molecule should be a sufficient risk factor for developing RA. However, many normal individuals carry the QKRAA motif and do not develop RA; and conversely, newly-diagnosed community-based patients with RA demonstrate no increase in DR4 frequency [21]. Using antigen genotype frequency, the distribution of shared-epitope DRB-1 alleles among RA patients in population-based studies predicted a recessive mode of inheritance whereas an additive (dominant) mode was rejected [22, 23].

A number of studies have demonstrated that the cumulative gene dosage effect of susceptibility alleles may correlate with the severity of RA [24–26]. Weyand and colleagues have shown that the second HLA-DRB1 allele in HLA-DR4 patients correlates with disease severity, as defined by extra-articular manifestations and the necessity for joint surgery. In this study, 100% of patients who inherited two DRB*04 genes had rheumatoid nodules compared to 59% of patients with only one gene [26]. Major organ involvement was observed in 61% and 11% of these patients, respectively. These data suggest a "dose response" effect of the HLA genes and imply that severity, rather than susceptibility, is a major contribution of HLA-DR to the disease.

Alternative explanations for the existence of a strong genetic association between RA and HLA-D genes have been proposed. First, the correlation between disease manifestations and HLA-DRB1 alleles might reflect the influence of HLA-DQ alleles in linkage disequilibrium with DR4. For example, DQw7 has been cited as an important marker gene in RA [27]. The concept that the HLA-DRB1 locus is associated with protection from RA and that the actual arthritogenic peptide-presenting molecule is HLA-DQ was proposed by Zanelli and David [28]. This was based on the observation that the presentation of type II collagen peptide by the H-2Aq molecule (equivalent to DQB1) determined the susceptibility to collagen arthritis, but polymorphic expression of the functional H-2Eb gene (equivalent to DRB1) conferred protection. Perhaps the DQ/DR haplotype is responsible for RA predisposition in humans and the polymorphism of the HLA-DR4 allele determines the degree of protection. This observation is supported by the fact that HLA-DQB1*0302 (DQw8) and HLA-DQB1*0301 (DQw7) are in linkage disequilibrium with most DR4 haplotypes and most HLA-DR4$^+$ RA patients express one of these alleles [29].

To demonstrate that the molecular basis for this protection is through the presentation of DRB1 HV3 peptide by RA-associated DQ molecules, Zanelli and colleagues constructed a DQ8.Ab^0 transgenic mouse model expressing a functional DQB1*0302/DQA1*0301 dimeric molecule in the absence of endogenous mouse class II molecules [30]. These mice were immunized with a series of DRB1 HV3 peptides corresponding to most HLA-DRB1 alleles, and in vitro T cell responses against the immunizing peptides were assessed. While HV3 peptides derived from non-associated DRB1 molecules were highly immunogenic in DQ8 transgenic mice, the HV3 peptides derived from RA-associated DRB1 alleles failed to induce a DQ8-restricted T cell response.

The shared-epitope in RA might therefore shape the T cell repertoire with positive selection of potentially autoreactive T cells due to unsuccessful presentation of the disease-associated DRB1 peptide by DQ8. HLA molecules have served as ligands for immature T cells and are critically involved in thymic education processes

[31]. Current thinking suggests that the importance of the shared-epitope is related to the way in which the HLA-DR-antigen complex is presented to T cells and is ultimately responsible for shaping T cell repertoire, rather than to binding of a specific antigen in the DR molecule groove [32]. There are no data to show that antigen recognition would be enhanced by possession of two HLA-DR alleles. However, peptide selection during thymus education could be greatly affected since the density of MHC molecules critically influences positive selection processes in the thymic environment [33]. While these studies certainly do not obviate a role for HLA-DR and T cells, they do suggest that the traditional T cell hypotheses in RA are simplistic.

An alternative approach to demonstrating local T cell activation involves determining T cell receptor gene utilization. Selective increases in specific T cell genes in the synovium might support the concept of local T cell expansion. This approach has successfully implicated T cells in a variety of immune-mediated diseases in humans and in animal models. For instance, specific Vβ and Vα gene segments are preferentially used in rodent experimental-allergic encephalomyelitis and collagen-induced arthritis models [34, 35]. Numerous studies have attempted to define specific T cell receptor gene utilization in RA patients, with conflicting results. TCR gene usage has been examined in synovial fluid, synovial tissue, and peripheral blood. Several studies have found variable usage of different Vα or Vβ family, but a pattern appears to be emerging that suggests an increased number of T cells express Vβ3, 14, and 17, especially in synovial tissue [36–39]. These particular Vβ genes are structurally related and are susceptible to activation by superantigens. This supports the hypothesis that specific T cells can be activated by bacterial or mycoplasma superantigens, leading to oligoclonal expansion and release of cytokines. Many studies, however, have not found evidence for restricted clonality of T cells in RA samples [40, 41].

In any case, the approach to study TCR gene usage or clonality may be doomed to failure in long standing disease due to "antigen-spread" or responses to secondary or irrelevant antigens. In animal models of autoimmunity, one must look at the earliest stages to identify relevant T cell receptor genes because the analysis becomes hopelessly complex within days. Study of the experimental allergic encephalitis model in rats in the early phase has identified a strong bias in the central nervous system for a few antigen-specific pathogenic TCR genes [42]. As the disease progresses, this bias is rapidly overwhelmed by the continued influx of non-specific cells recruited into the brain by chemokines and adhesion molecules.

Among the most interesting question facing a T cell driven model is why T cell products such as interferon (IFN)-γ, interleukin (IL)-4, or IL-2 are present in such low amounts in the inflamed joint. The first studies of cytokines in rheumatic disease were reported in the late 1970's when IFN bioassays were performed on serum and synovial effusions of patients with RA. Using viral cytopathic protection assays, high titers of IFN-like activity were identified [43]. The presence of IFN-γ activity in these samples appeared to confirm its putative role in inflammatory synovitis. At the time, IFN-γ was the only cytokine known to induce HLA-DR expression on cells, and high expression of this marker on many kinds of synovial cells is a cardinal finding of RA. The detection of IFN-γ in joint samples was not surprising and seemed to explain the elevated class II MHC antigen expression. However, these bioassays were later found to lack specificity and also detected non-IFN factors (like tumor necrosis factor (TNF) and IL-6) [44].

Specific immunoassays were subsequently used to help clarify the question of how much IFN-γ is in the inflamed joint. Only small amounts of immunoreactive IFN-γ (generally less than 0.2 U/ml) were detected in the joint effusions of patients with RA and in frozen sections of synovial tissue [45]. The difficulty detecting IFN-γ in RA did not appear to be due to methodological problems since it was easily measured in other diseases known to be mediated by T cells, such as tuberculous pleuritis [46]. Moreover, functional studies showed that the HLA-DR-inducing activity in joint samples was not neutralized by anti-IFN-γ activity. Later, macrophage-derived granulocyte-macrophage colony-stimulating factor (GM-CSF), not IFN-γ, was determined to be the major HLA-DR-inducing activation factor in the joint [47]. Similar observations were seen for other T cell products like IL-2, TNF-beta, and IL-4 [48, 49]. The concentrations detected using sensitive methods like reverse transcription-polymerase chain reaction (RT-PCR), when present, are very low. Normally, one might expect antigen presentation and T cell activation to be accompanied by the production of T cell cytokines. The question in RA is whether the trace amounts present are sufficient to feed the chronic inflammatory response. One possible exception is the recently described cytokine IL-17. This factor appears to be produced by synovial T cells and can mimic many activities of macrophage-derived IL-1 [50].

There are a number of potential explanations for the relatively low levels of T cell products in RA. For instance, the cytokines are produced in the microenvironment and can be present in functionally active concentrations that are too low to detect. An example of this phenomenon is the nonobese diabetic (NOD) mouse model, where systemic administration of antibodies to IFN-γ leads to amelioration of glucose intolerance even though only small amounts of IFN-γ are produced by islet cells [51]. Second, ultrastructural studies of RA synovium show that T lymphocytes interdigitate with HLA-DR-positive antigen-presenting cells, suggesting the importance of cell-to-cell contact [52]. Such membrane interactions can be functionally very important. For instance, transgenic mice over-expressing membrane-bound TNF on T cells develop severe inflammatory arthritis [53]. In addition, membrane interactions between T cells and fibroblasts can also regulate collagenase production. These data suggest that T cell cytokines can play a role even if they are not released into the synovial milieu as soluble proteins.

It is also possible that suppressive factors such as transforming growth factor (TGF)-β, IL-1Ra, or IL-10 down-regulate T cell cytokine production [54, 55]. This possibility is supported by studies demonstrating that neutralizing anti-IL-10 antibodies sometimes increase endogenous IFN-γ production by cultured synovial cells [56]. Finally, RA synovial T cells exhibit functional disability. These T cells respond poorly to cytokines and mitogenic stimulation. T cells in synovial fluid also do not respond normally in the autologous mixed leukocyte reaction (AMLR) [57]. Proliferative responses of RA peripheral blood T cells to phytohemagglutinin-P or anti-CD3 were impaired and correlated with the reduction of early intracellular calcium levels [58]. This hyporesponsive state of synovial T cells in RA might be due to impaired TCR-mediated signal transduction. Maurice and colleagues have shown that tyrosine phosphorylation of the TCR zeta chain, one of the most proximal events in TCR signaling, is diminished in RA synovial fluid T cells [59]. In addition, the decrease in tyrosine phosphorylation was accompanied by a decrease in zeta protein concentration. Finally, the important role of an altered redox state in T cell hyporesponsiveness has been suggested based on the observation that restoration of the intracellular glutathion (GSH) level enhanced mitogen-induced proliferative responses and IL-2 production in RA synovial fluid T cells [60].

While the products of T cell activation are difficult to detect in RA, an interesting alternative view for the role of T cells suggests that relative deficiency of specific T cell subsets actually contributes to synovial inflammation. The concept that T cells possess distinct subsets was first demonstrated in mice where T cell clones have at least two different cytokine profiles [61]. The Th1 subset produces IFN-γ and IL-2 whereas the Th2 phenotype produces IL-4, IL-5, and IL-10. Th1 and Th2 cells mediate distinct functions of the immune system. The former primarily regulates cytotoxicity and delayed-type hypersensitivity reactions [62–64]. The latter regulates antibody production and isotype switching and is more prominent in allergic responses [65, 66]. In most animal models of autoimmune disease, Th1 overactivity predominates while Th2 cytokines mediate disease suppression [67]. For example, IFN-γ and Th1 cells appear to be critical in collagen-induced arthritis in mice. Administration of anti-IFN-γ antibody early in the disease markedly reduces severity, while treatment with recombinant IFN-γ increases inflammation [68]. In contrast, IL-4 and IL-10 treatment ameliorates arthritis [69].

Although the precise role of Th1 and Th2 cells in RA has not been elucidated, the small amounts of T cell cytokines present are biased toward the Th1 phenotype [70]. *In situ* hybridization studies have detected a small amount of IFN-γ in the rheumatoid synovium and its mRNA can sometimes be identified using RT-PCR [71–73]. In contrast, Th2 cytokines (especially IL-4 and IL-13) are undetectable in the joint, even using sensitive techniques like nested RT-PCR [48]. Some IL-10 is present, but it is derived mainly from macrophages and the amount is not sufficient to suppress Th1 cytokine production [56]. Thus, the relative lack of Th2 cytokines in RA relative to Th1 cytokines may very well contribute to the pathogenesis of rheumatoid synovitis. Increasing Th2 cell activity could have beneficial effects by suppressing Th1 cells.

The fact that therapeutic interventions aimed at T cells have met with moderate success argues against a central role for T cells in chronic RA. For instance, only 25–30% of patients have a 50% response to cyclosporin even though this drug is an effective therapy for allogeneic transplantation [74]. Therapeutic strategies employing anti-CD4, anti-CD5, and anti-CDw52 antibodies have also been disappointing, despite severe and persistent lymphopenia [75–77]. In an open-label study using monoclonal antibody specific for CDw52 antigen, no change in the degree of infiltrating T cells in synovial tissue was observed in treated or control RA patients despite significant peripheral lymphopenia, suggesting that the lack of local depletion accounted for the clinical findings [78]. Perhaps this is due to the relative sparing of the memory T cell subset and the inability to lower T cell numbers below a certain threshold required for improvement. However, marked synovial T cell depletion has been observed after anti-CD4 treatment despite a lack of clinical efficacy [79]. An excellent example of "anti-T cell therapy" occurred in patients with AIDS who developed profound CD4 lymphopenia. Although the inflammatory aspect of the disease was ameliorated, histopathological and immunohistological examination of the joints at autopsy demonstrated continued cartilage destruction in the absence of T cells [80].

In light of the relative lack of T cell products in the joint, persistent T cell hyporesponsiveness, and the incomplete clinical response to therapy targeted at T cells, it is reasonable to reevaluate the T cell dogma. This does not necessarily undermine the likely contribution of T cells in the initial stages of RA, but rather suggests that we reconsider the complexity of the synovial response in chronic disease. A variety of hypotheses that potentially explain persistent synovial inflammation have been postulated (see Tab. 2). For instance, one obvious possibility is that an infectious agent such as a retrovirus or lentivirus infects synovial cells and alters local cell function. This situation has been described in the caprine encephalomyelitis-arthritis model [81]. Despite valiant efforts, however, similar infectious agents have not been discovered in RA.

Alternative hypotheses designed to explain chronic RA include paracrine cytokine networks in the synovial lining and the possibility that RA synoviocytes achieve a degree of autonomy and become "transformed". The "cytokine" model was proposed after it became clear that macrophage and fibroblast-like synoviocyte (FLS) cytokines are abundant in both synovial fluid and synovial tissues [82]. Cytokines such as IL-1, TNF-α, IL-6, GM-CSF, chemokines, as well as other mediators (prostaglandins, complement proteins, stromelysin, and collagenase), are readily detected. Among these, IL-1 and TNF-α are probably the two key factors in the inflammatory cascade that perpetuate the disease. Both IL-1 and TNF-α are produced by macrophage-like synoviocytes and are arthritogenic in animals [83, 84]. In RA, they stimulate fibroblast proliferation and increase secretion of IL-6 and GM-CSF as well as chemokines that recruit additional cells into the synovium. GM-CSF, particularly in combination with TNF-α, also increases HLA-DR expression on macrophages [47].

Table 2 - Alternative models for disease perpetuation in chronic rheumatoid arthritis

• Paracrine/autocrine cytokine networks
• Uncontrolled synovial infection (e.g. lentivirus)
• Synoviocyte transformation

Fibroblast-like cells are also involved in autocrine loops and can contribute to their own dysregulation through the elaboration of growth factors such as TGF-β and fibroblast growth factor. In addition, IL-1 and TNF-α are potent inducers of adhesion molecules like ICAM-1, E-selectin, and VCAM-1 on endothelial cells. Hence, the elaboration of chemokines and the expression of adhesion molecules recruits cells to the joint in an antigen-independent manner. What is not known is whether the accumulating T cells are activated by a synovial antigen after arrival. If not, then various T cell directed approaches are likely to have only modest efficacy. Alternative pathways involving T cells, such as direct activation of synoviocytes or macrophages by membrane-bound cytokines, beg the issue of an antigen-specific response. Such non-specific interactions might help feed the cytokine fire, but probably do not initiate it.

In addition, some so-called "back-up" cytokines can mimic the role of T cells in the inflamed synovium. For example, IL-15, which shares secondary structure with IL-2, is produced in substantial amounts mainly by macrophages and fibroblast-like synoviocytes [85]. It can serve as a potent T-lymphocyte chemoattractant and activator. Injection of recombinant IL-15 into mice induced a local tissue inflammatory infiltrate consisting predominantly of T lymphocytes. Synovial T lymphocytes stimulated by IL-15 proliferate, increase their ability to migrate into collagen gels, and express high amounts of CD69. The IL-15-stimulated T cells, in turn, directly activate macrophages to release interleukin-1 and TNF-alpha. T cells are thus called to the synovium by the macrophages to participate secondarily in the inflammatory event.

Another explanation for T cell-independent perpetuation of RA implicates autonomous, aggressive synoviocytes. In this scenario, synoviocytes are "transformed" by the rheumatoid process and ultimately make a distinct contribution to the pathology. Unlike fibroblasts originating from the skin, synovial fibroblasts constitutively express vascular cell adhesion molecule (VCAM-1) and stain positively for the enzyme unidine diphosphoglucose dehydrogenase (UDPGD) [86]. They also possess some features that are frequently associated with transformed cells. Under some conditions in culture, fibroblast-like synoviocytes (FLS) demonstrate loss of contact inhibition. In addition, cultured synovial fibroblasts, like the transformed cell lines, can grow in an anchorage-independent manner and express several oncogenes. Hence, the cellular transformation and loss of growth inhibition in FLS might contribute to synovial lining hyperplasia and the local invasion.

The notion that rheumatoid synoviocytes are permanently altered was recently examined *in vivo* in a severe combine immunodeficiency (SCID) mouse model where cartilage and purified FLS were co-transplanted into the renal capsule [87]. The explanted RA fibroblast-like synoviocytes proliferated and invaded into cartilage 30 to 60 days post transplantation. In addition, the fibroblast-like cells at the immediate site of cartilage destruction expressed messenger RNA for the cysteine proteinase cathepsin L, a major *ras*-induced protein. Invasion of the cartilage explant, however, was not seen if animals were given normal or osteoarthritis synoviocytes. These data provide evidence that synoviocytes are irreversibly altered in RA and that they remain activated even after removal from the articular inflammatory cytokine milieu.

Despite the fact that FLS proliferate in tissue culture, only a very small percentage of synovial lining cells show evidence of active cell division in RA as measured by tritiated thymidine incorporation [12]. The percentage of cells expressing the cell cycle-specific nuclear antigen Ki67 is also very low [10]. It is possible that synoviocyte proliferation in RA might be a feature of very early synovitis rather than established disease. However, given the relatively low level of active cell division, an alternative explanation for persistent synovial lining hyperplasia could be the failure of residential cells to undergo programmed cell death.

Abnormal apoptosis, or programmed cell death, plays a role in other autoimmune diseases. A defect of the *fas* gene (which regulates apoptosis) in MRL-lpr mice has been linked to lymphoproliferative disorders, arthritis, and lupus-like syndrome [88]. Defects in the regulation of the Fas/APO1 gene in humans has also been associated with abnormal apoptosis in systemic lupus erythematosus (SLE) in humans [89]. Fas protein is constitutively expressed by cultured synoviocytes and anti-Fas antibody can lead to cell death under some culture conditions [90]. However, little or no Fas-L, the natural Fas ligand, is present in RA synovium [91]. Hence, this normal mechanism for deleting cells may not be utilized in the RA intimal lining.

Using the histochemical techniques or ultrastructural methods, only a limited number of intimal lining cells appear to complete the apoptosis process [91]. However, extensive DNA fragmentation occurs in RA synovium as determined by less specific techniques for detecting DNA damage, especially in the intimal lining [90]. This suggests that the final pathway to cell death may be defective and that cells with DNA strand breaks can either recover or persist for prolonged periods of time.

A mechanism of abnormal apoptosis in RA could involve defects in a variety of proteins known to be involved in the regulation of cell proliferation and death, including the oncogene *c-myc*, *ras*, *bcl-2* or the *p53* tumor suppressor gene. The DNA damage could be induced by local oxygen radicals or nitric oxide (NO), both of which subsequently induce oncogene and p53 expression. If the damage is extensive, the p53 protein directs the cell towards apoptosis as a type of 'fail-safe' mechanism to prevent excessive cell accumulation or transformation. A defect in this pathway, either due to somatic mutations or other functional alterations, can potentially lead to arrested apoptosis.

Due to the discrepancy between DNA fragmentation and cell death, the role of p53 as a potential key regulator of DNA repair, cell replication, and apoptosis in RA was examined. Marked overexpression of the p53 protein was noted in rheumatoid synovium and in resting RA fibroblast-like synoviocytes [92]. Using RNA mismatch detection assays, somatic mutations in the *p53* gene were subsequently identified in RA synovium and cultured FLS but not in matched skin or blood [93]. In contrast, no p53 mismatches were detected in synovium, skin, or blood from patients with osteoarthritis (OA).

The genotoxic environment of the joint is most likely responsible for the mutations. Greater than 80% of the mutations identified are G/A and T/C transitions, which are typical features of oxidative deamination by NO or oxygen radicals [94, 95]. Hence, specific mutations of the *p53* gene arising from a genotoxic environment in chronic RA might contribute to the autonomy of synoviocytes and perpetuation of disease. The process whereby chronic inflammation promotes local *p53* mutations is probably not unique to RA, but might be a common feature of many diseases. By way of example, long-standing inflammation in ulcerative colitis is associated with p53 mutations and probably contributes to neoplasia [96, 97].

It is important to recognize that p53 mutations do not cause RA; rather, they are the result of local chronic inflammatory responses. The same genotoxic local environment causing specific p53 mutations can also lead to subsequent mutagenic exposure of other genes involved in apoptosis or regulation of the cell cycle. Overexpression of many proto-oncogenes has been reported in the rheumatoid synovium including *c-myc*, *c-fos*, and *c-H-ras* [98, 99]. Recently, Roivainen and colleagues have examined mutational activation of *ras* proto-oncogenes in RA synovial tissues and found that activation of H-ras by point mutations in codons 13 and 14 occurred in the synovial tissue of patients with RA, OA, and other arthropathies [100]. Such oncogenic mutations can up-regulate cell proliferation and induce cellular transformation.

In conclusion, considerable progress has been made in the understanding of RA. However, the dominant "T-cell" hypothesis that has dictated the direction of numerous therapeutic trials and research efforts probably requires re-evaluation. The role of T cells and antigen specific stimulation might be most important in the early phase of RA but the new paradigms suggest that the chronic inflammatory process might achieve a certain degree of autonomy that permits inflammation to persist after a T cell response has been down-regulated. The paracrine and autocrine networks of cytokines produced by the macrophages and FLS can sustain the inflammation. This, in turn, can lead to somatic mutations of the genes regulating apoptosis and the cell cycle. Such gene defects can lead to synovial autonomy, transformation, and invasion. These novel hypotheses establish a variety of novel therapeutic targets that will hopefully have greater success than T cell ablative therapy.

References

1 Wolfe AM (1968) The epidemiology of rheumatoid arthritis: A review. *Bull Rheum Dis* 19: 518–530
2 Zvaifler NJ (1996) A retrospective analysis of the pathogenesis of rheumatoid arthritis. *Revue De Rhumatisme* 63: 791–796
3 Zvaifler NJ (1965) A speculation on the pathogenesis of joint inflammation in rheumatoid arthritis. *Arthritis Rheum* 8: 289–293
4 Ziff M (1965) Heberden Oration, 1964: Some immunologic aspects of the connective tissue diseases. *Ann Rheumatic Dis* 24: 103–115
5 Hollander JL, McCarty JD, Astorga C, Castro-Murillo E (1965) Studies on the pathogenesis of rheumatoid joint inflammation. I. The "R.A. cell" and a working hypothesis. *Ann Intern Med* 62: 271–280
6 Weissmann G (1972) Lysosomal mechanisms of tissue injury in arthritis. *N Engl J Med* 286: 141–147
7 Cush JJ, Lipsky PE (1988) Phenotypic analysis of synovial tissue and peripheral blood lynphocytes isolated from patients with rheumatoid arthritis. *Arthritis Rheum* 31: 1230–1238
8 Laffon A, Garcia-Vicuna R, Humbria A, Postigo AA, Corbi AL, de Landazuri MO, Sanchez-Madrid F (1991) Upregulated expression and function of VLA-4 fibronectin receptors on human activated T cells in rheumatoid arthritis. *J Clin Invest* 88: 546–552
9 Postigo AA, Garcia-Vicuna R, Diaz-Gonzalez F, Arroyo AG, De Landazuri MO, Chi-Rosso G, Lobb RR, Laffon A, Sanchez-Madrid F (1992) Increased binding of synovial T lymphocytes from rheumatoid arthritis to endothelial-leukocyte adhesion molecule-1 (ELAM-1) and vascular cell adhesion molecule-1 (VCAM-1). *J Clin Invest* 89: 1445–1452
10 Lalor PA, Mapp PL, Hall PA, Revell PA (1987) Proliferative activity of cells in the synovium as demonstrated by a monoclonal antibody, Ki67. *Rheumatol Int* 7: 183–186
11 Krenn V, Schalhorn N, Greiner A, Molitoris R, Konig A, Gohlke F, Muller-Hermelink HK (1996) Immunohistochemical analysis of proliferating and antigen-presenting cells in rheumatoid synovial tissue. *Rheumatol Intl* 15: 239–247
12 Nykanen P, Bergroth V, Raunio P, Nordstrom D, Konttinen VT (1986) Phenotypic characterization of 3H-thymidine incorporating cells in rheumatoid arthritis synovial membrane. *Rheumatol Intl* 6: 269–271
13 Iannone F, Corrigall VM, Kingsley GH, Panayi GS (1994) Evidence for the continuous recruitment and activation of T cells into the joints of patients with rheumatoid arthritis. *Eur J Immunol* 24: 2706–2713
14 Sugiyama M, Tsukazaki T, Yonekura A, Matsuzaki S, Yamashita S, Iwasaki K (1996) Localization of apoptosis and expression of apoptosis related proteins in the synovium of patients with rheumatoid arthritis. *Ann Rheum Dis* 55: 442–449
15 Stastny P (1978) Association of the B-cell alloantigen DRw4 with rheumatoid arthritis. *N Engl J Med* 298: 869–871

16 Wordsworth BP (1990) The immunogenetics of rheumatoid arthritis. *Curr Opin Rheumatol* 2: 423–429
17 Gregersen PK, Silver J, Winchester RJ (1987) The shared epitope hypothesis. An approach to understanding the molecular genetic of susceptibility to rheumatoid arthritis. *Arthritis Rheum* 30: 1205–1213
18 Weetman AP, McGregor AM (1984) Autoimmune thyroid disease: developments in our understanding. *Endocrine Rev* 5: 309–321
19 Honeyman MC, Cram DS, Harrison LC (1993) Glutamic acid decarboxylase 67-reactive T cells: a marker of insulin-dependent diabetes. *J Exp Med* 177: 535–540
20 Penzotti JE, Doherty D, Lybrand TP, Nepom GT (1996) A structural model for TCR recognition of the HLA class II shared epitope sequence implicated in susceptibility to rheumatoid arthritis. *J Autoimmunity* 9: 287–293
21 Thomson W, Pepper L, Payton A, Carthy D, Scott D, Ollier W, Silman A, Symmons D (1993) Absence of an association between HLA-DRB1*04 and rheumatoid arthritis in newly diagnosed cases from the community. *Ann Rheumatic Dis* 32: 539–541
22 Rigby AS, Silman AJ, Voelm L, Gregory JC, Ollier WER, Khan MA, Nepom GT, Thomson G (1991) Investigating the HLA component in rheumatoid arthritis: An additive (dominant) mode of inheritance is rejected, a recessive mode is preferred. *Genetic Epidemiol* 8: 153–175
23 Evans TI, Han J, Singh R, Moxley G (1995) The genotypic distribution of shared-epitope DRB1 alleles suggests a recessive mode of inheritance of the rheumatoid arthritis disease-susceptibility gene. *Arthritis Rheum* 38: 1754–1761
24 Wordsworth P, Pile KD, Buckely JD, Lanchbury JS, Ollier B, Lathrop M, Bell JI (1992) HLA heterozygosity contributes to susceptibility to rheumatoid arthritis. *Am J Hum Genet* 51: 585–591
25 Nepom GT, Nepom BS (1992) Prediction of susceptibility to rheumatoid arthritis by human leukocyte antigen genotyping. *Rheum Dis Clin North Am* 18: 785–792
26 Weyand CM, Hicok KC, Conn DL, Goronzy JJ (1992) The influence of HLA–DRB1 genes on disease severity in rheumatoid arthritis. *Ann Intern Med* 117: 801–806
27 McCusker CT, Reid B, Green D, Gladman DD, Buchanan WW, Singal DP (1991) HLA-D region antigens in patients with rheumatoid arthritis. *Arthritis Rheum* 34: 192–197
28 Zanelli E, Gonzalez-Gay MA, David CS (1995) Could HLA-DRB1 be the protective locus in rheumatoid arthritis? *Immunol Today* 16: 274–278
29 Doherty DG, Vaughan RW, Donalson PT, Mowat AP (1992) HLA DQA, DQB, and DRB genotyping by oligonucleotide analysis: distribution of alleles and haplotypes in British caucasoids. *Hum Immunol* 34: 53–63
30 Zanelli E, Krco CJ, Baisch JM, Cheng S, David CS (1996) Immune response of HLA-DQ8 transgenic mice to peptides from the third hypervariable region of HLA-DRB1 correlates with predisposition to rheumatoid arthritis. *Proc Natl Acad Sci USA* 93: 1814–1819
31 Blackman M, Kappler J, Marrack P (1990) The role of the T cell receptor in positive and negative selection of developing T cells. *Science* 248: 1335–1341

32 Weyand CM, Goronzy JJ (1994) Disease mechanisms in rheumatoid arthritis: Gene dosage effect of HLA-DR haplotypes. *J Lab Clin Med* 124: 335–338

33 Berg LJ, Frank G, Davis M (1990) The effects of MHC gene dosage and allelic variations on T-cell receptor selection. *Cell* 60: 1043–1053

34 Zamvil SS, Steinman L (1990) The T lymphocyte in experimental allergic encephalomyelitis. *Ann Rev Immunol* 8: 579–621

35 Osman GE, Toda M, Kanagawa O, Hood LE (1993) Characterization of the T cell receptor repertoire causing collagen arthritis in mice. *J Exp Med* 177: 387–395

36 Paliard X, West SG, Lafferty JA, Clements JR, Kappler JW, Marrack P, Kotzin BL (1991) Evidence for the effects of a superantigen in rheumatoid arthritis. *Science* 253: 325–329

37 Howell MD, Diveley JP, Lundeen KA, Esty A, Winters ST, Carlo DJ, Brostoff SW (1991) Limited T-cell receptor beta-chain heterogeneity among interleukin 2 receptor-positive synovial T cells suggests a role for superantigen in rheumatoid arthritis. *Proc Natl Acad Sci USA* 88: 10921–10925

38 Grom AA, Thomson SD, Luyrink L, Passo M, Choi E, Glass DN (1993) Dominant T-cell receptor beta chain variable region V beta 14+ clones in juvenile rheumatoid arthritis. *Proc Natl Acad Sci USA* 90: 11104–11108

39 Jenkins RN, Nikaein A, Zimmermann A, Meek K, Lipsky PE (1993) T cell receptor V beta gene bias in rheumatoid arthritis. *J Clin Invest* 92: 2688–2701

40 Uematsu Y, Wege H, Strauss A, Ott M, Bannwarth W, Lanchbury J, Panayi G, Steinmetz M (1991) The T-cell-receptor repertoire in the synovial fluid of a patient with rheumatoid arthritis is polyclonal. *Proc Natl Acad Sci USA* 88: 8534–8538

41 Olive C, Gatenby PA, Serjeantson SW (1991) Analysis of T cell receptor V alpha and V beta gene usage in synovia of patients with rheumatoid arthritis. *Immunol Cell Biol* 69: 349–354

42 Karin N, Szafer F, Mitchell D, Gold DP, Steiman L (1993) Selective and nonselective stages in homing of T lymphocytes to the central nervous system during experimental allergic encephalomyelitis. *J Immunol* 150: 4116–4124

43 Hooks JJ, Moutsopoulos HM, Geis SA, Stahl NI, Decker JL, Notkins AL (1979) Immune interferon in the circulation of patients with autoimmune diseases. *N Engl J Med* 301: 5–8

44 Kohase M, Henriksen-deStefano D, May LT, Vilcek J, Sehgal PB (1986) Induction of β_2 interferon by tumor necrosis factor: a homeostatic mechanism in the control of cell proliferation. *Cell* 45: 659–666

45 Firestein GS, Zvaifler NJ (1987) Peripheral blood and synovial fluid monocyte activation in inflammatory arthritis: II. Low levels of synovial fluid and synovial tissue interferon suggest that γ-interferon is not the primary macrophage activating factor. *Arthritis Rheum* 30: 864–871

46 Barnes PF, Fong SJ, Brennan PJ, Twomey PE, Mazumder A, Modin RL (1990) Local production of tumor necrosis factor and IFN-γ in tuberculous pleuritis. *J Immunol* 145: 149–154

47 Alvaro-Gracia JM, Zvaifler NJ, Firestein GS (1989) Cytokines in chronic inflammatory

arthritis: IV. Granulocyte/macrophage colony-stimulating factor-mediated induction of class II MHC antigen on human monocytes: A possible role in rheumatoid arthritis. *J Exp Med* 170: 865–875

48 Miossec P, Navillat M, Dupuy d'Angeac A, Sany J, Banchereau J (1990) Low levels of interleukin-4 and high levels of transforming growth factor beta in rheumatoid arthritis. *Arthritis Rheum* 33: 1180–1187

49 Firestein GS, Xu WD, Townsend K, Broide D, Alvaro-Gracia J, Glase-Brook A, Zvaifler NJ (1988) Cytokines in chronic inflammatory arthritis: I. Failure to detect T cell lymphokines (interleukin 2 and interleukin 3) and presence of macrophage colony-stimulating factor (CSF-1) and a novel mast cell growth factor in rheumatoid synovitis. *J Exp Med* 168: 1573–1586

50 Chabeaud M, Fossiez F, Miossec P (1997) Regulation of the effects of IL 17 on IL 6 and LIF production by RA synoviocytes. *Arthritis Rheum* 40: S1449

51 Campbell IL, Kay TWH, Oxbrow L, Harrision LC (1991) Essential role for interferon-gamma and interleukin 6 in autoimmune insulin-dependent diabetes in NOD/Wehi mice. *J Clin Invest* 87: 739–742

52 Kurosaka M, Ziff M (1983) Immunoelectron microscopic study of the distribution of T cell subsets in rheumatoid synovium. *J Exp Med* 158: 1191–1210

53 Georgopoulos S, Plows D, Kollias G (1996) Transmembrane TNF is sufficient to induce localized tissue toxicity and chronic inflammatory arthritis in transgenic mice. *J Inflammation* 46: 86–97

54 Firestein GS, Berger AE, Tracey DE, Chosay JG, Chapman DL, Paine MM, Yu C, Zvaifler NJ (1992) IL-1 receptor antagonist protein production and gene expression in rheumatoid arthritis and osteoarthritis synovium. *J Immunol* 149: 1054–1062

55 Wahl SM, Allen JB, Wong HL, Dougherty SF, Ellingsworth LR (1990) Antagonistic and agonistic effects of transforming growth factor-beta and IL-1 in rheumatoid synovium. *J Immunol* 145: 2514–2519

56 Katsikis KD, Chu CQ, Brennan FM, Maini RN, Feldmann M (1994) Immunoregulatory role of interleukin-10 in rheumatoid arthritis. J Exp Med 179: 1517–1527

57 Bergroth V, Tsai V, Zvaifler NJ (1989) Differences in responses of normal and rheumatoid arthritis peripheral blood T cells to synovial fluid and peripheral blood dendritic cells in allogeneic mixed leukocyte reactions. Arthritis Rheum 32: 1381–1389

58 Allen ME, Young SP, Mechell RH, Bacon PA (1995) Altered T lymphocyte signaling in rheumatoid arthritis. *Eur J Immunol* 25: 1547–1554

59 Maurice MM, Lankester AC, Bezemer AC, Geertsma MF, Tak PP, Breedveld FC, van Lier RA, Verweij CL (1997) Defective TCR-mediated signaling in synovial T cells in rheumatoid arthritis. *J Immunol* 159: 2973–2978

60 Maurice MM, Nakamura H, van der Voort EA, van Vliet AI, Staal FJ, Tak PP, Breedveld FC, Verweij CL (1997) Evidence for the role of an altered redox state in hyporesponsiveness of synovial T cells in rheumatoid arthritis. *J Immunol* 158(3): 1458–1465

61 Mosmann TR, Cherwinski H, Bond MW, Giedlin MA, Coffman RL (1986) Two types

of murine helper T cell clone. I. Definition according to profiles of lymphokine activities and secreted proteins. *J Immunology* 136: 2348–2357

62 Yamamura M, Uyemura K, Deans RJ, Weinberg K, Rea Th, Bloom BR, Modlin RL (1991) Defining protective responses to pathogens: cytokines profiles in leprosy lesions. *Science* 254: 277–279

63 Tsicopoulos A, Hamid Q, Varney V, Ying S, Moqbel R, Durham SR, Kay AB (1992) Preferential messenger RNA expression of Th1-type cells (IFN-gamma^{+}, IL-2^{+}) in classical delayed-type (tuberculin) hypersensitivity reactions in human skin. *J Immunol* 148: 2058–2061

64 Cher DJ, Mosmann TR (1987) Two types of murine helper T cell clone. II. Delayed-type hypersensitivity is mediated by Th1 clones. *J Immunol* 138: 3688–3694

65 Lebman DA, Coffman RL (1988) Interleukin 4 causes isotype switching to IgE in T cell-stimulated clonal B cell cultures. *J Exp Med* 168: 853–862

66 Stevens TL, Bossie A, Sanders VM, Fernandez-Botran R, Coffman RL, Mosmann TR, Vitetta ES (1988) Regulation of antibody isotype secretion by subsets of antigen-specific helper T cells. *Nature* 334: 255–258

67 Liblau RS, Singer SM, McDevitt HO (1995) Th1 and Th2 CD4+ T cells in the pathogenesis of organ-specific autoimmune diseases. *Immunol Today* 16: 34–38

68 Boissier MC, Chiocchia G, Bessis N, Hajnal J, Garotta G, Nicoletti F, Fournier C. (1995) Biphasic effect of interferon-gamma in murine collagen-induced arthritis. *Eur J Immunol* 25: 1184–1190

69 Walmsley M, Katsikis PD, Abney E, Parry S, Williams RO, Maini RN, Feldmann M (1996) Interleukin-10 inhibition of the progression of established collagen-induced arthritis. *Arthritis Rheum* 39: 495–503

70 Fava R, Olsen N, Keski-Oja J, Moses H, Pincus T (1989) Active and latent forms of transforming growth factor beta activity in synovial effusions. *J Exp Med* 169: 291

71 Simon AK, Seipelt E, Sieper J (1994) Divergent T-cell cytokine patterns in inflammatory arthritis. *Proc Nat Acad Sci USA* 91: 8562–8566

72 Kotake S, Schumacher HR, Jr., Yarboro CH, Arayssi TK, Pando JA, Kanik KS, Gourley MF, Klippel JH, Wilder RL (1996) In vivo gene expression of type 1 and type 2 cytokines in synovial tissues from patients in early stages of rheumatoid, reactive and undifferentiated arthritis. *Arthritis Rheum* 39: S117

73 Bucht A, Larsson P, Weisbrot L, Thorne L, Pisa P, Smedegard G, Keystone EC, Gronberg A (1996) Expresion of interferon-gamma (IFN-gamma), IL-10, IL-12, and transforming growth factor-beta (TGF-beta) mRNA in synovial fluid cells from patients in the early and late phases of rheumatoid arthritis (RA). *Clin Exp Immunol* 103: 357–367

74 Wells G, Tugwell P (1993) Cyclosporin A in rheumatoid arthritis: Overview of efficacy. *Br J Rheumatol* 32: 51–56

75 Watts RA, Isaacs JD, Hale G, Hazleman BL, Waldmann H (1993) CAMPATH-1H in inflammatory arthritis. Clin Exp Rheumatol 11: S165–S167

76 Strand V, Lipsky PE, Cannon GW, Calabrese LH, Wiesenhutter C, Cohen SB, Olsen NJ,

Lee ML, Lorenz TJ, Nelson B (1993) Effects of administration of an anti-CD5 plus immunoconjugate in rheumatoid arthritis. Results of two phase II studies. The CD5 Plus Rheumatoid Arthritis Investigators Group. *Arthritis Rheum* 36: 620–630

77 Moreland LW, Pratt PW, Bucy RP, Jackson BS, Feldman JW, Koopman WJ (1994) Treatment of refractory rheumatoid arthritis with a chimeric anti-CD4 monoclonal antibody: Long-term followup of CD4+ T cell counts. *Arthritis Rheum* 37: 834–838

78 Jendro MC, Ganten T, Matteson EL, Weyand CM, Goronzy JJ (1995) Emergence of oligoclonal T cell populations following therapeutic T cell depletion in rheumatoid arthritis. *Arthritis Rheum* 38: 1242–1251

79 Tak PP, van der Lubbe PA, Cauli A, Daha MR, Smeets TJM, Kluin PM, Meinders AE, Yanni G, Panayi GS, Breedveld FC (1995) Reduction of synovial inflammation after anti-CD4 monoclonal antibody treatment in early rheumatoid arthritis. *Arthritis Rheum* 38: 1457–1465

80 Muller-Ladner U, Kriegsmann J, Gay RE, Koopman WJ, Gay S, Chatham WW (1995) Progressive joint destruction in a Human Immunodeficiency Virus-infected patient with rheumatoid arthritis. *Arthritis Rheum* 39: 1328–1332

81 Narayan O, Sheffer D, Clements JE, Tennekoon G (1985) Restricted replication of lentiviruses. Visna viruses induce a unique interferon during interaction between lymphocytes and infected macrophages. *J Exp Med* 162: 1954–1969

82 Firestein GS, Zvaifler NJ (1990) How important are T cells in chronic rheumatoid synovitis? *Arthritis Rheum* 33: 768–773

83 Chandrasekhar S, Harvey AK, Hrubey PS, Bendele AM, (1990) Arthritis induced by interleukin-1 is dependent on the site and frequency of intraarticular injection. *Clin Immunol Immunopathol* 55: 382–400

84 Henderson B, Pettipher ER (1989) Arthritogenic actions of recombinant IL-1 and tumour necrosis factor alpha in the rabbit: Evidence of synergistic interactions between cytokines *in vivo*. *Clin Exp Immunol* 75: 306–310

85 McInnes IB, Al-Mughales J, Field M, Leung BP, Huang FP, Dixon R, Sturrock RD, Wilkinson PC, Liew FY (1996) The role of interleukin-15 in T-cell migration and activation in rheumatoid arthritis. *Nature Med* 2: 175–182

86 Edwards JC, Wilkinson LS, Pitsillides AA (1993) Palisading cells of rheumatoid nodules: comparison with synovial intimal cells. *Ann Rheum Dis* 52: 801–805

87 Geiler T, Kriegsmann J, Keyszer GM, Gay RE, Gay S (1994) A new model for rheumatoid arthritis generated by engraftment of rheumatoid synovial tissue and normal human cartilage into SCID mice. *Arthritis Rheum* 37: 1664–1671

88 Nagata S, Golstein P (1995) The Fas death factor. *Science* 267: 1449–1456

89 Wu J, Wilson J, He J, Xiang L, Schur PH, Mountz JD (1996) Fas ligand mutation in a patient with systemic lupus erythematosus and lymphoproliferative disease. *J Clin Invest* 98: 1107–1113

90 Firestein GS, Yeo M, Zvaifler NJ (1995) Apoptosis in rheumatoid arthritis synovium. *J Clin Invest* 96: 1631–1638

91 Nakajima T, Aono H, Hasunuma T, Yamamoto K, Shirai T, Hirohata K, Nishioka K

(1995) Apoptosis and functional Fas antigen in rheumatoid arthritis synoviocytes. *Arthritis Rheum* 38: 485–491
92 Firestein GS, Nguyen K, Aupperle KR, Yeo M, Boyle DL, Zvaifler NJ (1996) Apoptosis in rheumatoid arthritis: p53 overexpression in rheumatoid arthritis synovium. *Am J Pathol* 149: 2143–2151
93 Firestein GS, Echeverri F, Yeo M, Zvaifler NJ, Green DR (1997) Somatic mutations in the p53 tumor suppressor gene in rheumatoid arthritis synovium. *Proc Natl Acad Sci USA* 94: 10895–10900
94 Nguyen T, Brunson D, Crespi CL, Penman BW, Wishnok JS, Tannenbaum SR (1992) DNA damage and mutation in human cells exposed to nitric oxide *in vitro*. *Proc Natl Acad Sci USA* 89: 3030–3034
95 Wink DA, Kasprzak KS, Maragos CM, Elespuru RK, Misra M, Dunams TM, Cebula TA, Koch WH, Andrews AW, Allen JS et al. (1991) DNA deaminating ability and genotoxicity of nitric oxide and its progenitors. *Science* 254: 1001–1003
96 Brentnall TA, Crispin DA, Rabinovitch PS, Haggitt RC, Rubin CE, Stevens AC, Burmer GC (1994) Mutations in the *p53* gene: an early marker of neoplastic progression in ulcerative colitis. *Gastroenterol* 107: 369–378
97 Harris CC (1995) 1995 Deichmann Lecture – *p53* tumor suppressor gene: at the crossroads of molecular carcinogenesis, molecular epidemiology and cancer risk assessment. *Toxicology Letters* 82–83: 1–7
98 Roivainen A, Isomaki P, Nikkari S, Saario R, Vuori K, Toivanen P (1995) Oncogene expression in synovial fluid cells in reactive and early rheumatoid arthritis: a brief report. *Br J Rheumatol* 34: 805–808
99 Roivainen A, Soderstrom KO, Pirila L, Aro H, Kortekangas P, Merilahti-Palo R, Yli-Jama T, Toivanen A, Toivanen P (1996) Oncoprotein expression in human synovial tissue: an immunohistochemical study of different types of arthritis. *Br J Rheumatol* 35: 933–942
100 Roivainen A, Jalava J, Pirila L, Yli-Jama T, Tiusanen H, Toivanen P (1997) H-ras oncogene point mutations in arthritic synovium. *Arthritis Rheum* 40: 1636–1643

T cell receptor rearrangements in arthritis

David E. Fox[1] *and Nora G. Singer*[2]

[1]Division of Rheumatology, Specialized Center of Research in Rheumatoid Arthritis and Multipurpose Arthritis and Musculoskeletal Diseases Center, University of Michigan, 3918 Taubman Center, Ann Arbor, MI 48109-0358, USA; [2]Department of Pediatrics, Division of Immunology, Allergy and Rheumatology and Department of Internal Medicine Division of Rheumatic Diseases, Case Western Reserve University Medical School, 11100 Rainbow Babies & Childrens Hospital, Cleveland, OH 44106, USA

Introduction

Investigation of T cell receptor usage in human inflammatory arthritis, particularly rheumatoid arthritis (RA), has been a focus of intense interest over the past decade. This interest is predicated on several underlying observations and assumptions [1]. First, well-studied animal models of inflammatory arthritis depend upon T cell recognition of specific antigen, often foreign antigen that may share cross-reactive determinants with components of the joint. Transfer of disease to non-arthritic animals by T cells of appropriate antigen specificity has provided a clear demonstration that events initiated through the T cell receptor can cause joint destruction. Similar conclusions can be reached from other animal models for autoimmune diseases, such as experimental allergic encephalomyelitis (EAE).

Second, T cells seem to be important in human arthritis, especially RA, and are certainly abundant in synovial tissue and fluid, along with a variety of antigen-presenting cells with which T lymphocytes can interact. Many of these T cells display a surface phenotype consistent with immunologic memory and activation.

Third, human RA is associated with genetic risk factors, of which the best defined is a set of alleles within the polymorphic class II major histocompatibility complex (MHC) loci. It has been proposed that RA associated class II alleles such as HLA-DR4, could predispose to disease by presenting arthritogenic peptides to T lymphocytes. This hypothesis has not yet been proven, and a variety of other models can be proposed to explain the MHC association with RA or other autoimmune diseases. However, if the peptide presentation model is correct, T lymphocytes with specific T cell receptors capable of recognizing such MHC-peptide complexes could be critical in initiation and/or maintenance of disease, analogous to observations in animal models.

This chapter will analyze the current understanding of T cell receptor (TCR) usage in RA and other forms of human inflammatory arthritis. In order to understand the expressed T cell repertoire in arthritic diseases, the biology of the TCR and methods for determining TCR usage will be briefly reviewed. Expression of both the

T Cells in Arthritis, edited by P. Miossec, W.B. van den Berg and G.S. Firestein

αβ and γδ TCR in RA will be discussed, in both articular and non-articular locations. TCR usage in juvenile chronic arthritis and psoriatic arthritis will also be reviewed. The potential for TCR directed therapeutic approaches to arthritis is considered in another chapter of this volume.

Biology of the T cell receptor

The human T cell receptor plays a critical role in initiating and regulating most immune responses. The dimeric antigen recognition components of the TCR (αβ or γδ) are expressed in the T cell membrane in strict association with a complex signal transduction apparatus collectively termed CD3, which is in turn linked with an array of intracellular signalling molecules and pathways. Some key rules for the formation and function of T cell receptors are displayed in Table 1. The extraordinary clonal diversity of the expressed T cell receptor repertoire is achieved through a variety of mechanisms. These include both rearrangement and modification of a limited number of germline gene segments, including no more than a few dozen α and β variable segment genes and somewhat fewer γ and δ segment variable genes. The most highly variable portion of the expressed T cell receptor, termed CDR3 (complimentarity determining region 3), interacts directly with processed antigen presented by MHC molecules in specialized antigen binding clefts.

Most positive and negative selection of T cells occurs in the thymus. Current understanding of these processes emphasizes the avidity of interaction between specific immature T lineage cells in the thymus and thymic antigen-presenting cells. High avidity interactions lead to deletion of autoreactive cells, while lower avidity interactions lead to positive selection of cells that are later able to recognize exogenous antigen in association with self MHC. The avidity of these interactions, and therefore the outcome of the selection process is controlled by a number of variables including antigen concentration, the specific MHC molecules presenting a given antigen, the direct interaction between individual expressed TCR's and antigenic peptides, and other factors controlling the adhesion and accessory signalling events that occur between thymocytes and thymic antigen-presenting cells. The T cell repertoire that emerges following thymic selection may be subject to further modification over time, influenced substantially by the many encounters of the immune system with conventional antigens and superantigens of microbial origin. Although the immune system depends upon specificity of antigenic recognition to properly focus immune effector function and formation of immunologic memory, T lymphocyte clones with unique TCR's do not generally dominate antigen directed immune responses. Instead, a heterogeneous variety of lymphocytes, which cannot be demonstrated to bear specificity for the relevant target antigen, typically greatly outnumber antigen-specific T cells in normal interactions of the immune system with pathogenic microorganisms.

Table 1 - Rules for TCR expression and function

- Most circulating mature T cells (usually >95%) express the αβ TCR. The remainder express the γδ TCR
- TCR diversity is achieved by
  1) Combinatorial rearrangement of germline gene segments (V, J and C for α and γ; V, D, J and C for β and δ)
  2) Addition and deletion of nucleotides at the VDJ junctions
  3) Ability of each α chain to form heterodimers with multiple β chains (and vice versa)
- Most T cells express only one TCR but rare T cells with two distinct TCR's have been detected
- Positive and negative selection occur primarily in the thymus and are regulated in part by the specific MHC molecules expressed by an individual
- Most T cells recognize processed peptide antigens presented in a specialized peptide-binding cleft by MHC molecules; in general $CD4^+$ T cells recognize antigen on class II MHC and $CD8^+$ T cells recognize antigen on class I MHC
- Some T cells recognize non-peptide antigens, including lipid and carbohydrate-containing molecules; presentation of such antigens may be MHC independent, involving CD1 or other molecules
- Superantigens activate entire Vβ families of T cells; superantigens are presented to the TCR by MHC molecules through binding sites distinct from those used by processed peptide antigens
- Activation of T cells requires one or more co-stimulatory signals in addition to antigen/MHC; such second signals are transduced through surface structures distinct from the TCR

Genetic factors that regulate the TCR repertoire in RA

TCR gene polymorphisms in RA

There is no evidence to indicate inheritance and expression of unique TCR genes in RA, or lack of inheritance and expression of any of the known TCR genes. Several studies have, however, investigated whether detectable polymorphisms in the four known TCR gene regions are statistically associated with clinical RA, or with subsets of RA [2–17]. Interpretation of such studies is complex, due to the various gene subregions analyzed, which represent only a portion of the large TCR gene loci. A variety of techniques have been employed, including restriction fragment length polymorphism analysis, and PCR-based analysis of specific microsatellites or regions of TCR gene sequences. A few reports suggest that susceptibility to RA is associated with TCR gene polymorphisms [2, 4, 10, 11, 13, 15, 16], while other studies find no linkage [3, 5–9, 12, 14, 17]. This evidence appears to be most convincing for the TCRA (α chain) locus, and the closely linked TCRD (δ) locus [4, 10, 13, 16] with somewhat less convincing data to suggest an association with alleles in the B (β) locus [2, 4, 11, 13, 15]. The largest of these studies examined 766 patients with erosive, seropositive RA and 813 controls from three northern European populations. Of four TCRA and two TCRB loci investigated, a single locus, termed TCRAV8S1, showed a greater incidence of the genotype 2 allele compared with the genotype 1 allele in RA patients [16]. However the overall odds ratio was only 1.3 (95% confidence interval 1.1 to 1.7). No influence of HLA-DR genotypes on this TCRA association could be detected. This finding needs to be confirmed by family studies and in other racial groups. Association of this polymorphism with specific features of the expressed TCRα repertoire and to immunological phenomena relevant to RA is not understood at this time.

Of the reports that have failed to show linkage of RA to polymorphisms in the TCR loci, the findings appear to be most convincing for the TCRB locus, for which a variety of polymorphisms have been investigated in several different ethnic groups [3, 5–9, 14, 17]. One report, which requires confirmation, has suggested that a TCR Vβ8 polymorphism could be a prognostic marker within the RA patient group, with more rapid radiographic progression associated with one of the alleles [5]. Negative data regarding an association of RA with TCRA or D gene polymorphisms also exist [9, 17], although neither of these studies includes as many subjects as the study of Cornelis [16] which did find a weak TCRA association.

In juvenile chronic arthritis, there is controversy concerning a possible association with a TCRB polymorphism [18–21]. Two independent studies found association with a TCRBV6.1 allele [19, 21] in pauciarticular disease, while a third study showed no association [20]. In a study of patients with rheumatic fever from two distinct racial groups, no association was found with TCRA or TCRB alleles [22]. Furthermore, polymorphisms of the CD3ε chain, part of the CD3 complex associated with the TCR in the T cell membrane, showed no association with susceptibility to juvenile chronic arthritis [23].

Effects of disease associated MHC polymorphisms on the TCR repertoire in arthritis

The association of RA with class II MHC polymorphisms is well known, and probably accounts for about 50% of the genetic component of susceptibility to RA. In Caucasian patients with seropositive disease, HLA-DR4 and related DR alleles that contain the "shared epitope" (including amino acids QKRAA or QRRAA at residues 70 to 74 of the DR beta chain), has been associated both with susceptibility to RA and severity of disease [1, 24–30]. There is also evidence for a role for other genes in the class II locus, particularly HLA-DQ [31, 32], but also HLA-DM genes [33] and closely linked genes that encode for molecules other than MHC structures [34]. Linkage disequilibrium between various genes in the MHC locus complicates these analyses. Within the shared epitope susceptibility locus, presence of arginine at position 71 has been associated with milder, rheumatoid factor negative disease, while a lysine at this position correlates with more severe, rheumatoid factor positive disease [35].

The functions of class II MHC molecules include control of positive and negative selection of developing $CD4^+$ T cells in the thymus, and presentation of both processed peptide antigens and superantigens to mature $CD4^+$ T cells in lymphoid organs and inflammatory lesions. Therefore, reasonable explanations for association of class II MHC alleles with immune mediated disease, such as RA, include (1) selection of a TCR repertoire that predisposes to RA and (2) presentation of arthritogenic peptides to mature T cells [36]. Either of these mechanisms might be expected to alter the expressed repertoire. At this point, conclusive evidence proving or disproving either of these mechanisms is not available, and a variety of other possibilities exist to explain the association between MHC alleles and RA (reviewed in [37, 38]). One model proposes that the shared epitope functions like an endogenous superantigen, selecting or activating T cells with an appropriate TCRβ that uses residues in CDR1 and CDR2, as well as CDR3, to recognize the shared epitope [39]. Under some circumstances HLR-DR peptides might induce or regulate autoimmune responses by being presented to T cells on other MHC molecules, such as HLA-DQ [40].

The strength of the gene dosage effect of the shared epitope in RA [25–30] tends to argue against a key role for HLA-DR in presentation of an arthritogenic antigen, since the shared epitope should behave in a generally dominant fashion if this mechanism is paramount. These findings are more consistent with absence of the shared epitope as a protective factor, rather than presence of the shared epitope as a susceptibility factor for RA. Clarification of this point will be of considerable importance for understanding the expressed T cell repertoire in RA and the potential utility of treatment strategies directed against the TCR.

Evidence for a role of MHC polymorphisms in selection of the TCR repertoire RA is somewhat stronger at this point, although not definitively established [41–44]. In healthy individuals, presence of the shared epitope does not appear to alter the expression of TCRB variable region gene families, but does affect expression of some of the TCRB region J gene families, in association with the Vβ3, Vβ14 and Vβ17 genes [42, 43]. This effect was evident in naive T cells as well as in the total T cell population [42, 43]. Furthermore, shared epitope positive normal individuals showed a different pattern of Jβ usage than patients with RA [42]. Although this latter finding was interpreted to indicate unique thymic selection events in RA, no data to directly substantiate this point is yet available. Furthermore, the findings regarding unique TCRBJ expression in RA (versus normal individuals with the shared epitope) were not confirmed in a study from another group, which included analysis of monozygotic twins discordant for RA [44]. The issue of whether monozygotic twins discordant for RA have distinct TCR repertoires remains controversial [45, 46].

At this point, therefore, the hypothesis that the mechanism by which MHC alleles predispose to RA involves interaction between MHC (with or without antigen) and the TCR is not yet proven. That such interactions can cause arthritis is well supported by various animal models, including a spontaneous arthritis model in a TCR-transgenic mouse [47], but whether any of these models reflect the same fundamental mechanisms that produce human RA remains uncertain.

Methods for determining TCR usage

Approaches to determining T cell receptor usage in a variety of immune responses, including autoimmune diseases, have evolved over time with a series of improvements in resolution, precision, comprehensiveness, and scope of information obtained. Table 2 outlines several of the methods that have been applied to analysis of TCR usage in human arthritis, particularly RA. Some approaches, such as Southern blotting, are now less useful, given the relatively low level of sensitivity in detecting T cell subpopulations and the imprecise nature of the information obtained. Methods that involve analysis of TCR sequence data clearly give the most direct definition of clonality within heterogeneous T cell populations. Nevertheless, the goal of precisely documenting the T cell repertoire used *in vivo* in human arthritis, peripherally or in lesions, remains elusive, since collection and interpretation of precise sequence information within all TCR gene families expressed in an arthritic lesion is a technically formidable task that has not yet been accomplished.

The TCR αβ repertoire in RA

A large number of studies over the past ten years have examined the usage of T cell receptor gene segments in RA, both in peripheral blood and in the joint. The hypothesis that initially prompted much of this work was that T cell clones of pathogenic significance would be expanded and detectable amidst polyclonal populations, especially in synovial lesions. TCRB gene rearrangements have received the greatest attention, but some information on TCRA gene usage is also available. Several recent reviews consider the numerous studies of the RA TCR repertoire [48–51]. Some of the issues important in analyzing the large body of work in this area are outlined in Table 3.

Early studies did not attempt to detect changes in individual Vβ families, but instead used Southern blotting to look for expanded (but uncharacterized) clones

Table 2 - Methods for analysis of T cell receptor (TCR) repertoire usage

Technique	Advantage(s)	Disadvantage(s)
Monoclonal antibody surface staining (by FACS or immuno-histochemistry)	Results not affected by T cell activation state, only expressed TCR's detected	Specificity of some antibodies for individual TCR families is not always firmly established. Complete TCR phenotyping difficult with small tissue samples.
Southern blot	Not affected by TCR mRNA stability or abundance, or by T cell activation state	Apparent clonal bands can be polyclonal and/or can be due to common Dβ-Jβ rearrangements (false +). May not be sensitive enough to detect biologically significant clonal expansions within polyclonal populations (false –).
Polymerase chain reaction (PCR) amplification of TCR V gene families	Suitable for analysis of α, β, γ or δ TCR gene usage, feasible with small samples	Equivalent, quantitative amplification of all TCR families is technically difficult; results do not provide direct evidence of clonality.
Gel electrophoresis of PCR products (SSCP-single strand conformational polymorphism)	Can estimate degree of heterogeneity or clonality within individual V region families	Heterogeneous transcripts of different sizes can co-migrate as a single band.
Sequence analysis of V region segments (especially CDR3-compementarity determining region 3), following PCR amplification of expressed TCR genes	Can suggest whether repertoire skewing reflects effects of conventional (nominal) peptide antigen or superantigen	Laborious, fidelity of the results depends on avoiding pitfalls inherent in PCR amplification of TCR transcripts. Cycling cells that are transcriptionally activated will be over-represented.
Sequencing of TCR genes expressed by cloned T cells	Concurrent analyses of antigen specificity, autoreactivity, cytokine production and effector function are feasible	T cell cloning is laborious, inefficient, and variably successful depending upon T cell subset and activation state.

Table 3 - Issues in analysis of TCR repertoire in arthritis

- Patient characteristics: age, gender, genetic composition (especially MHC), concurrent diseases
- Stage of disease
- Source of T cells – blood, synovial tissue, synovial fluid
- Subset of cells examined
  - CD4 or CD8
  - TCR αβ or TCR γδ
  - activated or resting
  - naive or memory
  - cultured or freshly isolated
- Possible skewing of TCR repertoire by infectious agents in combination with the immunosuppressive effects of inflammatory disease and/or its treatment
- Methodology used (Table 2)
- Significance of TCR repertoire perturbations usually not clear since target antigen for specific TCR generally not known; amplified clones could be pathogenic, regulatory, or irrelevant to the disease.

among synovial fluid or synovial tissue T cells, or in panels of T cell clones generated from the RA synovial compartment [52–64]. Results of these studies were not entirely consistent, but in general oligoclonality was most readily detected when T cells were first cultured with IL-2 [53, 59, 63, 64]. Among random T cell clones grown from RA synovial fluid [55] or tissue [56], almost all used different TCRB gene rearrangements. Nevertheless, patients could be identified who appeared to have identical expanded clones in multiple joints [57, 61, 64].

Subsequently a large number of studies have asked whether certain TCRβ (or α) families were expressed by RA T cells at a different frequency than would be expected in the absence of RA, and/or whether distinct TCR sequences were favored within particular Vβ families. The methods used and the problems inherent in such studies have been summarized in Tables 2 and 3. Results of a cross-section of this work [65–110] are summarized in Table 4. While many earlier studies, especially those using antibodies to selected TCR V gene products, examined expression of only a subset of the TCRA and B genes, other studies (generally using PCR-based techniques) have comprehensively studied the Vβ repertoire. The TCRA genes and α chains have been more difficult to completely analyze for technical reasons. Most reports include analysis of matched PB T cell samples as controls for SF or ST T cell samples. Control samples from lymphoid organs of RA patients might be even more appropriate, but obtaining such samples is unlikely to be practical.

Inspection of Table 4 yields the following observations:

1. Skewing (also termed bias) in TCR V region usage has been frequently observed, but the specific V genes thought to be overexpressed differ among the various studies.
2. For each Vβ family found to be overexpressed in one or more studies, contradictory findings exist in other studies. (Not shown are the many instances in which neither over nor under expression of specific V genes was found). Data for Vα expression is less extensive than for Vβ.
3. Some of the larger studies tend to find fewer differences between RA joint and RA PB T cells, or between RA and normal PB T cells, than is seen in smaller studies. This highlights the complexities in appropriate statistical analysis of this type of data.
4. Most studies that use control SF or ST samples from other forms of arthritis find few, if any, features of the lesional TCR repertoire unique to RA, when V region usage is quantitated.
5. A pattern of TCR αβ usage that is distinctive for early versus late RA has not yet emerged from these studies.
6. Several studies have examined whether the expressed TCR repertoire *within* specific V region families is clonally restricted or uses special motifs within the hypervariable antigen-recognition CDR3 domain. This involves cloning and sequencing of PCR-amplified transcripts spanning the region of interest. In general, clonal restriction has been found when sought by this approach, both in PB and in SF or ST. Evidence for unique CDR3 motifs from lesional T cells (reviewed in ref 51) could imply local expansion of antigen-reactive T cells, but direct confirmation of such a hypothesis is not available. Although Vβ clonality of $CD4^+$ cells defined by this approach seems to be greater in the joint than in PB [111, 112] it is readily demonstrable in some studies in RA PB [112, 113], and to a far greater degree than in $DR4^+$ controls or patients with psoriatic arthritis [113]. Within the RA joint, different areas of tissue contain similar expanded clones [114]. On the other hand, PB $CD8^+$ cells from normal individuals frequently display TCRα clonal expansion, which is exaggerated in RA [80]. Many of these findings suggested altered control of expansion and persistence of activated T cells in patients with RA.

The TCR γδ repertoire in RA

In adult peripheral blood and lymphoid organs, a small minority of T lymphocytes bear the γδ receptor, and most of these cells are $CD4^-CD8^-$. According to several reports, this subset is expanded in most RA patients, in PB, ST and SF [115–119], although other studies have not found this subset to be expanded in RA PB [120–123]. It is possible that contradictory findings may be explained by differences in

Table 4 - TCRα and TCRβ chain usage in RA

Reference	Year	Number of patients	RA sample source	Subset	Controls	Vβ	1	2	3	4	5	6	7
65	1988	10	SF,ST		RA PB	x					↑		
66	1991	7	SF		RA and nl PB	x							
66	1991	7	PB		nl PB	x							
67	1991	5	ST	CD25+	RA PB	x			↑C				
68	1991	2	SF		RA PB								
69	1991	5	ST		RA and nl PB	x							
70	1991	3	SF		RA PB	x						↓	↑
71	1991	1	SF		RA PB	x		↑	↑				
72	1992	9	ST		RA PB	x							
73	1992	35	SF, ST	CD4+, CD8+	RA and nl PB	x							
74	1992	4	SF		RA PB	x		↑				↑	
75	1992	8	SF		RA PB	x				↑C	↑		
76	1992	10	ST		non-RA ST, SF	x	↓	↓	↓	↓	↓		
77	1993	14	SF		RA PB								
78	1993	5	SF		RA PB	x		↑	↑				
79	1993	8	SF, ST	CD4+	RA and nl PB	x							
80	1993	46	PB	CD8+	nl PB								
81	1993	24	SF, ST		RA PB	x	↓			↓	↓	↑	
82	1993	6	RN	IL-2 responsive	RA and nl PB	x					↑	↑	
83	1993	6	SF		RA PB	x						↑C	
84	1993	3	SF, ST		RA and nl PB	x		↑C					
85	1993	2	SF	CD4+	RA PB	x		↑		↑			
85	1993	2	SF	CD8+	RA PB	x				↑C			
86	1993	12	SF		RA PB, non-RA SF and PB	x						↓	
87	1994	7	SF		RA PB	x		↑				↑	
87	1994	7	SF	CD4+	SF CD8+	x		↑				↑	
88	1994	5	SF, PB	CD4+	nl PB	x			C				
89	1994	49	SF, ST, PB		nl and SLE PB, non-RA SF	x							
90	1994	1	PB		nl PB	x						↑	
91	1994	1	SF, ST, PB		nl PB	x							
92	1995	13	ST, PB		nl PB	x			↑	↓			
93	1995	31	PB	CD8+	nl PB	x			↑				
94	1995	12	SF, PB		nl PB	x						↑	
95	1995	3	SF			x							
96	1995	22	SF		RA PB	x						↑	
97	1995	8	ST		non-RA ST	x							↑
98	1995	4	ST		RA PB	x							
99	1995	3	PB		nl PB	x							
100	1995	3	ST		RA PB, non-RA SF	x							
101	1995	33	PB		nl PB	x							
101	1995	11	ST		RA PB	x	↓		↓	↓	↓	↑	
101	1995	19	SF		RA PB	x				↓	↓	↑	
102	1995	28	PB		nl PB	x	C		C	C		C	
103	1995	7	SF		RA PB	x		↑			↓	↑	
104	1995	13	ST		RA PB	x			↑	↓			
105	1995	4	ST	CD4+CD45RO+	RA PB	x							
106	1996	6	ST, SF		RA and nl PB	x	C	C		C		C	C
107	1996	2	ST		RA PB	x		C	C	C			
108	1996	8	SF		non-RA SF, RA and nl PB								
109	1996	14	SF, PB		nl PB	x	C	C	C	C			C
110	1996	32	PB	CD8+	nl PB	x			C				

PB - peripheral blood
SF - synovial fluid
ST - synovial tissue
RN - rheumatoid nodule
↑ - *expansion of V family*
↓ - *reduction of V family*

9	10	11	12	13	14	15	16	17	18	19	20	21	22	23	24	Vα	2	5	6	7	10	11	12	14	15	17	18	23	28	Subfamilies
					↑																									
					↓																									
					↑C			↑C																						
																x								↑	↑			↑		↑Vα14.2
																x														
↓	↓	↓														x														
																x														↑Vβ2.1, ↑Vβ3.1
																x										↓	↓			
																x														
↓																x								↑	↑			↑		
				↑C	C											x					↑				↑		↑			Vβ13.1 oligoclonal
									↓							x	↓	↓												
																x	↑C													
					↑	↑																								
																x							↑							↑Vα12.1
	↓				↑	↑	↓			↓																				↓Vβ5.1
			↑																											
																x						↑								
↓																														
					↑C			↑C																						
																x														
				↓								↑																		
					C			C																						
								↑																						
				↑																										↑Vβ6.7
								C																						
								↑					↑																	
																x							↑							↑Vα12.1
				↑	↑																									
			C		C																									
										↑																				↑Vβ6.7
								↑								x									↑					
↓																														
				↓	↓																									↓Vβ513.2
						↑																								↓Vβ5.1
					↑		↓																							↓Vβ5.1
				C					C																					C in Vβ 13.2
				↓				↓				↑	↓																	↓Vβ5.1, 13.1, 13.2
↓								↑		↓			↑																	
		↑														x														
																x				↑										
C								C																						
																x										↑				
		C	C	C		C		C	C	C	C			C																C in Vβ13.1

- *clonal expansion within V family*

X - indicates which TCR chains (α or β) were examined in each study

nl - normal individuals without arthritis

disease activity, as has been documented in Still's disease, in which elevation of the PB γδ TCR subset is seen only during active disease [124]. A surface phenotype indicating activation of γδ T cells was found to correlate with disease activity in RA [123]. SF and ST T cells from patients with spondylarthropathies [118, 121] or osteoarthritis [119] contained a smaller percentage of γδ cells than RA specimens.

The number of variable chain genes in the TCRG and TCRD loci is much smaller than is the case for TCRA and TCRB. Numerous reports have found that the predominant δ variable chain used in the joint is distinct from that found in peripheral blood [125–129]. Most synovial T cells use Vδ1 while most PB T cells use Vδ2. The Vδ1 cells in the joint are activated, and sequence analysis shows these cells to be polyclonal [129], although RA PB γδ cells were found to be oligoclonal [130–133]. Age matching of normal controls is important in such studies, since γδ cell oligoclonality increases with age both in normal individuals and in RA patients [134]. However, the proportion of PB T cells bearing the γδ TCR has been reported to be higher in young compared to old RA patients [135].

Of 11 different Vγ chains, Vγ9 is expressed by about 44% of normal PB γδ cells, but only one-third of RA PB γδ cells [136]. The Vγ3 subset is slightly expanded in RA PB and markedly expanded in RA SF, accounting for 60% of SF γδ cells [136]. However Vγ8 is the primary Vγ chain expressed in RA ST [137]. T cells bearing Vγ8 and Vδ1 also comprise a major subset of human IEL (intra-epithelial lymphocytes). Synovial fluid T cells show evidence of distinct Jγ segment usage and oligoclonal sequences [138, 139], but additional data is required to determine if this finding is specific for RA. Furthermore, the expressed γ chain repertoire appears to be very diverse in different individuals, even in monozygotic twins, whether they are concordant or discordant for RA [140]. It therefore appears unlikely that a prototypic γδ cell repertoire can be identified that either predisposes to RA or is generated by RA [140].

These conclusions do not, of course, exclude an important role for clones or larger subsets of γδ cells in RA, in pathogenic antigen-specific or autoreactive responses, or in regulatory networks. Cloned γδ cells can respond to both peptide antigen in an MHC-restricted fashion and to non-conventional microbial antigens [141], which are small non-peptide molecules that are often phosphorylated [142]. Clones of γδ T cells responsive to mycobacterial antigens have been isolated from RA SF [143], but controversy exists as to whether γδ cells are important [144] or unimportant [145] in responses of RA SF cells to mycobacterial antigens. In a different study, SF γδ T cells from both psoriatic arthritis and RA were found to respond to a crude streptococcal antigen [146]. Indirect evidence also suggests that Vδ1$^+$ γδ lines from RA SF recognize an unknown antigen on RA synovial tissue cells [147]. One potential mechanism for an immunoregulatory role of γδ cells in synovial inflammation has been elucidated in Lyme disease, in which it is proposed that γδ cells bearing Fas-ligand induce apoptosis of pathogenic Fas (CD95)$^+$ CD4$^+$ T cells in synovial tissue [148]. In murine collagen-induced arthritis, appropriately-timed injection of an activating monoclonal antibody specific for $\gamma\delta$ cells can worsen disease [149]. In contrast, *in vivo* depletion of $\gamma\delta$ cells worsens rat adjuvant arthritis [150].

Felty's Syndrome and large granular lymphocyte clonal expansions in RA

Felty's syndrome is a term commonly used to describe the entity of rheumatoid arthritis and neutropenia, and is usually associated with splenomegaly. A subset of patients with Felty's Syndrome appear to have a clonal, low grade neoplasm that is characterized by the presence of large granular lymphocytes (LGL) [151]. These cells generally express the cytotoxic T-cell surface marker CD8 [151] and one or more natural killer cell antigens such as CD16, CD56 or CD57 on their surface [151– 153]. Occasionaly, such patients may have a detectable rearrangement in the γ-chain of the $\gamma\delta$ TCR [154], but $\alpha\beta$ clonality is probably more common [155]. Large granular lymphocyte (LGL) leukemia is by definition a clonal proliferation of lymphocytes, which phenotypically resemble those seen in Felty's Syndrome, and many patients who have LGL leukemia also have RA [156]. In Table 5, the available data on LGL leukemia and Felty's Syndrome is summarized, including the type of patients studied, techniques used, and general conclusions. Overall the findings support the conclusion that in these entities the T cell repertoire is restricted. In addition, one report indicates that the $CD4^+CD57^+$ subset is expanded in RA PB, and has a restricted repertoire that overlaps with the repertoire of the $CD4\text{-}CD57^+$ subset [159].

Juvenile chronic arthritis

Juvenile chronic arthritis (JCA) is a group of arthritides which includes both the triad of diseases falling under the category of juvenile rheumatoid arthritis (JRA) and seronegative spondyloarthropathy presenting in childhood. JRA encompasses the diagnoses of systemic onset JRA or Still's disease, the "adult-like" polyarticular JRA which is often antinuclear antibody (ANA) and/or rheumatoid factor $(RF)^+$ (>4 joints in first 6 months), and the pauciarticular or oligoarticular form of JRA (4 or fewer joints in first 6 months), which is also frequently ANA^+. Because of the difficulty distinguishing clinically in children between pauciarticular JRA and the HLA-B27 associated seronegative spondyloarthropathies (which frequently present with peripheral joint rather than axial symptoms), the European pediatric rheumatology community uses the term JCA, which includes both pauciarticular JRA and juvenile-onset spondyloarthritis. If causative factors for individual diseases can be identified then reevaluation of this nomenclature system may be undertaken.

Hypotheses regarding causes of the subtypes of JRA should take into account the following factors: (1) children are generally healthy but are frequently exposed to

Table 5 - Studies in LGL/Felty's Syndrome

Study	Year	Techniques used	Patients	Conclusions
Gonzales-Chambers et al (151)	1992	Southern blot for TCR re-arrangement	23 patients with RA and/or neutropenia; 17 controls with chronic RA and no neutropenia	8/23 clonal B-chain re-arrangement no re-arrangement in controls
Meliconi et al (155)	1992	Southern blot	19 RA and neutropenia, 17 without neutropenia	3 patients with TCRB re-arrangement
Toussirot et al (157)	1993	Southern blot of PBLs	2 RA and "pseudo-Felty's"	polyclonal usage of TCR in PBLs
Bowman et al (153)	1995	RT-PCR from RNA of $CD8^+$ T cells	10 RA and LGL, 1 control	unique TCRBD1 and TCRBD2, D region sequence in reverse orientation
Davey et al (156)	1995	RT-PCR from PBMC RNA, Southern blot, sequence analysis of subcloned PCR products	12 patients with LGL leukemia, 7 of whom also had RA; 5 normal controls	3/7 LGL-RA patients used Vβ6 in the leukemic LGLs; Vβ6 usage not seen in non-RA leukemic LGL's
Bowman et al (158)	1997	RT-PCR from RNA of clonal CD8+ T-cells, sequencing PCR products from CD8+ T cells	10 RA and LGL patients	expanded clones with specific Vα and Vβ usage found in most patients, but different TCR's used in each patient; β junctional motif LG or RG 7/14, GXG 8/14

multiple infectious stimuli (2) HLA associations for JRA have been described and appear to be specific to the particular JRA subtypes (3) patients with JRA frequently have a limited course and remit with medical therapy (4) an autoantibody (and possible autoantigen) has been identified in association with uveitis in ANA^{+} pauciarticular JRA patients [160]. Investigation of possible causative agents in JRA has thus focused on defining the T cell populations in JRA, in hopes of identifying expanded populations of T cells, which may be responding to inciting antigens.

Current experimental evidence indicates that oligoclonal expansion of synovial T cells occurs during the course of JCA in children. These oligoclonal populations occur in a wide variety of TCR Vβ clones, but may occur more frequently in the Vβ8 and Vβ20 subsets [161, 162]. The data does not support the hypothesis that a single oligoclonal population of T cells is responding to a single antigen, but more studies are needed to determine if distinct Vβ clones (e.g. Vβ20 and Vβ2) share similar CDR3 motifs, and if children who are of different HLA types use distinct Vβ clones but common CDR3 motifs during oligoclonal expansion of synovial T cells.

Other controversial issues in TCR usage in JRA include conflicting observations about the presence of a VB6 genomic polymorphism [19–21, 167]. Some patients with early onset pauci- or polyarticular JRA, especially HLA-DR1^{+} patients, have a higher carrier rate of a VB6 allele which is less likely to undergo productive TCR rearrangement [167]. Speculation that such patients actually have a skew in their T cell repertoire which then causes increased susceptibility to JRA has not yet been substantiated by experimental data.

Summarized in Table 6 are studies of the T-cell repertoire in JRA, including the numbers of patients studied, techniques used and general conclusions.

Psoriatic arthritis

Psoriasis is a chronic inflammatory skin disease in which abnormal accumulations of T cells are found juxtaposed to activated keratinocytes. Patients with psoriatic arthritis may have an associated spondyloarthropathy resembling other HLA-B27 positive conditions, and/or a peripheral asymmetric or symmetric erosive arthritis. Joint and/or skin inflammation has been hypothesized to result from a common antigenic stimulus. However, evidence supporting this hypothesis such as (1) identification of a single immunogenic antigen or (2) identification of oligoclonal T cells that are found in psoriatic joints and psoriatic skin has been elusive. Recently, two published abstracts suggest the presence of psoriatic skin and joint T-cells [171] which share similar CDR3 motifs, and oligoclonal expansion of CD8^{+} T cells in psoriatic joints. A single publication utilizing the Southern blotting method of detecting TCRVB rearrangements shows oligoclonal expansion of T cells from the joint of a patient with psoriatic arthritis [172]. Full length publications have not yet

Table 6 - Studies in JRA of TCR usage

Study	Year	Techniques used	Patients	Conclusions
Horneff (163)	1992	flow cytometry to detect selected Vβ	24	detected increased usage in PB of Vβ5 and Vβ6 in patients with active JRA and increased usage in PB of Vβ8 in a patient with HLA-B27 associated disease.
Sioud et al. (162)	1992	PCR, subcloning and sequencing of Vβ20 clones	18 patients: 10 with pauciarticular onset, 7 with poly-articular onset, one with systemic onset; 3 control patients	SF repertoire restricted compared with PB; similar Vβ usage in PB CD4 and CD8 cells, increased usage of Vβ 2,18, and 20 in SFMC; within Vβ20 SF population is oligo clonal; restricted use of Vα in SF of 4/6 patients tested
Doherty et al. (164)	1992	RT-PCR using mRNA derived from PB and SF	5 patients with seronegative arthritis, 4 of whom were HLA-B27$^+$	differences noted comparing PB and SF of some patients (↑Vβ2,6,8,14 or 20)
Bernstein et al. (165)	1993	Southern blot	9 patients (7 pauci, 1 poly, 1 systemic)	Evidence of TCR rearrangement in SF of 2 patients
Grom et al. (166)	1993	PCR, Southern blotting, sequencing Vβ14 subclones	27 patients (12 poly, 10 pauci, 5 systemic), extensive analysis of samples from 1 polyarticular patient	6/27 (all polyarticular, 3 RF$^+$) had overexpression of Vβ14 in SF compared with PB, within Vβ14 had repeated use of a CDR3 region

Ostenstad et al. (168)	1995	RT-PCR of mRNA from SFMC, PBMC, or T cell antigen-specific lines or clones	JRA and RA patients with extensive analysis of 1 patient	Increased usage Vα2.2 and Vβ5.5 in 1 patient; predominance of one clone within the Vα3 population, in contrast to the Vα6 which was polyclonal.
Thompson et al. (161)	1995	PCR, cDNA sequencing	36 patients (14 poly, 18 pauci, 4 systemic) cDNA sequencing of subcloned PCR fragments in 32/36 patients	Evidence of SFMC oligoclonality in Vβ2, Vβ3, (pauci/poly), Vβ4, Vβ8, Vβ11, Vβ12, VB13.1, VB14, VB16, Vβ17, Vβ18, Vβ20 (poly, pauci, systemic onset); Vβ5.1, Vβ5.2, Vβ6, Vβ7, Vβ13.2, Vβ20 (poly); Vβ2,14,17 most commonly used in polyarticular JRA
Zhang et al. (169)	1996	RT-PCR	3 patients with JRA analyzed at multiple time points	SF oligoclonal with variability between patients but persistence of some T cell clones over time.
Thompson et al. (170)	1998	PCR, cDNA sequencing of paired PB and SF or ST; limited sequencing of Vβ8 cells in polyarticular JRA and Vβ20 cells in pauci-articular JRA (includes juvenile spondyloarthropathies)	Vβ20 sequencing from 41 patients, with total of 57 samples; Vβ8 sequencing from 17 patients with total of 30 samples; includes analysis of CD4$^+$ and CD4$^-$ T cell subsets	Vβ20: 36/42 SF/ST samples and 2/13 PBMC samples were clonally expanded as evidenced by presence of similar CDR3 motifs. Expansion occurs in all 3 types of JRA, with higher frequency of expanded Vβ20 clones in pauci-JRA. Vβ8: 19/23 SF/ST and 4/19 PB samples had clonal expansion. Expanded clones use distinct CDR3 sequence for TCR in CD4$^+$ and CD4$^-$ populations. Certain Jβ segments used more frequently in Vβ8 clones and others in Vβ20 clones.

employed the more sensitive PCR based technology (SSCP) in psoriatic arthritis, as has been performed using patient samples from RA and JRA. Although data have not yet been published that fully support the concept that psoriatic arthritis is an antigen-driven process, cautious optimism about the utility of such studies is appropriate.

Relationship between the expressed TCR repertoire and antigen-specific T cell responses in RA

Although a variety of antigen-directed responses can be demonstrated using peripheral and synovial T cells in RA, the antigenic responses that are important in initiation of disease and joint destruction are not yet clear. Furthermore, it has been difficult to link observations about skewing of the T cell repertoire in RA to antigen-directed responses. Antigens of potential interest include autoantigens, conventional microbial peptide antigens, and superantigens. Although strong evidence for effects of a superantigen recognized by Vβ14 was observed in one study [66], most subsequent studies have been unable to confirm these findings, and the identity of the specific superantigen that affected the $V\beta14^{+}$ population in RA has not been clarified. Since rheumatoid arthritis synovial fibroblasts, as well as professional antigen presenting cells, can present superantigen to T cells [173], any superantigens present in the synovial compartment should generate strong T cell responses.

In contrast to activation of an entire Vβ family by superantigens, conventional peptide antigens can activate small subsets of clones from many different Vβ families. For example, T cells from at least 13 different Vβ families can respond to purified protein derivative (PPD) presented by HLA-DR4 or DR14.1 [174]. It is apparent, therefore, that a diverse T cell repertoire is not incompatible with an antigen-specific T cell response.

A variety of bacterial antigens, particularly mycobacterial antigens, have been investigated as targets of the immune response in RA. In addition to studies of the responses of γδ T cells (mentioned in the section on the TCR γδ repertoire in RA), responses of αβ T cells have been demonstrated in synovial fluid or synovial tissue [175–185]. The 65 kDa mycobacterial heat shock protein was shown to stimulate proliferative responses of synovial fluid but not peripheral blood T cells from patients with reactive arthritis, as well as some patients with rheumatoid arthritis [175–177], and these responses were accentuated in early disease [176]. The epitopes recognized by hsp65 reactive T cells do not cross react with a homologous human heat shock protein [177, 178]. Clones of such cells appear to show preferential usage of specific TCRA and TCRB V genes, including the combinations of AV13/BV3 and AV6/BV13 [177]. However, when T cell clones specific for the crude BCG antigen are generated from RA synovial fluid, there is an overrepresentation of Vβ8 [179]. Immune responses to other specific mycobacterial antigens have also been found in the synovial compartment in RA and JRA [180–182]. T cells reactive against the 18.6 and 30 kDa mycobacterial antigens are heterogeneous, and use at least 8 different Vβ families in their T cell receptors [181].

The functional importance of synovial T cells that can respond to mycobacterial proteins is unclear at present [183–185]. At most there is only partial overlap between T cells that respond to human hsp60 and those reactive with the 65 kDa mycobacterial heat shock protein [183, 184]. Although generation of cytotoxic T lymphocytes during the course of such response has been demonstrated [183], responses to human hsp60 can also be dominated by Th2 cells which secrete cytokines capable of suppressing joint inflammation [185].

Another series of observations regarding responses to microbial antigens in RA has focused on antigens cross reactive with the QKRAA "shared epitope" sequence expressed by RA associated HLA-DR alleles [24, 186, 187]. This sequence is contained in a variety of bacterial and viral antigens [186, 187]. Studies of monozygotic twins discordant for RA demonstrate T cell responses to such peptides independent of the presence of RA, suggesting control of such responses by either genetic or shared environmental factors [186]. Synovial fluid T cells from early RA patients have particularly strong responses to such antigens, that are relatively specific for RA [187]. Whether such responses are pathogenic or an epiphenomena of disordered control of lymphocyte reactivity remains unclear. Additional information is needed about the TCR repertoire used by T cells that recognize such antigens.

In addition to possible reactivity against self Class II, other autoreactive responses are of potential interest in RA. Synovial dendritic cells have been proposed as the key antigen presenting cells capable of initiating responses to autoantigens in the joint [188]. Type II collagen has been extensively studied as a target antigen in both animal models and human disease [189–194]. Even in inbred mice, the TCR αβ repertoire of collagen-reactive T cells is rather complex [189, 190]. Nevertheless, large deletions within the Vβ locus can markedly influence susceptibility to arthritis [189]. Although antigen-specific T cells reactive with Type II collagen can be found in the joint and peripheral blood of patients with RA [191–194], such responses are also found in control subjects [193]. In synovial fluid, predominance of three of the Vβ types was found by PCR analysis among T cells responding to Type II collagen, Vβ14, Vβ17 and Vβ8 [194]. Whether this pattern is restricted to RA and is pathogenic remains unclear at this time. Other potential autoantigens in the joint include proteoglycan [191, 194], unidentified substances in autologous but not allogeneic synovial fluid [195, 196], and immunoglobulin heavy chains or immunoglobulin binding proteins [197]. In addition, the clonally expanded $V\alpha 12^+$ T cells from peripheral blood of some patients with rheumatoid arthritis can recognize autologous Epstein-Barr virus transformed lymphoid cell lines [198].

Beyond the T cell receptor – Co-stimulatory molecules and signalling abnormalities involved in activation of synovial T cells

The polyclonal synovial T cell population is clearly distinct from peripheral blood T cells in subjects with arthritis or in control individuals. T cells found in the joint express memory and activation markers, including Class II MHC, CD45RO, and the CD40 ligand [199, 200]. The $CD60^{+}$ subset dominates the synovial T cell infiltrate and CD60 can deliver an activating signal to these cells [199]. Certain phenotypic characteristics of both $CD4^{+}$ and $CD8^{+}$ peripheral blood T cells also appear to be unusual in patients with RA [201–203]. Among $CD4^{+}$ T cells, the $CD28^{-}$ subset is expanded and is characterized by autoreactivity [201, 202]. Among $CD8^{+}$ cells, a higher than normal proportion express CD57, and this subset tends to contain clonally expanded Vβ populations [203]. There is evidence for altered signalling properties of RA T cells [204–206], perhaps in part due to chronic effects of cytokines [206]. Understanding antigen-specific responses in RA and other forms of arthritis, and the significance of apparent TCR oligoclonality, will undoubtedly require integration of relevant information about function and abnormalities of costimulatory molecules and signalling structures on these T cells. At this time the conceptual basis for targeting specific T cell populations in the treatment of RA is incomplete. Empiric approaches to T cell depletion can generate a new distribution of T cell clones with the potential for increased oligoclonality and/or pathogenicity [207]. Better understanding of the relationship between the expressed TCR repertoire and the pathogenic sequence of events in RA (and other forms of arthritis) is required to provide a rational basis for TCR-directed therapeutic approaches.

Acknowledgements
We are grateful to Jennifer Dunn, Matthew Hollenbeck and Nancy Elslager for assistance in preparation of the manuscript. Supported in part by NIH grants AR38477, AR01955, AR20557

References

1 Alsalameh S, GR Burmester, JR Kalden (1994) Basic mechanisms in rheumatoid arthritis: The role of T lymphocytes in rheumatoid synovitis. In: S-E Dahlen (ed): *Adv Prostaglandin Thromboxane Leukot Res*, Vol 22 1994, Raven Press, Ltd New York, 289-394
2 McDermott M, DL Kastner, JD Holloman, G Schmidt-Wolf, AS Lundberg, AA Sinha, C Hsu, P Cashin, MG Molloy, B Mulcahy (1995) The role of T-cell receptor β chain genes in the susceptibility to rheumatoid arthritis. *Ann N Y Acad Sci* 756: 173–175
3 Wallin J, J Hillert, O Olerup, B Carlsson, H Strom (1991) Association of rheumatoid

arthritis with a dominant DR1/Dw4/Dw14 sequence motif, but not with T cell receptor β chain gene alleles or haplotypes. *Arthritis Rheum* 34: 1416–1424

4 Funkhouser, SW, P Concannon, P Charmley, DL Vredevoe, L Hood (1992) Differences in T cell receptor restriction fragment length polymorphisms in patients with rheumatoid arthritis. *Arthritis Rheum* 35(4): 465–471

5 de Vries N, CFM Prinsen, EBJM Mensink, PLCM van Riel, MA van't Hof, LBA van de Putte (1993) A T cell receptor β chain variable region polymorphism associated with radiographic progression in rheumatoid arthritis. *Ann Rheum Dis* 52: 327–331

6 Pile K, P Wordsworth, F Liote, T Bardin, J Bell, F Cornelis (1993) Analysis of a T-cell receptor Vβ segment implicated in susceptibility to rheumatoid arthritis: Vβ2 germline polymorphism does not encode susceptibility. *Ann Rheum Dis* 52: 891–894

7 Lunardi D, M Ibberson, S Zeminian, G De Sandre, AK So (1994) Lack of association of T cell receptor Vβ8 polymorphism with rheumatoid arthritis in United Kingdom and Italian white patients. *Ann Rheum Dis* 53: 341–343

8 Vandevyver C, XX Gu, P Geusens, M Spaepen, L Philippaerts, J Cassiman, J Raus (1994) HLA class II and T-cell receptor β chain polymorphisms in Belgian patients with rheumatoid arthritis: no evidence for disease association with the TCRBC2, TCRBV8 and TCRBV11 polymorphisms. *Ann Rheum Dis* 53: 580–586

9 Charmley P, JL Nelson, JA Hansen, A Branchaud, RA Barrington, D Templin, G Boyer, AP Lanier, P Concannon (1994) T-cell receptor polymorphisms in Tlingit Indians with rheumatoid arthritis. *Autoimmunity* 19: 247–251

10 Vandevyver C, P Geusens, JJ Cassiman and J Raus (1994) T cell receptor delta locus polymorphism in rheumatoid arthritis. *Eur J Immunogen* 21: 479–483

11 McDermott M, DL Kastner, JD Holloman, G Schmidt-Wolf, AS Lundberg, AA Sinha, C Hsu, P Cashin, MG Molloy, B Mulcahy et al (1995) The role of T cell receptor β chain genes in the susceptibility to rheumatoid arthritis. *Arthritis Rheum* 38(1): 91–95

12 McDermott M, C Hsu, MG Molloy, B Mulcahy, M Phelan, F Shanahan, F O'Gara, C Adams, LA Rubin, DO Clegg et al (1995) Non-linkage of a T-cell receptor gamma chain microsatellite (D7S485) to rheumatoid arthritis in multiplex families. *Journal of Autoimmunity* 8: 131–138

13 Gomolka M, H Menninger, JE Saal, EM Lemmel, ED Albert, O Niwa, JT Epplen, C Epplen (1995) Immunoprinting: various genes are associated with increased risk to develop rheumatoid arthritis in different groups of adult patients. *J Mol Med* 73: 19–29

14 Li Y, G Sun, Q Zhen, D-H Yoo, N Bhardwaj, DN Posnett, MK Crow, SM Friedman (1996) Allelic variants of human TCR BV17S1 defined by restriction fragment length polymorphism, single strand conformation polymorphism, and amplification refractory mutation system analyses. *Hum Immunol* 49: 85–95

15 Mu H, P Charmley, M-C King, LA Criswell (1996) Synergy between T cell receptor β gene polymorphism and HLA-DR4 in susceptibility to rheumatoid arthritis. *Arthritis Rheum* 39(6): 931–937

16 Cornelis F, L Hardwick, RM Flipo, M Martinez, S Lasbleiz, JF Prud'Homme, TH Tran,

S Walsh, A Delaye, A Nicod et al (1997) Association of rheumatoid arthritis with an amino acid allelic variation of the T cell receptor. *Arthritis Rheum* 40(8): 1387–1390

17 Hall FC, MA Brown, DE Weeks, S Walsh, A Nicod, S Butcher, LJ Andrews, BP Wordsworth (1997) A linkage study across the T cell receptor A and T cell receptor B loci in families with rheumatoid arthritis. *Arthritis Rheum* 40(10): 1798–1802

18 Nepom BS, U Malhotra, DA Schwarz, JW Nettles, JG Schaller, P Concannon (1991) HLA and T cell receptor polymorphisms in pauciarticular-onset juvenile rheumatoid arthritis. *Arthritis Rheum* 34: 1260–1267

19 Maksymowych WP, CA Gabriel, L Luyrink, H Melin-Aldana, M Elma, EH Giannini, DJ Lovell, C VanKerckhove, J Leiden, E Choi, DN Glass (1992) Polymorphism in a T-cell receptor variable gene is associated with susceptibility to a juvenile rheumatoid arthritis subset. *Immunogenetics* 35: 257–262

20 Ploski R, T Hansen, O Forre (1993) Lack of association with T-cell receptor TCRBV6S1*2 allele in HLA-DQA1*0101-positive Norwegian juvenile chronic arthritis patients. *Immunogenetics* 38: 444–445

21 Charmley P, BS Nepom, P Concannon (1994) HLA and T cell receptor β-chain DNA polymorphisms identify a distinct subset of patients with pauciarticular-onset juvenile rheumatoid arthritis. *Arthritis Rheum* 37(5): 695–701

22 Abbott WGH, A Geursen, JS Peake, IJ Simpson, MA Skinner, PLJ Tan (1995) Search for linkage disequilibrium between alleles in the T cell receptor α and β chain loci and susceptibility to rheumatic fever. *Immunology and Cell Biology* 73: 369–371

23 Timon M, A Arnaiz-Villena, P Perez-Aciego, P Morales, D Benmamar, J Regueiro (1991) A diallelic RFLP of the CD3-epsilon chain of the clonotypic T-lymphocyte receptor is not associated with certain autoimmune diseases. *Hum Genet* 86(4): 363–364

24 Gregersen PK, J Silver, RJ Winchester (1987) The shared epitope hypothesis: an approach to understanding the molecular genetics of susceptibility to rheumatoid arthritis. *Arthritis Rheum* 30: 1205–1213

25 Walport MJ, WE Ollier, AJ Silman (1992) Immunogenetics of rheumatoid arthritis and the Arthritis and Rheumatism Council's National Repository. *Br J Rheumatol* 31(10): 701–705

26 Weyand CM, C Xie, JJ Goronzy (1992) Homozygosity for the HLA-DRB1 allele selects for extra-articular manifestations in rheumatoid arthritis. *J Clin Invest* 89: 2033–2039

27 Weyand CM, C Hicok, D Conn, JJ Goronzy (1992) The influence of HLA-DRB1 genes on disease severity in rheumatoid arthritis. *Ann Intern Med* 117: 801–806

28 Evans TI, J Han, R Singh, G Moxley (1995) The genotypic distribution of shared-epitope DRB1 alleles suggests a recessive mode of inheritance of the rheumatoid arthritis disease-susceptibility gene. *Arthritis Rheum* 38: 1754–1761

29 Moreno I, A Valenzuela, A Garcia, J Yelamos, B Sanchez, W Hernanz (1996) Association of the shared epitope with radiological severity of rheumatoid arthritis. *J Rheumatol* 23: 6–9

30 Wagner U, S Kaltenhauser, H Sauer, S Arnold, W Seidel, H Hantzschel, JR Kalden, R

Wassmuth (1997) HLA markers and prediction of clinical course and outcome in rheumatoid arthritis. *Arthritis Rheum* 40(2): 341–351
31 Singal DP, D Green, B Reid, D Gladman, WW Buchanan (1992) HLA-D region genes and rheumatoid arthritis (RA): importance of DR and DQ genes in conferring susceptibility to RA. *Ann Rheum Dis* 51: 23–28
32 Zanelli E, CJ Krco, JM Baisch, S Cheng, CS David (1996) Immune response of HLA-DQ8 transgenic mice to peptides from the third hypervariable region of HLA-DRB1 correlates with predisposition to rheumatoid arthritis. *Proc Natl Acad Sci USA* 93: 1814–1819
33 Pinet V, B Combe, O Avinens, S Caillat-Zuchman, J Sany, J Clot, J-F Eliaou (1997) Polymorphism of the HLA-DMA genes in rheumatoid arthritis. *Arthritis Rheum* 40(5): 854–858
34 Brennan P, B Ollier, J Worthington, A Hajeer, A Silman (1996) Are both genetic and reproductive associations with rheumatoid arthritis linked to prolactin? *Lancet* 348: 106–109
35 Weyand CM, TG McCarthy, J Goronzy (1995) Correlation between disease phenotype and genetic heterogeneity in rheumatoid arthritis. *J Clin Invest* 95: 2120–2126
36 Gregersen PK (1992) T-cell receptor-major histocompatibility complex genetic interactions in rheumatoid arthritis. *Rheum Dis Clin North Am* 18(4): 793–807
37 Fox DA (1997) The role of T cells in immunopathogenesis of rheumatoid arthritis. *Arthritis Rheum* 40(4): 598–609
38 Fox DA (1997) Rheumatoid arthritis – heresies and speculations. *Perspect Biol Med* 40(4): 479–491
39 Penzotti JE, GT Nepom, TP Lybrand (1997) Use of T cell receptor/HLA-DRB1*04 molecular modeling to predict site-specific interactions for the DR shared epitope associated with rheumatoid arthritis. *Arthritis Rheum* 40(7): 1316–1326
40 Zanelli E, CJ Krco, CS David (1997) Critical residues on HLA-DRB1*0402 HV3 peptide for HLA-DQ8-restricted immunogenicity. *J Immunol* 158: 3545–3551
41 Walser-Kuntz DR, C Weyand, JW Fulbright, SB Moore, J Goronzy (1995) HLA-DRB1 molecules and antigenic experience shape the repertoire of CD4 T cells. *Hum Immunol* 44: 203–209
42 Walser-Kuntz DR, CM Weyand, AJ Weaver, WM O'Fallon, JJ Goronzy (1995) Mechanisms underlying the formation of the T cell receptor repertoire in rheumatoid arthritis. *Immunity* 2(6): 597–605
43 Kohsaka H, T Nanki, WE Ollier, N Miyasaka, DA Carson (1996) Influence of the rheumatoid arthritis-associated shared epitope on T-cell receptor repertoire formation. *Proc Assoc Am Physicians* 108(4): 323–328
44 Nanki T, H Kohsaka, N Mizushima, WE Ollier, DA Carson, N Miyasaka (1996) Genetic control of T cell receptor BJ gene expression in peripheral lymphocytes of normal and rheumatoid arthritis monozygotic twins. *J Clin Invest* 98(7): 1594–1601
45 Kohsaka H, A Taniguchi, PP Chen, WE Ollier, DA Carson (1993) The expressed T cell receptor V gene repertoire of rheumatoid arthritis monozygotic twins: rapid analysis by

anchored polymerase chain reaction and enzyme-linked immunosorbent assay. *Eur J Immunol* 23(8): 1895–1901
46 Mizushima N, H Kohsaka, T Nanki, WER Ollier, DA Carson, N Miyasaka (1997) HLA-dependent peripheral T cell receptor (TCR) repertoire formation, its modification by rheumatoid arthritis. *Clin Exp Immunol* 110: 428–433
47 Kouskoff V, AS Korganow, V Duchatelle, C Degott, C Benoist, D Mathis (1996) Organ-specific disease provoked by systemic autoimmunity. *Cell* 87(5): 811–822
48 Sakkas LI, PF Chen, CD Platsoucas (1994) T-cell antigen receptors in rheumatoid arthritis. *Immunol Res* 13(2–3): 117–138
49 Zwillich SH, DB Weiner, WV Williams (1994) T cell receptor analysis in rheumatoid arthritis: what have we learnt? *Immunol Res* 13(1): 29–41
50 Goronzy JJ, CM Weyand (1995) T cells in rheumatoid arthritis Paradigms and facts. *Rheum Dis Clin North Am* 21(3): 655–674
51 Struyk L, GE Hawes, MK Chatila, FC Breedveld, JT Kurnick, PJ van den Elsen (1995) T cell receptors in rheumatoid arthritis. *Arthritis Rheum* 38(5): 577–589
52 Savill CM, PJ Delves, D Kioussis, P Walker, PM Lydyard, B Colaco, M Shipley, IM Roitt (1987) A minority of patients with rheumatoid arthritis show a dominant rearrangement of T-cell receptor β chain genes in synovial lymphocytes. *Scand J Immunol* 25: 629–635
53 Stamenkovic I, M Stegagno, KA Wright, SM Krane, EP Amento, RB Colvin, RJ Duquesnoy, JT Kurnick (1988) Clonal dominance among T-lymphocyte infiltrates in arthritis. *Proc Natl Acad Sci USA* 85: 1179–1183
54 Keystone EC, M Minden, R Klock, L Poplonski, J Zalcberg, T Takadera, TW Mak (1988) Structure of T cell antigen receptor β chain in synovial fluid cells from patients with rheumatoid arthritis. *Arthritis Rheum* 31: 1555–1557
55 Duby AD, AK Sinclair, SL Osborne-Lawrence, W Zeldes, L Kan, DA Fox (1989) Clonal heterogeneity of synovial fluid T lymphocytes from patients with rheumatoid arthritis. *Proc Natl Acad Sci USA* 86: 6206–6210
56 Hakoda M, T Ishimoto, K Yamamoto, K Inoue, N Kamatani, N Miyasaka, K Nishioka (1990) Clonal analysis of T cell infiltrates in synovial tissue of patients with rheumatoid arthritis. *Clin Immunol Immunopathol* 57(3): 387–398
57 Chatila MK, F Pandolfi, I Stamenkovic, JT Kurnick (1990) Clonal dominance among synovial tissue-infiltrating lymphocytes in arthritis. *Hum Immunol* 28: 252–257
58 Miltenburg AMM, JM van Laar, MR Daha, RRP de Vries, PJ van den Elsen, FC Breedveld (1990) Dominant T-cell receptor β-chain gene rearrangements indicate clonal expansion in the rheumatoid joint. *Scand J Immunol* 31: 121–126
59 van Laar JM, AMM Miltenburg, MJA Verdonk, MR Daha, RRP de Vries, PJ van den Elsen, FC Breedveld (1991) Lack of T cell oligoclonality in enzyme-digested synovial tissue and in synovial fluid in most patients with rheumatoid arthritis. *Clin Exp Immunol* 83: 352–358
60 Hylton W, C Smith-Burchnell, BK Pelton, RG Palmer, AM Denman, M Malkovsky (1992) Polyclonal origin of rheumatoid synovial T-lymphocytes. *Br J Rheumatol* 31(1): 55–57

61 van Laar JM, AM Miltenburg, MJ Verdonk, MR Daha, RR de Vries, PJ van den Elsen, FC Breedveld (1992) T-cell receptor β-chain gene rearrangements of T-cell populations expanded from multiple sites of synovial tissue obtained from a patient with rheumatoid arthritis. *Scand J Immunol* 35(2): 187–194

62 Lu Y, BS Kim, RM Pope (1992) Clonal heterogeneity of synovial fluid T lymphocytes in inflammatory synovitis. *Clin Immunol Immunopathol* 63(1): 28–33

63 Korthauer U, B Hennerkes, H Menninger, HW Mages, J Zacher, AJ Potocnik, F Emmrich, RA Kroczek (1992) Oligoclonal T cells in rheumatoid arthritis: identification strategy and molecular characterization of a clonal T-cell receptor. *Scand J Immunol* 36(6): 855–863

64 Cantagrel A, A Alam, HL Coppin, B Mazieres, C De Preval (1993) Clonality of T lymphocytes expanded with IL-2 from rheumatoid arthritis peripheral blood, synovial fluid and synovial membrane. *Clin Exp Immunol* 91(1): 83–89

65 Brennan FM, S Allard, M Londei, C Savill, A Boylston, S Carrel, RN Maini, M Feldmann (1988) Heterogeneity of T cell receptor idiotypes in rheumatoid arthritis. *Clin Exp Immunol* 73: 417–423

66 Paliard X, SG West, JA Lafferty, JR Clements, JW Kappler, P Marrack, BL Kotzin (1991) Evidence for the effects of a superantigen in rheumatoid arthritis. *Science* 253: 325–329

67 Howell MD, JP Diveley, KA Lundeen, A Esty, ST Winters, DJ Carlo, SW Brostoff (1991) Limited T-cell receptor β-chain heterogeneity among interleukin 2 receptor-positive synovial T cells suggests a role for superantigen in rheumatoid arthritis. *Proc Natl Acad Sci USA* 88: 10921–10925

68 Pluschke G, G Ricken, H Taube, S Kroninger, I Melchers, HH Peter, K Eichmann, U Krawinkel (1991) Biased T cell receptor Vα region repertoire in the synovial fluid of rheumatoid arthritis patients. *Eur J Immunol* 21(11): 2749–2754

69 Olive C, PA Gatenby, SW Serjeantson (1991) Analysis of T cell receptor Vα and Vβ gene usage in synovia of patients with rheumatoid arthritis. *Immunol Cell Biol* 69: 349– 354

70 Sottini A, L Imberti, R Gorla, R Cattaneo, D Primi (1991) Restricted expression of T cell receptor Vβ but not Vα genes in rheumatoid arthritis. *Eur J Immunol* 21: 461–466

71 Uematsu Y, H Wege, A Straus, M Ott, W Bannwarth, J Lanchbury, G Panayi, M Steinmetz (1991) The T-cell-receptor repertoire in the synovial fluid of a patient with rheumatoid arthritis is polyclonal. *Proc Natl Acad Sci USA* 88: 8534–8538

72 Bucht A, JR Oksenberg, S Lindblad, A Gronberg, L Steinman, L Klareskog (1992) Characterization of T-cell receptor αβ repertoire in synovial tissue from different temporal phases of rheumatoid arthritis. *Scand J Immunol* 35(2): 159–165

73 Gudmundsson S, J Ronnelid, A Karlsson-Parra, J Lysholm, B Gudbjornsson, B Widenfalk, CH Janson, L Klareskog (1992) T-cell receptor V-gene usage in synovial fluid and synovial tissue from RA patients. *Scand J Immunol* 36(5): 681–688

74 Krawinkel U, G Pluschke (1992) T cell receptor variable region repertoire in lymphocytes from rheumatoid arthritis patients. *Immunobio* 185(5): 483–491

75 Lunardi C, C Marguerie, AK So (1992) An altered repertoire of T cell receptor V gene

expression by rheumatoid synovial fluid T lymphocytes. *Clin Exp Immunol* 90(3): 440–446

76 Williams, WV, Q Fang, D Demarco, J VonFeldt, RB Zurier, DB Weiner (1992) Restricted heterogeneity of T cell receptor transcripts in rheumatoid synovium. *J Clin Invest* 90(2): 326–333

77 Broker BM, U Korthauer, P Heppt, G Weseloh, R de la Camp, RA Kroczek, F Emmrich (1993) Biased T cell receptor V gene usage in rheumatoid arthritis Oligoclonal expansion of T cells expressing Vα2 genes in synovial fluid but not in peripheral blood. *Arthritis Rheum* 36(9): 1234–1243

78 Davey MP, DD Munkirs (1993) Patterns of T-cell receptor variable β gene expression by synovial fluid and peripheral blood T-cells in rheumatoid arthritis. *Clin Immunol Immunopathol* 68(1): 79–87

79 Dedeoglu F, H Kaymaz, N Seaver, SF Schluter, DE Yocum, JJ Marchalonis (1993) Lack of preferential Vb usage in synovial T cells of rheumatoid arthritis patients. *Immunol Res* 12(1): 12–20

80 DerSimonian H, M Sugita, DN Glass, AL Maier, ME Weinblatt, T Reme, MB Brenner (1993) Clonal Vα 12.1$^+$ T cell expansions in the peripheral blood of rheumatoid arthritis patients. *J Exp Med* 177(6): 1623–1631

81 Jenkins RN, A Nikaein, A Zimmermann, K Meek, PE Lipsky (1993) T cell receptor Vβ gene bias in rheumatoid arthritis. *J Clin Invest* 92(6): 2688–2701

82 De Keyser F, G Verbruggen, EM Veys, C Cuvelier, AM Malfait, D Benoit, D Elewaut, J Vermeersch, A Heirwegh (1993) T cell receptor Vβ usage in rheumatoid nodules: marked oligoclonality among IL-2 expanded lymphocytes. *Clin Immunol Immunopathol* 68(1): 29–34

83 Maruyama T, I Saito, S Miyake, H Hashimoto, K Sato, H Yagita, K Okumura, N Miyasaki (1993) A possible role of two hydrophobic amino acids in antigen recognition by synovial T cells in rheumatoid arthritis. *Eur J Immunol* 23(9): 2059–2065

84 Pluschke G, A Ginter, H Taube, I Melchers, HH Peter, U Krawinkel (1993) Analysis of T cell receptor Vβ regions expressed by rheumatoid synovial T lymphocytes. *Immunobiology* 188(4–5): 330–9

85 Sottini A, L Imberti, A Bettinardi, C Mazza, R Gorla, D Primi (1993) Selection of T lymphocytes in two rheumatoid arthritis patients defines different T-cell receptor Vβ repertoires in CD4$^+$ and CD8$^+$ T-cell subsets. *J Autoimmun* 6(5): 621–637

86 Struyk L, JT Kurnick, GE Hawes, JM van Laar, R Schipper, JR Oksenberg, L Steinman, RR de Vries, FC Breedveld, P van den Elsen (1993) T-cell receptor V-gene usage in synovial fluid lymphocytes of patients with chronic arthritis. *Hum Immunol* 37(4): 237– 251

87 Cooper SM, KD Roessner, M Naito-Hoopes, DB Howard, LK Gaur, RC Budd (1994) Increased usage of Vβ2 and Vβ6 in rheumatoid synovial fluid T cells. *Arthritis Rheum* 37(11): 1627–1636

88 Goronzy JJ, P Bartz-Bazzanella, W Hu, MC Jendro, DR Walser-Kuntz (1994) Dominant clonotypes in the repertoire of peripheral CD4$^+$ T cells in rheumatoid arthritis. *J Clin Invest* 94(5): 2068–76

89 Zagon G, JR Tumang, Y Li, SM Friedman, MK Crow (1994) Increased frequency of Vβ17-positive T cells in patients with rheumatoid arthritis. *Arthritis Rheum* 37(10): 1431–1440

90 Travaglio-Encinoza A, JM Anaya, AD d'Angeac, J Sany, T Reme (1994) TCR Vβ selection from a DRB1*401*0101 patient with rheumatoid arthritis complicated by a CD8+ T cell infiltrated rheumatoid pericarditis [letter]. *J Rheumatol* 21(7): 1373–1375

91 Li Y, G-R Sun, JR Tumang, MK Crow, SM Friedman (1994) CDR3 sequence motifs shared by oligoclonal rheumatoid arthritis synovial T cells. Evidence for an antigen-driven response. *J Clin Invest* 94: 2525–2531

92 Alam A, J Lule, H Coppin, N Lambert, B Mazieres, C De Preval, A Cantagrel (1995) T-cell receptor variable region of the β-chain gene use in peripheral blood and multiple synovial membranes during rheumatoid arthritis. *Hum Immunol* 42(4): 331–339

93 Fitzgerald JE, NS Ricalton, AC Meyer, SG West, H Kaplan, C Behrendt, BL Kotzin (1995) Analysis of clonal CD8+ T cell expansions in normal individuals and patients with rheumatoid arthritis. *J Immunol* 154(7): 3538–3547

94 Hucheng A, E Champagne, J Sevin, J Riond, J Tkaczuck, B Mazieres, A Cambon-Thomsen, A Cantagrel (1995) Abnormal T cell receptor Vβ gene expression in the peripheral blood and synovial fluid of rheumatoid arthritis patients. *Clin Exp Rheumatol* 13(1): 29–36

95 Khazaei HA, C Lunardi, AK So (1995) CD4 T cells in the rheumatoid joint are oligoclonally activated and change during the course of disease. *Ann Rheum Dis* 54(4): 314–317

96 Melchers I, HH Peter, H Eibel (1995) The T and B cell repertoire of patients with rheumatoid arthritis. *Scand J Rheumatol Suppl* 101: 153–162

97 Ramanujam T, M Luchi, HR Schumacher, S Zwillich, CP Chang, PE Callegari, JM Von Feldt, Q Fang, DB Weiner, WV Williams (1995) Detection of T cell receptors in early rheumatoid arthritis synovial tissue. *Pathobiology* 63(2): 100–108

98 Travaglio-Encinoza A, I Chaouni, H Dersimonian, C Jorgensen, J Simony-Lafontaine, F Romagne, J Sany, AD Dupuy d'Angeac, MB Brenner, T Reme (1995) T cell receptor distribution in rheumatoid synovial follicles. *J Rheumatol* 22(3): 394–399

99 Silver J, B Gulwani-Akolkar, PN Akolkar (1995) The influence of genetics, environment, and disease state on the human T-cell receptor repertoire. *Ann NY Acad Sci* 756: 28–52

100 Padula SJ, A Sampieri (1995) T-cell receptor use in early rheumatoid arthritis. *Ann NY Acad Sci* 756: 147–158

101 Jenkins RN, DE McGinnis (1995) T-cell receptor Vβ gene utilization in rheumatoid arthritis. *Ann NY Acad Sci* 756: 159–172

102 Hingorani R, J Monteiro, R Pergolizzi, R Furie, E Chartash, PK Gregersen (1995) CDR3 length restriction of T-cell receptor β chains in CD8+ T-cells of rheumatoid arthritis patients. *Ann NY Acad Sci* 756: 179–182

103 Cooper, SM, KD Roessner, M Naito-Hoopes, C Dobbs, JA Nicklas, DB Howard, LK Gaur, RC Budd (1995) Unstimulated rheumatoid synovial T-cells have a consistent Vβ gene bias when compared to peripheral blood T-cells. *Ann NY Acad Sci* 756: 186–189

104 Alam A, J Lule, N Lambert, H Coppin, B Mazieres, C De Preval, A Cantagrel (1995) Use of T-cell receptor V genes in synovial membrane in rheumatoid arthritis. *Ann NY Acad Sci* 756: 199–200

105 Struyk L, GE Hawes, RJ Dolhain, A van Scherpenzeel, B Godthelp, FC Breedveld, PJ van den Elsen (1995) Evidence for selective *in vivo* expansion of synovial tissue-infiltrating $CD4^+CD45RO^+$ T-lymphocytes on the basis of CDR3 diversity. *Ann NY Acad Sci* 756: 204–207

106 Ikeda Y, K Masuko, Y Nakai, T Kato, T Hasanuma, SI Yoshino, Y Mizushima, K Nishioka, K Yamamoto (1996) High frequencies of identical T cell clonotypes in synovial tissues of rheumatoid arthritis patients suggest the occurrence of common antigen driven immune responses. *Arth Rheum* 39(3): 446–453

107 Alam A, N Lambert, J Lule, H Coppin, B Mazieres, C de Preval, A Cantagrel (1996) Persistence of dominant T cell clones in synovial tissues during rheumatoid arthritis. *J Immunol* 156(9): 3480–3485

108 Fischer DC, B Opalka, A Hoffmann, W Mayr, HD Haubeck (1996) Limited heterogeneity of rearranged T cell receptor Vα and Vβ transcripts in synovial fluid T cells in early stages of rheumatoid arthritis. *Arthritis Rheum* 39(3): 454–462

109 Gonzalez-Quintial R, R Baccala, RM Pope, AN Theofilopoulos (1996) Identification of clonally expanded T cells in rheumatoid arthritis using a sequence enrichment nuclease assay. *J Clin Invest* 97(5): 1335–1343

110 Hingorani R, J Monteiro, R Furie, E Chartash, C Navarrete, R Pergolizzi, PK Gregersen (1996) Oligoclonality of Vβ3 TCR chains in the $CD8^+$ T cell population of rheumatoid arthritis patients. *J Immunol* 156(2): 852–858

111 Struyk L, GE Hawes, HM Mikkers, PP Tak, FC Breedveld, PJ van den Elsen (1996) Molecular analysis of the T-cell receptor β-chain repertoire in early rheumatoid arthritis: heterogeneous TCRBV gene usage with shared amino acid profiles in CDR3 regions of T lymphocytes in multiple synovial tissue needle biopsies from the same joint *Eur. J Clin Invest* 26(12): 1092–1102

112 Lim A, A Toubert, C Pannetier, M Dougados, D Charron, P Kourilsky, J Even (1996) Spread of clonal T-cell expansions in rheumatoid arthritis patients. *Hum Immunol* 48(1–2): 77–83

113 Waase I, C Kayser, PJ Carlson, JJ Goronzy, CM Weyand (1996) Oligoclonal T cell proliferation in patients with rheumatoid arthritis and their unaffected siblings. *Arthritis Rheum* 39(6): 904–913

114 Yamamoto K, Y Ikeda, K Masuko, Y Nakai, T Kato, T Hasunuma, Y Mizushima, K Nishioka (1995) High frequencies of identical T-cell clonotypes accumulating in different areas of synovial lesions of rheumatoid arthritis patients. *Ann NY Acad Sci* 756: 208–210

115 Brennan F, C Plater-Zyberk, RN Maini, M Feldmann (1989) Coordinate expansion of 'fetal type' lymphocytes (TCR $\gamma\delta^+$T and $CD5^+$B) in rheumatoid arthritis and primary Sjogren's syndrome. *Clin Exp Immunol* 77: 175–178

116 Reme T, M Portier, F Frayssinoux, B Combe, P Miossec, F Favier, J Sany (1990) T cell

receptor expression and activation of synovial lymphocyte subsets in patients with rheumatoid arthritis Phenotyping of multiple synovial sites. *Arthritis Rheum* 33: 485–492

117 Chaouni I, M Radal, J Simony-Lafontaine, B Combe, J Sany, T Reme (1990) Distribution of T-cell receptor-bearing lymphocytes in the synovial membrane from patients with rheumatoid arthritis. *J Autoimmun* 3: 737–745

118 Keystone EC, C Rittershaus, N Wood, KM Snow, J Flatow, JC Purvis, L Poplonski, PC Kung (1991) Elevation of a γδ T cell subset in peripheral blood and synovial fluid of patients with rheumatoid arthritis. *Clin Exp Immunol* 84: 78–82

119 Meliconi R, M Uguccioni, A D'Errico, C A, L Frizziero, A Facchini (1992) T-cell receptor γδ positive lymphocytes in synovial membrane. *Br J Rheumatol* 31(1): 59–61

120 Smith MD, B Broker, L Moretta, E Ciccone, CE Grossi, JC Edwards, F Yuksel, B Colaco, C Worman, L Mackenzie, R Kinner, G Weseloh, K Gluckert, PM Lydyard (1990) T γδ cells and their subsets in blood and synovial tissue from rheumatoid arthritis patients. *Scand J Immunol* 32: 585–593

121 Meliconi R, C Pitzalis, GH Kingsley, GS Panayi (1991) γ/δ T cells and their subpopulations in blood and synovial fluid from rheumatoid arthritis and spondyloarthritis. *Clin Immunol Immunopathol* 59(1): 165–172

122 Lunardi C, C Marguerie, MJ Walport, AK So (1992) T γδ cells and their subsets in blood and synovial fluid from patients with rheumatoid arthritis. *Br J Rheumatol* 31(8): 527–530

123 Lamour A, F Jouen-Beades, O Lees, D Gilbert, X Le Loet, F Tron (1992) Analysis of T cell receptors in rheumatoid arthritis: the increased expression of HLA-DR antigen on circulating $\gamma\delta^+$ T cells is correlated with disease activity. *Clin Exp Immunol* 89(2): 217–222

124 Hoshino T, A Ohta, M Nakao, T Ota, T Inokuchi, S Matsueda, R Gouhara, A Yamada, K Itoh, K Oizumi (1996) TCR $\gamma\delta^+$ T cells in peripheral blood of patients with adult Still's disease. *J Rheumatol* 23(1): 124–129

125 Sioud M, J Kjeldsen-Kragh, A Quayle, C Kalvenes, K Waalen, O Forre, JB Natvig (1990) The Vδ gene usage by freshly isolated T lymphocytes from synovial fluids in rheumatoid synovitis: a preliminary report. *Scand J Immunol* 31: 415–421

126 Andreu JL, A Trujillo, JM Alonso, J Mulero, C Martinez (1991) Selective expansion of T cells bearing the γ/δ receptor and expressing an unusual repertoire in the synovial membrane of patients with rheumatoid arthritis. *Arthritis Rheum* 34: 808–814

127 Sioud M, O Forre, JB Natvig (1991) T cell receptor delta diversity of freshly isolated T lymphocytes in rheumatoid synovitis. *Eur J Immunol* 21: 239–241

128 Shen Y, S Li, AJ Quayle, OJ Mellbye, JB Natvig, O Forre (1992) TCR $\gamma\delta^+$ cell subsets in the synovial membranes of patients with rheumatoid arthritis and juvenile rheumatoid arthritis. *Scand J Immunol* 36(4): 533–540

129 Bucht A, K Soderstrom, T Hultman, M Uhlen, E Nilsson, R Kiessling, A Gronberg (1992) T cell receptor diversity and activation markers in the Vδ1 subset of rheumatoid synovial fluid and peripheral blood T lymphocytes. *Eur J Immunol* 22(2): 567–574

130 Olive C, PA Gatenby, SW Serjeantson (1992) Evidence for oligoclonality of T cell receptor d chain transcripts expressed in rheumatoid arthritis patients. *Eur J Immunol* 22(10): 2587–2593

131 Olive C, PA Gatenby, SW Serjeantson (1994) Persistence of γ/δ T cell oligoclonality in the peripheral blood of rheumatoid arthritis patients. *Immunol Cell Biol* 72(1): 7–11

132 Olive C, PA Gatenby, SW Serjeantson (1992) Molecular characterization of the Vγ9 T cell receptor repertoire expressed in patients with rheumatoid arthritis. *Eur J Immunol* 22(11): 2901–2906

133 Olive C, P Gatenby, S Serjeantson (1995) T cell receptor γ/δ usage in rheumatoid arthritis. *Ann NY Acad Sci*: 183–185

134 Giachino C, L Granziero, V Modena, V Maiocco, C Lomater, F Fantini, A Lanzavecchia, N Migone (1994) Clonal expansions of Vδ1+ and Vδ2+ cells increase with age and limit the repertoire of human γ/δ T cells. *Eur J Immunol* 24(8): 1914–1918

135 Hassan J, G Yanni, V Hegarty, C Feighery, B Bresnihan, A Whelan (1996) Increased numbers of CD5+ B cells and T cell receptor (TCR) γδ+ T cells are associated with younger age of onset in rheumatoid arthritis (RA). *Clin Exp Immunol* 103(3): 353–356

136 Kageyama Y, Y Koide, S Miyamoto, T Inoue, TO Yoshida (1994) The biased Vγ gene usage in the synovial fluid of patients with rheumatoid arthritis. *Eur J Immunol* 24(5): 1122–1129

137 Soderstrom K, A Bucht, E Halapi, C Lundqvist, A Gronberg, E Nilsson, DL Orsini, Y van de Wal, F Koning, ML Hammarstrom, R Kiessling (1994) High expression of Vγ8 is a shared feature of human γδ T cells in the epithelium of the gut and in the inflamed synovial tissue. *J Immunol* 152(12): 6017–6027

138 Kageyama Y, Y Koide, S Miyamoto, K Kushida, T Inoue, TO Yoshida (1995) Analysis of junctional sequences of T cell receptor g chain transcripts in γδ T cells from rheumatoid synovial fluid. *J Rheumatol* 22(5): 812–816

139 Doherty PJ, RD Inman, RM Laxer, ED Silverman, SX Yang, I Suurmann, S Pan (1996) Analysis of T cell receptor γ transcripts in right and left knee synovial fluids of patients with rheumatoid arthritis. *J Rheumatol* 23(7): 1143–1150

140 Kohsaka H, PP Chen, A Taniguchi, WE Ollier, DA Carson (1993) Divergent T cell receptor γ repertoires in rheumatoid arthritis monozygotic twins. *Arthritis Rheum* 36(2): 213–221

141 Holoshitz J, LM Vila, BJ Keroack, DR McKinley, NK Bayne (1992) Dual antigenic recognition by cloned γδ T cells. *J Clin Invest* 89: 308–314

142 Tanaka Y, S Sano, E Nieves, G De Libero, D Rosa, RL Modlin, MB Brenner, BR Bloom, CT Morita (1994) Nonpeptide ligands for human γδ T cells. *Proc Natl Acad Sci USA* 91(17): 8175–8179

143 Holoshitz J, F Koning, JE Coligan, J De Bruyn, S Strober (1989) Isolation of CD4− CD8− mycobacteria-reactive T lymphocyte clones from rheumatoid arthritis synovial fluid. *Nature* 339: 226–229

144 Soderstrom K, E Halapi, E Nilsson, A Gronberg, J van Embden, L Klareskog, R Kiessling (1990) Synovial cells responding to a 65-kDa mycobacterial heat shock pro-

tein have a high proportion of a TcR gamma delta subtype uncommon in peripheral blood. *Scand J Immunol* 32: 503–515

145 Pope RM, A Landay, RL Modlin, J Lessard, AE Koch (1991) γ/δ T cell receptor positive T cells in the inflammatory joint: lack of association with response to soluble antigens. *Cell Immunol* 137(1): 127–138

146 Grinlinton FM, MA Skinner, NM Birchall, PL Tan (1993) $\gamma\delta^+$ T cells from patients with psoriatic and rheumatoid arthritis respond to streptococcal antigen. *J Rheumatol* 20(6): 982–987

147 Ohta M, N Sato (1994) The cytotoxic analysis of T cell receptor $V\delta1^+$ T cell lines derived from the synovial fluid of rheumatoid arthritis patients. *Clin Exp Immunol* 97(2): 193–199

148 Vincent MS, K Roessner, D Lynch, D Wilson, SM Cooper, J Tschopp, LH Sigal, RC Budd (1996) Apoptosis of Fas^{high} $CD4^+$ synovial T cells by borrelia-reactive Fas-$ligand^{high}$ γδ T cells in Lyme arthritis. *J Exp Med* 184(6): 2109–2117

149 Peterman GM, C Spencer, AI Sperling, JA Bluestone (1993) Role of γδ T cells in murine collagen-induced arthritis. *J Immunol* 151(11): 6546–6558

150 Pelegri C, P Kuhnlein, E Buchner, CB Schmidt, A Franch, M Castell, T Hunig, F Emmrich, RW Kinne (1996) Depletion of γδ T cells does not prevent or ameliorate, but rather aggravates, rat adjuvant arthritis. *Arthritis Rheum* 39(2): 204–215

151 Gonzales-Chambers R, D Przepiorka, A Winkelstein, A Agarwal, TW Starz, WE Kline, H Hawk (1992) Lymphocyte subsets associated with T cell receptor β-chain gene rearrangement in patients with rheumatoid arthritis and neutropenia. *Arthritis Rheum* 35(5): 516–520

152 Bray RA, RM Pope, AL Landay (1991) Identification of a population of large granular lymphocytes obtained from the rheumatoid joint coexpressing the CD3 and CD16 antigens. *Clin Immunol Immunopathol* 58(3): 409–418

153 Bowman SJ, JS Lanchbury (1995) Non-standard D region usage by human TCRB sequences. *Immunogenetics* 43: 110–111

154 Vie H, S Chevalier, R Garand, JP Moisan, V Praloran, MC Devilder, JF Moreau, JP Soulillou (1989) Clonal expansion of lymphocytes bearing the γδ T-cell receptor in a patient with large granular lymphocyte disorder. *Blood* 74(1): 285–290

155 Meliconi R, GH Kingsley, C Pitzalis, L Sakkas, GS Panayi (1992) Analysis of lymphocyte phenotype and T cell receptor genotype in Felty's syndrome. *J Rheumatol* 19(7): 1058–1064

156 Davey MP, G Starkebaum, TP Loughran, Jr (1995) $CD3^+$ leukemic large granular lymphocytes utilize diverse T-cell receptor Vβ genes. *Blood* 85(1): 146–150

157 Toussirot E, P Lafforgue, JR Harle, S Kaplanski, P Mannoni, PC Acquaviva (1993) Pseudo Felty's syndrome. A polyclonal disease with a favorable prognosis. Report of two cases with Southern blot analysis of TCR. *Clin Exp Rheumatol* 11(6): 591–595

158 Bowman SJ, MA Hall, GS Panayi, JS Lanchbury (1997) T cell receptor α-chain and β-chain junctional region homology in clonal $CD3^+$, $CD8^+$ T lymphocyte expansions in Felty's Syndrome. *Arthritis Rheum* 40(4): 615–623

159 Imberti L, A Sottini, S Signorini, R Gorla, D Primi (1997) Oligoclonal CD4+ CD57+ T-cell expansions contribute to the imbalanced T-cell receptor repertoire of rheumatoid arthritis patients. *Blood* 89(8): 2822–2832
160 Murray K, W Szer, A Grom, P Donnelly, J Levinson, E Giannini, D Glass, I Szer (1997) Antibodies to the 45 kDa DEK nuclear antigen in pauciarticular onset juvenile rheumatoid arthritis and iridocyclitis: Selective association with MHC gene. *J Rheumatol* 24(3): 560–567
161 Thompson S, A Grom, S Bailey, L Luyrink, E Giannini, K Murray, M Passo, D Lovell, E Choi, D Glass (1995) Patterns of T lymphocyte clonal expansion in HLA-typed patients with juvenile rheumatoid arthritis. *J Rheumatol* 22(7): 1356–1364
162 Sioud M, J Kjeldsen-Kragh, S Suleyman, O Vinje, J Natvig, O Forre (1992) Limited heterogeneity of T cell receptor variable region gene usage in juvenile rheumatoid arthritis synovial T cells. *Eur J Rheumatol* 22(9): 2413–2418
163 Horneff G, M Hanson, V Wahn (1992) T-cell receptor V beta chain expression in patients with juvenile rheumatoid arthritis. *Rheumatol Int* 12: 221–226
164 Doherty P, E Silverman, R Laxer, S Yang, S Pan (1992) T cell receptor Vβ usage in synovial fluid of children with arthritis. *J Rheumatol* 19(3): 463–468
165 Bernstein B, A Miltenburg, J van Laar, R Hertzberger, F Breedveld, T cell receptor rearrangements in juvenile rheumatoid arthritis: a search for oligoclonality. *Clin Exp Rheumatol* 1993 11(2): 209–213
166 Grom AA, SD Thompson, L Luyrink, M Passo, E Choi, DN Glass (1993) Dominant T-cell-receptor β chain variable region Vβ14+ clones in juvenile rheumatoid arthritis. *Proc Natl Acad Sci USA* 90(23): 11104–11108
167 Charmley P, P Concannon (1995) PCR-based genotyping and haplotype analysis of human TCRGV gene segment polymorphisms. *Immunogenetics* 42(4): 254–261
168 Ostenstad B, A Dybwad, T Lea, O Forre, O Vinje, M Sioud (1995) Evidence for monoclonal expansion of synovial T cells bearing Vα2.1/ Vβ5.5 gene segments and recognizing synthetic peptide that shares homology with a number of putative autoantigens. *Immunology* 86(2): 168–175
169 Zhang H, D Phang, R Laxer, E Silverman, S Pan, P Doherty (1997) Evolution of the T cell receptor β repertoire from synovial fluid T cells of patients with juvenile onset rheumatoid arthritis. *J Rheumatol* 24(7): 1396–1402
170 Thompson SD, KJ Murray, AA Grom, MH Passo, E Choi, DN Glass (1998) Comparative sequence analysis of the human T cell receptor β chain in juvenile rheumatoid arthritis and juvenile spondyloarthropathies: Evidence for antigenic selection of T cells in the synovium. *Arthritis Rheum* 41(3): 482–497
171 Tasslulas IO, SR Duncan, M Centola, AN Theofilopoulos, DT Boumpas (1997) Concordant T cell receptor Vβ expansions in synovial tissue and skin of patients with psoriatic arthritis. *Arthritis Rheum* 40(9): S260
172 Costello P, K Peterson, B Bresnihan, R Winchester, O FitzGerald (1997) Repertoire of synovial fluid CD8+ T cells in psoriatic arthritis appears antigen-driven. *Arthritis Rheum* 40(9): S36

173 Tsai C, J Diaz, LA, NG Singer, LL Li, AH Kirsch, R Mitra, BJ Nickoloff, LJ Crofford, DA Fox (1996) Responsiveness of human T lymphocytes to bacterial superantigens presented by cultured rheumatoid arthritis synoviocytes. *Arthritis Rheum* 39(1): 125–136
174 Hansen T, E Qvigstad, KE Lundin, E Thorsby (1992) T-cell receptor β usage by 35 different antigen-specific T-cell clones restricted by HLA-Dw4 or -Dw14.1. *Hum Immunol* 35(3): 149–156
175 Gaston JS, PF Life, LC Bailey, PA Bacon (1989) *In vitro* responses to a 65-kilodalton mycobacterial protein by synovial T cells from inflammatory arthritis patients. *J Immunol* 143: 2494–2500
176 Res PC, CG Schaar, FC Breedveld, W van Eden, JD van Embden, IR Cohen, RR de Vries (1988) Synovial fluid T cell reactivity against 65 kD heat shock protein of mycobacteria in early chronic arthritis. *Lancet* 2: 478–480
177 Celis L, C Vandevyver, P Geusens, J Dequeker, J Raus, J Zhang (1997) Clonal expansion of mycobacterial heat-shock protein-reactive T lymphocytes in the synovial fluid and blood of rheumatoid arthritis patients. *Arthritis Rheum* 40(3): 510–519
178 Gaston JS, PF Life, PJ Jenner, MJ Colston, PA Bacon (1990) Recognition of a mycobacteria-specific epitope in the 65-kD heat- shock protein by synovial fluid-derived T cell clones. *J Exp Med* 171: 831–841
179 Wilson KB, AJ Quayle, S Suleyman, J Kjeldsen-Kragh, O Forre, JB Natvig, JD Capra (1993) Heterogeneity of the TCR repertoire in synovial fluid T lymphocytes responding to BCG in a patient with early rheumatoid arthritis. *Scand J Immunol* 38(1): 102–112
180 Natvig JB, AJ Quayle (1995) V-genes of T-cell receptors in rheumatoid arthritis. *Ann NY Acad Sci* 756: 138–146
181 Sioud M, J Kjeldsen-Kragh, AJ Quayle, HG Wiker, D Sorskaar, JB Natvig, O Forre (1991) Immune responses to 186 and 30-kDa mycobacterial antigens in rheumatoid patients, and Vβ usage by specific synovial T-cell lines and fresh T cells. *Scand J Immunol* 34(6): 803–812
182 Pope RM, MA Pahlavani, E LaCour, S Sambol, BV Desai (1989) Antigenic specificity of rheumatoid synovial fluid lymphocytes [see comments]. *Arthritis Rheum* 32: 1371–1380
183 Li SG, AJ Quayle, Y Shen, J Kjeldsen-Kragh, F Oftung, RS Gupta, JB Natvig, OT Forre (1992) Mycobacteria and human heat shock protein-specific cytotoxic T lymphocytes in rheumatoid synovial inflammation. *Arthritis Rheum* 35(3): 270–281
184 Quayle AJ, KB Wilson, SG Li, J Kjeldsen-Kragh, F Oftung, T Shinnick, M Sioud, O Forre, JD Capra, JB Natvig (1992) Peptide recognition, T cell receptor usage and HLA restriction elements of human heat-shock protein (hsp) 60 and mycobacterial 65-kDa hsp-reactive T cell clones from rheumatoid synovial fluid. *Eur J Immunol* 22(5): 1315–1322
185 van Roon JAG, W van Eden, JLAM van Roy, FJPG Lafeber, JWJ Bijlsma (1997) Stimulation of suppressive T cell responses by human but not bacterial 60-kD heat-shock protein in synovial fluid of patients with rheumatoid arthritis. *J Clin Invest* 100(2): 459–463

186 La Cava A, JL Nelson, WER Ollier, A MacGregor, EC Keystone, JC Thorne, JF Scavulli, CC Berry, DA Carson, S Albani (1997) Genetic bias in immune responses to a cassette shared by different microorganisms in patients with rheumatoid arthritis. *J Clin Invest* 100(3): 658–663
187 Albani S, EC Keystone, JL Nelson, WER Ollier, A La Cava, AC Montemayor, DA Weber, C Montecucco, A Martini, DA Carson (1995) Positive selection in autoimmunity: Abnormal immune responses to a bacterial dnaJ antigenic determinant in patients with early rheumatoid arthritis. *Nat Med* 1(5): 448–452
188 Thomas R, PE Lipsky (1996) Could endogenous self-peptides presented by dendritic cells initiate rheumatoid arthritis. *Immunol Today* 17(12): 559–564
189 Nabozny GH, MJ Bull, J Hanson, MM Griffiths, HS Luthra, CS David (1994) Collagen-induced arthritis in T cell receptor Vβ congenic B10Q mice. *J Exp Med* 180(2): 517–524
190 Osman GE, M Toda, O Kanagawa, LE Hood (1993) Characterization of the T cell receptor repertoire causing collagen arthritis in mice. *J Exp Med* 177(2): 387–395
191 Wooley PH, IA Cuesta, S Sud, Z Song, JA Affholter, RL Karvonen, F Fernandez-Madrid (1995) Oligoclonal T-receptor (Vβ) use in the response to connective tissue antigens by synovial fluid T-cells from rheumatoid arthritis patients. *Ann NY Acad Sci* 756: 195–198
192 Londei M, CM Savill, A Verhoef, F Brennan, ZA Leech, V Duance, RN Maini, M Feldmann (1989) Persistence of collagen type II-specific T-cell clones in the synovial membrane of a patient with rheumatoid arthritis. *Proc Natl Acad Sci USA* 86: 636–640
193 Snowden N, I Reynolds, K Morgan, L Holt (1997) T cell responses to human type II collagen in patients with rheumatoid arthritis and healthy controls. *Arthritis Rheum* 40(7): 1210–1218
194 Cuesta IA, S Sud, Z Song, JA Affholter, RL Karvonen, F Fernandez-Madrid, PH Wooley (1997) T cell receptor (Vβ) bias in the response of rheumatoid arthritis synovial fluid T cells to connective tissue antigens. *Scand J Rheumatol* 26(3): 166–173
195 Maurice MM, PC Res, A Leow, T van Hall, MR Daha, L Struyk, P van den Else, FC Breedveld, CL Verweij (1995) Joint-derived T cells in rheumatoid arthritis proliferate to antigens present in autologous synovial fluid. *Scand J Rheumatol Suppl* 101: 169–177
196 Res PC, L Struijk, A Leow, MR Daha, PC van den Elsen, FC Breedveld (1994) Inflamed joints of patients with rheumatoid arthritis contain T cells that display *in vitro* proliferation to antigens present in autologous synovial fluid. Functional analysis on the basis of synovial-fluid-reactive T-cell clones and lines. *Hum Immunol* 40(4): 291–298
197 van Schooten WC, D Devereux, CH Ho, J Quan, BA Aguilar, CJ Rust (1994) Joint-derived T cells in rheumatoid arthritis react with self-immunoglobulin heavy chains or immunoglobulin-binding proteins that copurify with immunoglobulin. *Eur J Immunol* 24(1): 93–98
198 Behar SM, C Roy, MB Brenner (1995) Expansions of Vα12 $CD8^+$ T-cells in rheumatoid arthritis. *Ann NY Acad Sci* 756: 130–137
199 Fox DA, JA Millard, L Kan, WS Zeldes, W Davis, J Higgs, F Emmrich, RW Kinne

(1990) Activation pathways of synovial T lymphocytes. Expression and function of the UM4D4/CDw60 antigen. *J Clin Invest* 86: 1124–1136
200 MacDonald KPA, Y Nishioka, PE Lipsky, R Thomas (1997) Functional CD40 ligand is expressed by T cells in rheumatoid arthritis. *J Clin Invest* 100(9): 2404–2414
201 Martens PB, JJ Goronzy, D Schaid, CM Weyand (1997) Expansion of unusual $CD4^+$ T cells in severe rheumatoid arthritis. *Arthritis Rheum* 40(6): 1106–1114
202 Schmidt D, J Goronzy, CM Weyand (1996) $CD4^+$ $CD7^-$ $CD28^-$ T cells are expanded in rheumatoid arthritis and are characterized by autoreactivity. *J Clin Invest* 97(9): 2027–2037
203 Wang EC, TM Lawson, K Vedhara, PA Moss, PJ Lehner, LK Borysiewicz (1997) $CD8high^+$ ($CD57^+$) T cells in patients with rheumatoid arthritis. *Arthritis Rheum* 40(2): 237–248
204 Allen ME, SP Young, RH Michell, PA Bacon (1995) Altered T lymphocyte signaling in rheumatoid arthritis. *Eur J Immunol* 25: 1547–1554
205 Carruthers DM, WG Naylor, ME Allen, GD Kitas, PA Bacon, SP Young (1996) Characterization of altered calcium signalling in T lymphocytes from patients with rheumatoid arthritis (RA). *Clin Exp Immunol* 105: 291–296
206 Cope AP, M Londie, NR Chu, SBA Cohen, MJ Elliott, FM Brennan, RN Maini, M Feldmann (1994) Chronic exposure to tumor necrosis factor (TNF) *in vitro* impairs the activation of T cells through the T cell receptor/CD3 complex; reversal *in vivo* by anti-TNF antibodies in patients with rheumatoid arthritis. *J Clin Invest* 94: 749–760
207 Jendro MD, T Ganten, EL Matteson, CM Weyand, JJ Goronzy (1995) Emergence of oligoclonal T cell populations following therapeutic T cell depletion in rheumatoid arthritis. *Arthritis Rheum* 38(9): 1242–1251

T cell-independent joint destruction

Juliane K. Franz[1,2], Thomas Pap[1], Ulf Müller-Ladner[1,3], Renate E. Gay[1], Gerd R. Burmester[2] and Steffen Gay[1]

[1] Center of Experimental Rheumatology, Department of Rheumatology, University Hospital Zürich, Gloriastr. 25, CH-8091 Zürich, Switzerland; [2] Department of Rheumatology and Clinical Immunology, Charité University Hospital, Humboldt University of Berlin, Schumannstr. 20–21, D-10117 Berlin, Germany; [3] Department of Internal Medicine, Division of Rheumatology and Clinical Immunology, University of Regensburg, Franz-Josef-Strauß-Allee 11, D-93042 Regensburg, Germany

Introduction

Rheumatoid arthritis (RA) is a chronic systemic disorder of unknown etiology. Although, early and late stages of the disease may be driven by different processes, affected joints are characterized by inflammation, synovial hyperplasia, and abnormal immune responses [1]. The abundance of T cells within the rheumatoid synovium as well as the association of certain major histocompatibility complex (MHC) class II molecules with RA [2] implied a central role for T cells in the pathophysiology of the disease. However, recent advances in molecular biology have fostered new concepts for the pathogenesis of RA. Specifically, the investigation of early stages of disease, the development of novel animal models, and the application of novel molecular biology techniques such as *in-situ hybridization* (ISH) and *polymerase chain reaction* (PCR) have identified "alternative", T cell-independent mechanisms involved in the initiation and perpetuation of the destructive synovitis characteristic of RA.

Synovial architecture in RA

RA synovial membrane consists of two distinct layers of cells. While the most superficial cells form the lining layer, those cells of the deeper region constitute the sublining layer. During the course of RA, both layers of the synovial membrane undergo dramatic changes. Histologically, the most prominent features are hyperplasia of the lining layer and infiltration of the sublining by mononuclear cells such as T cells, B cells, and macrophages, accompanied by an intensive neovascularization [1]. While the accumulation of inflammatory cells can also be found in other inflammatory joint diseases such as reactive arthritis, the synovial hyperplasia and activation of lining cells appears specific to RA. Thus, the normally thin lining can increase to up to 10 cell layers. It attaches to cartilage and bone and mediates progressive joint

T Cells in Arthritis, edited by P. Miossec, W.B. van den Berg and G.S. Firestein

destruction. This hyperplastic lining consists of macrophage-like type A and fibroblast-like type B synoviocytes. Type A synoviocytes express various macrophage-markers such as CD11b, CD14, and CD 68 and can be therefore identified by immunohistochemistry [3]. Fibroblast-like synoviocytes lack characteristic surface markers, but can be stained with antibodies recognizing prolyl 4-hydroxylase, an enzyme characteristic for collagen synthesis [4]. In RA, about two-third of the synoviocytes exhibit the macrophage-like phenotype, whereas one third are fibroblast-like type B synoviocytes [5]. Both cell types have been found to be highly activated in RA. Macrophage-like cells express large amounts of human leukocyte antigen (HLA) DR molecules and abundantly secrete cytokines and growth factors [5]. Fibroblast-like cells display a phenotype which appears transformed, differing from normal synovial fibroblasts both with respect to their morphology and to some characteristic tumor-like properties [6, 7]. They represent the predominant cell type at sites of cartilage and bone erosion by the RA synovium [8].

Synovial hyperplasia: proliferation versus defective apoptosis

The mechanisms leading to hyperplasia of RA synovium have not been fully elucidated yet. Studies by Aicher et al. have shown that synovial cells from patients with RA do not proliferate faster than those from osteoarthritis (OA) patients [9]. Moreover, the idea that an increased proliferation rate of synovial cells would be an explanation for the hyperplasia of rheumatoid synovium has been contradicted by the fact that only 1–5% of synovial cells are proliferating, as determined by thymidine incorporation [10]. Mitosis is also rarely found in RA synovial tissue [11] and immunohistochemistry for specific proliferation markers such as Ki-67 revealed only a very low number of positive cells within the RA synovium. Interestingly, Ki-67-positive cells were located predominantly within lymphocytic infiltrates, while no Ki-67- positive cells were detectable in the lining layer [12]. Furthermore, only 1% of fibroblast-like cells expressing proto-oncogenes such as *jun-B* and *c-fos* were also positive for Ki-67, indicating that the majority of RA synovial fibroblasts do not show an accelerated proliferation [13].

Therefore, the increased number of cells within RA synovium most likely results from cell migration into the synovium and alteration of apoptotic pathways. The number of cells within RA synovium exhibiting morphological features of apoptosis, or programmed cell death, is very low (<1%) when examined by ultrastructural methods [14, 15]. In contrast, applying *in-situ* nick-end labeling techniques, which detect DNA fragments, a much higher number of cells has been suggested to undergo apoptosis [16], especially within the lining layer. However, the latter results are most likely explained by DNA strand breaks within the inflamed synovium, which are caused by toxic stimuli such as oxygen radicals, and may not necessarily result in apoptosis. Data supporting an altered apoptosis in joint diseases, however, could be obtained from animal models. In the MRL/lpr mouse model, which resembles human RA to a certain extent [17], a mutation of the *Fas* gene has been identified to be responsible for the autoimmune disease in homozygous animals, caused by the insertion of a retrotransposon [18, 19]. To induce apoptosis, specific pathways have to be activated, e.g., the ligation of Fas to cell-bound or soluble Fas ligand. Several studies analyzed the expression of Fas and Fas ligand in human RA [14, 16, 20]. Although Fas has been shown to be expressed in RA synovial tissue as well as in cultured RA synovial fibroblast-like cells, its role remains unclear. Recent findings, indicating a dual function of the Fas molecule, may shed new light on the role of Fas in the balanced action of pro- and anti-apoptotic molecules. Apart from its pro-apoptotic function, Fas appears to be involved in pathways leading to proliferation [21]. Therefore, it is very likely that intracellular signaling pathways following Fas activation are modified by additional stimuli, thus determining whether the affected cell undergoes apoptosis or proliferates. In this context, these findings may explain the fact that cultured synovial fibroblasts are resistant to Fas-induced apoptosis, despite the surface expression of Fas molecules [22]. Interesting data were also obtained from a collagen-induced arthritis model [23]. In these animals, Fas expression was up-regulated throughout the synovium. Substitution of naturally low levels of Fas ligand could be achieved by retroviral gene transfer of Fas ligand, resulting in a substantial reduction of inflammatory cells in the sublining and of synovial cells in the lining layer [23].

Growing evidence implies an imbalance between apoptosis inhibiting and promoting pathways in rheumatoid synovium. Recently, the novel anti-apoptotic molecule sentrin has been demonstrated to be expressed strongly within RA synovium [24]. Sentrin, which was termed after its guardian function against cell death signaling, interacts with the signal competent forms of Fas/APO-1 and tumor necrosis factor (TNF) receptor-1 death-domains, and overexpression of sentrin in transfected BJAJ cells provides protection against apoptosis [25]. It is interesting to note that the majority of sentrin-expressing cells were located within the synovial lining layer and displayed the fibroblast-like phenotype [24]. Bcl-2, another potent inhibitor of apoptosis, has also been shown to be expressed by synovial lining cells [14]. A third line of evidence for an imbalance between cell death and survival in RA emerges from data demonstrating an overexpression of the tumor suppressor protein p53 both within RA synovial lining *in situ* and synovial fibroblast-like cells [26]. Somatic mutations of the *p53* gene are known to extend cellular survival in a variety of tumors. Recently, mutations of the *p53* gene within "hot spots" have also been detected in RA synovium [27].

Taken together, the current data on apoptosis-regulating molecules in RA suggest that apoptosis-suppressing signaling outweighs pro-apoptotic pathways in RA, leading to an extended life-span of synovial lining cells and resulting in a prolonged expression of matrix-degrading enzymes at sites of joint destruction (Fig. 1).

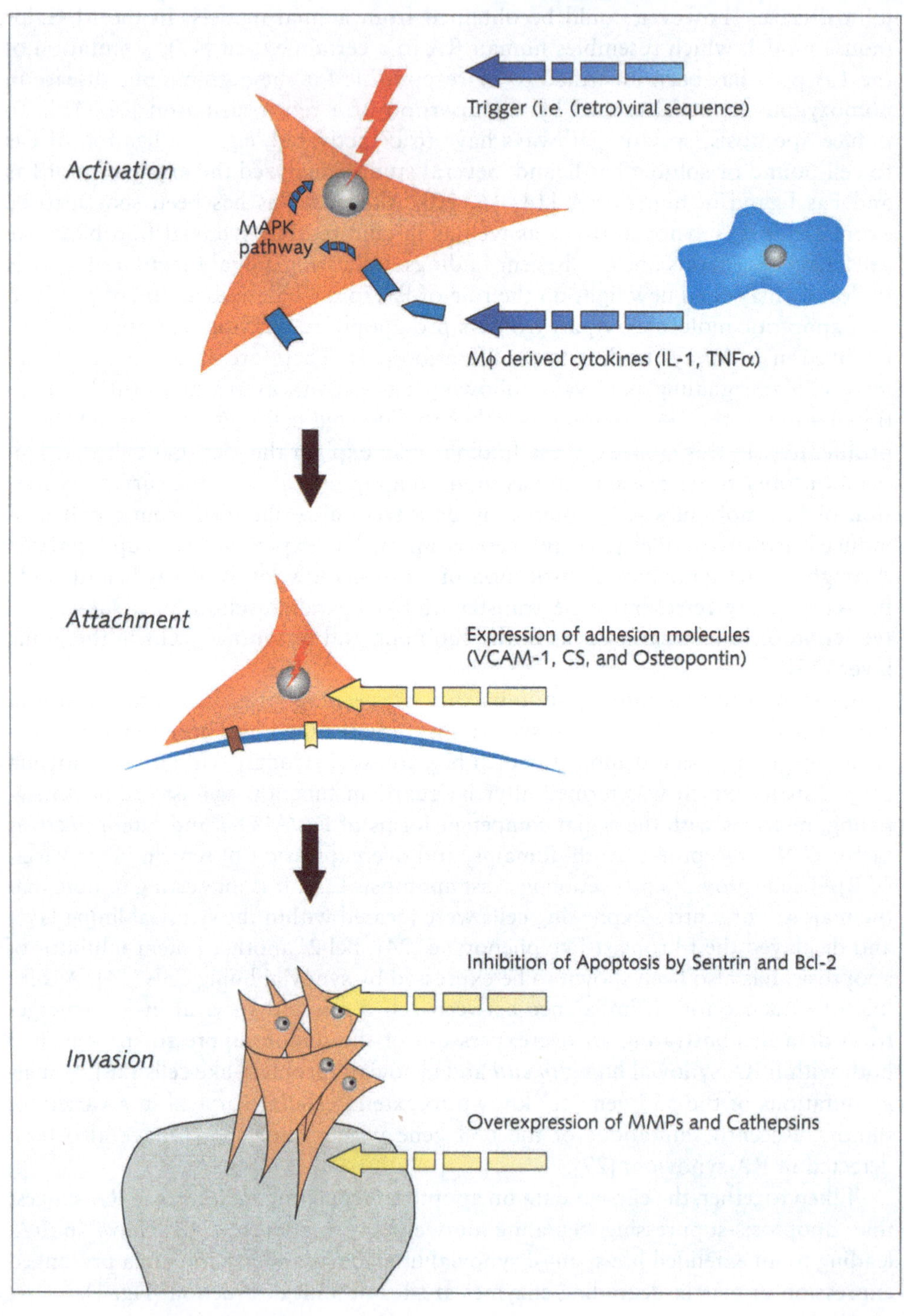

Trigger (i.e. (retro)viral sequence)
Activation
MAPK
pathway
Mφ derived cytokines (IL-1, TNFα)
Attachment
Expression of adhesion molecules
(VCAM-1, CS, and Osteopontin)
Inhibition of Apoptosis by Sentrin and Bcl-2
Invasion
Overexpression of MMPs and Cathepsins

Based on these experimental data, modulation of apoptosis-regulating pathways are currently being examined for potential novel therapeutic approaches. Rapamycin, an immunosuppressive agent that decreases growth-factor-dependent proliferation of synovial cells and diminishes the expression of the apoptosis-inhibiting molecule Bcl-2, was shown to enhance the susceptibility to Fas-mediated apoptosis of cultured RA synovial fibroblasts [28]. In addition, paclitaxel, an antineoplastic drug, selectively inhibited proliferation of synovial fibroblasts by blocking the cell cycle and inducing apoptosis [29]. Finally, intraarticular administration of monoclonal anti-Fas antibodies to human T cell leukemia virus type I tax transgenic mice induced apoptosis and led to a significant improvement of the arthritis [30].

The activated phenotype

The invasive growth of rheumatoid synovium into cartilage and bone similar to that seen in tumors supports the hypothesis of activation of normal synoviocytes into aggressively growing, invading, synovial cells. Synovial fibroblasts derived from RA patients reveal characteristic morphological alterations [6] such as abundant cytoplasm, a dense rough endoplasmatic reticulum, and large pale nuclei with several prominent nucleoli. The expression of several proto-oncogenes and transcription factors are also consistent with an activated phenotype [7, 8]. The early response gene *egr-1* (previously called Z 225), modulating the regulation of the proto-oncogenes *sis* and *ras*, is up-regulated in RA synovium [9, 31]. Another early response gene, *c-fos*, which is involved in control of matrix-degrading enzymes such as collagenase and stromelysin has also been found in synovial cells [31]. Most interestingly, in mice transgenic for *c-fos*, induction of antigen-induced arthritis leads to severe synovitis characterized by the predominant infiltration of fibroblast-like cells and

Figure 1
T cell-independent pathways in RA. Unidentified exogenous or endogenous stimuli activate synovial lining fibroblasts to express various adhesion molecules which enable the attachment of RA synovium to cartilage and bone. The activated synovial fibroblasts produce a broad array of metalloproteinases and cathepsins which mediate the invasive growth of RA synovium into cartilage and bone. Increasing evidence points towards alterations of apoptotic pathways in RA, leading to an extented life-span of synovial fibroblasts, accompanied by a prolonged expression of matrix-degrading enzymes. In addition, activated synovial fibroblasts produce chemokines/chemoattractant factors which contribute to the accumulation of inflammatory cells in the RA synovium in an antigen-independent manner.

the absence of lymphocytes [32]. Furthermore, the oncogenes *ras*, *raf*, *sis*, *myb* and *myc* have been detected in RA patients to various extents and were predominantly up-regulated in synovial cells attaching to cartilage and bone [33]. Somatic mutations of the tumor suppressor gene p53 in RA synovium outlined above [27] may also provide a non-functional "cell death suppressor" gene in activated synovial fibroblasts. Further evidence supporting the concept of an activated phenotype derives from *in-vitro* studies on synovial fibroblast-like cells. In contrast to normal fibroblasts, which do not proliferate in culture beyond confluency, RA synovial fibroblasts escape this control mechanism and grow even after contact has been established and are capable of proliferating in an anchorage-independent manner [34].

Data from several animal models suggest the involvement of activated fibroblasts in joint destruction. First experiments were carried out in nude BALB/c mice, where the injection of RA synovial cells resulted in the formation of a "pannus-like" tissue [35].

The most convincing evidence for the activation of synovial fibroblasts arises from the severe combined immunodeficiency (SCID) mouse model of RA. Grafting of synovial tissue from RA patients together with normal human cartilage under the renal capsule of SCID mice, which lack functional T, B, and NK cells, led to invasion of the co-implanted cartilage by the synovial tissue [36], resembling articular erosions found in human RA. Most strikingly, the use of isolated RA synovial fibroblasts instead of complete synovial tissue also resulted in cartilage erosions within at least 30 days, whereas control implantations with normal skin fibroblasts or fibroblasts from osteoarthritis patients did not cause erosions [37]. In these experiments, invading RA synovial fibroblasts maintain their capacity to express proto-oncogenes, cathepsins, cytokines (Fig. 2), and adhesion molecules [37]. Taken together, these data provide evidence that RA synovial fibroblasts are capable of mediating progressive joint destruction in the absence of T cells or other inflammatory cells.

In this context it is of interest that a patient suffering from long-term RA, and a more recent HIV-infection with subsequent AIDS, showed progressive joint destruction with aggressively growing fibroblast-like cells, despite lacking $CD4^+$ T cells [38].

The mechanisms leading to the aggressive phenotype of RA synovial fibroblast-like cells have not yet been fully elucidated. Two possible hypotheses are currently being discussed. According to the classical model, synovial fibroblast-like cells respond passively to factors produced by macrophages and T cells (mainly to the cytokines IL-1 and TNFα) which are abundant in RA synovial fluid and tissue [5, 39, 40, 41]. However, the results of the above mentioned SCID mouse model for RA have challenged this hypothesis (Fig. 2). In addition, the anti-inflammatory effect of currently administered anti-rheumatic therapies has not been proven to inhibit joint destruction, indicating an uncoupling of inflammation and destruction in RA [42, 43].

The second hypothesis favours activation of RA synovial fibroblasts by an independent stimulus which subsequently leads to an autonomous activation, e.g. by retroviral activation of specific gene sequences [1, 7, 44]. Initial data supporting this concept have been provided by the ultrastructural detection of type C retrovi-

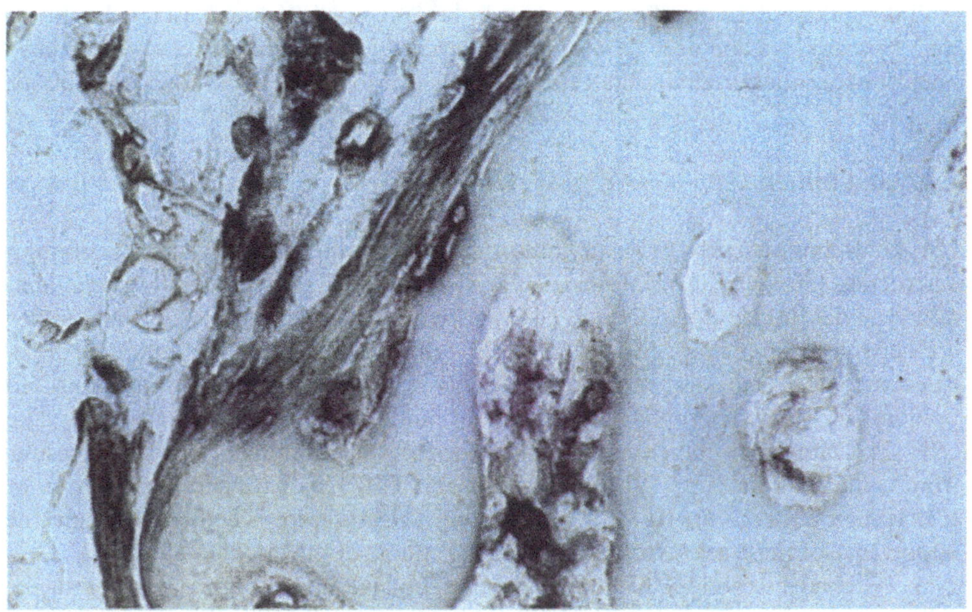

Figure 2
RA synovial fibroblasts co-implanted with normal human cartilage under the renal capsule of a SCID mouse. The RA fibroblasts invade into the cartilage and maintain their capacity to express IL-16 mRNA, as determined by in situ *hybridization (dark signal), for at least 60 days in the absence of exogenous stimuli.*

ral particles in synovial fluids of RA patients [45]. Furthermore, mRNA for a homolog of the transducin-like enhancer protein (TLE) has been detected within the RA synovial lining using highly conserved retroviral pol-primers [46]. As TLE proteins are involved in nuclear transcription, this may reflect the activated state of synovial lining cells. In other studies using normal synovial fibroblasts that were immortalized by transformation with the simian virus 40 (SV 40) large T antigen [47, 48, 49], the fibroblasts maintained the expression of surface receptors and adhesion molecules such as Fas, IL-1 receptor, and platelet-derived growth factor receptor 1 [47]. TNFα-dependent activation of the early response gene *egr-1* [47] and expression of transcription regulators such as AP-1 and NFκB were also preserved [48].

It is worth noting that in a patient infected with human T cell lymphotrophic virus (HTLV-I), a retrovirus that is known to cause a RA-like disease, hyperplastic synovium with fibrinoid masses containing high quantities of HTLV-I derived *tax/rex* mRNA could be found in numerous nodules along the tendon sheaths [50].

Taking these data together, it remains to be proven whether a "sustained imprinting" by cytokines and/or a "transforming" event by retroviral sequences of endogenous or exogenous origin results in the activated phenotype of RA synovial fibroblasts.

Cytokine milieu

Cytokines undoubtedly play an important role in the pathophysiology of joint destruction [39, 41, 51, 52]. In particular, IL-1 and TNFα are abundant in rheumatoid synovial fluid and tissue [5, 39, 41] and are considered to be key players as they are capable of inducing a variety of other cytokines, chemokines, adhesion molecules, metalloproteinases, and prostaglandins [5, 41]. Both cytokines are produced predominantly by macrophage-like synovial lining cells, but also by fibroblast-like cells [5]. Data from numerous animal studies as well as initially promising results from clinical studies aiming to inhibit IL-1 and TNFα by parenteral application of IL-1 receptor antagonist (IL-1Ra) and soluble TNF receptor (sTNFR), highlight the importance of these two cytokines during the course of the disease [40, 41, 43]. Utilising cellular interaction, neighbouring macrophage-like cells and fibroblast-like cells create paracrine and autocrine networks that contribute to the perpetuation of chronic synovitis. For example, IL-1 and TNFα, released by macrophages may activate fibroblast-like cells, which, in turn, induce class II MHC molecule antigen expression by macrophages (Fig. 3). Furthermore, growth factors such as fibroblast growth factor (FGF) may stimulate fibroblasts in an autocrine manner and enhance fibroblast activation [7].

IL-6, another fibroblast- and macrophage-derived cytokine, with both pro- and anti-inflammatory potential, appears also to play an important role in RA [41]. Interesting data emerged from IL-6 knock-out mice in which the cellular infiltrates within the knee joints were found to be reduced after induction of arthritis by zymosan [53]. However, the loss of cartilage proteoglycan was enhanced, implying an uncoupling of inflammatory and destructive pathways. Additional evidence supporting the latter observation emerges from the finding that cytokines have also been found to be elevated in non-destructive joint diseases [54–56].

The lack of substantial amounts of T cell cytokines such as IL-2, IL-4, and IFNγ in rheumatoid synovial fluid and tissue [56, 57] contrasts with the abundance of macrophage- and fibroblast-derived cytokines and growth factors and called the role of T cells in RA into question. Although synovial tissue resembles an ongoing autoimmune response [2], the responsible antigen(s) remain elusive. Therefore, additional, non-antigen-dependent processes have been proposed to explain T cell accumulation and activation in RA [58]. Several studies demonstrated elevated levels of chemokines/chemoattractant factors such as MIP-1α, MIP-1β, MCP-1, RANTES, and IL-8 in synovial fluids from RA patients [59–61]. These chemokines are produced by synovial fibroblasts and macrophages and mediate chemoattrac-

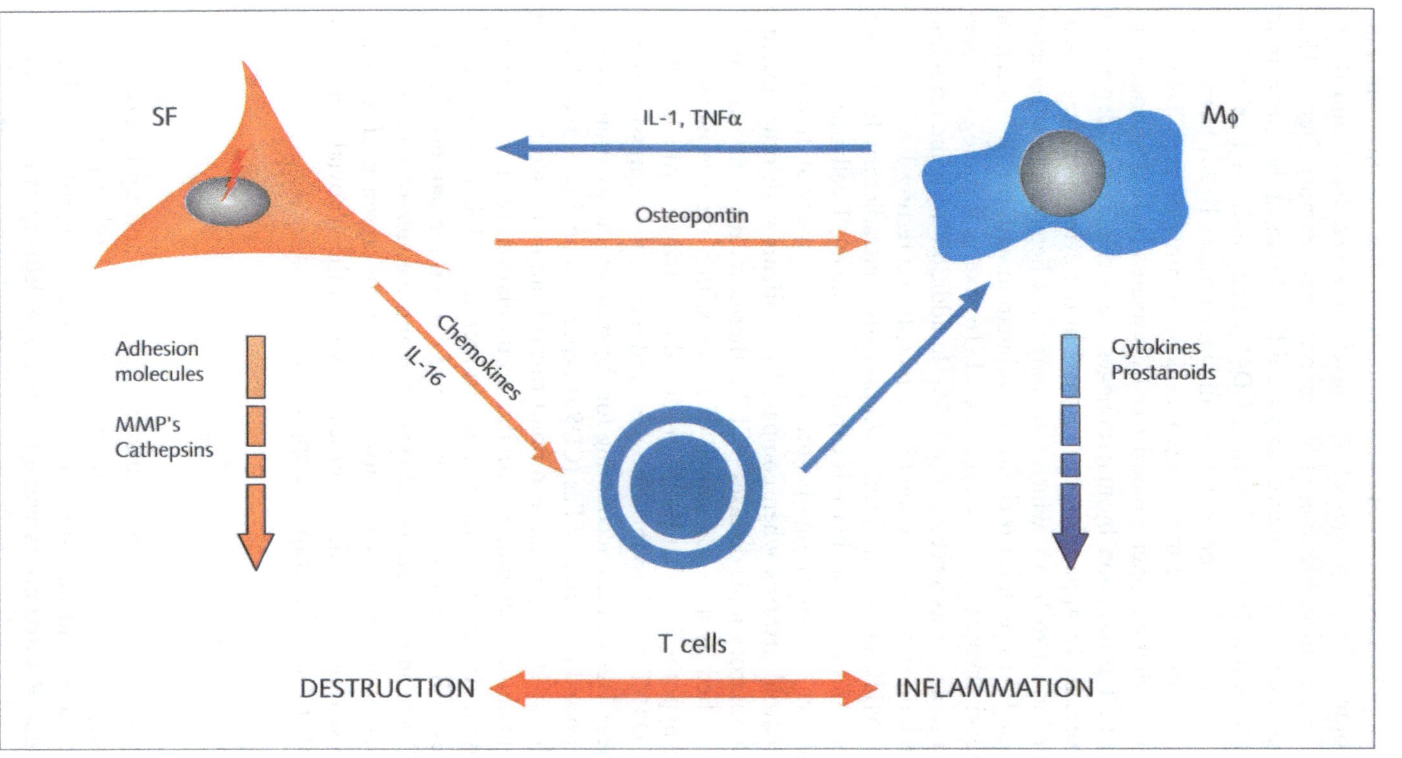

Figure 3

Interactions between synovial fibroblasts (SF), macrophages (MΦ) and T cells in RA. Macrophage-derived IL-1 and TNFα stimulate fibroblasts to produce matrix-degrading enzymes. Fibroblasts in turn secrete factors which may affect macrophages, such as GM-CSF, IL-6, IL-8, and MCP-1. Moreover, they secrete chemoattractant molecules for T cells such as IL-16. Whereas fibroblasts are predominantly responsible for joint destruction, macrophages mediate inflammatory responses. However, further potentiating events can occur as synovial fibroblasts also produce pro-inflammatory cytokines, and macrophages can release some MMPs at low levels [5].

tion of various cell populations into sites of inflammation using specific chemokine receptors. In this context the properties of two novel cytokines, IL-15 and IL-16, might be of crucial importance. McInnes et al. demonstrated recently that IL-15 is produced in substantial amounts by macrophages and fibroblasts in the rheumatoid synovial membrane [62]. Interleukin-15 attracts $CD4^+$ T cells, induces T cell proliferation, B cell maturation and isotype switching, and may protect T cells from apoptosis. Interestingly, the responding migratory T cells are mainly of the $CD45RO^+$ phenotype. It is thought that peripheral blood T cells, activated by IL-15, induce significant TNFα and IL-1 production by macrophages via a cell-contact-dependent mechanism. Therefore, IL-15 appears to be "higher" in the cytokine cascade than TNFα [62, 63]. In contrast to IL-15, which functions via a heterodimeric receptor consisting of a unique IL-15 receptor α chain in combination with the IL-2 receptor [62], the second novel chemoattractant cytokine, IL-16, exerts it biological functions using the CD4 molecule as a receptor [64, 65]. In addition to chemoattraction of $CD4^+$ cells, IL-16 induces the expression of IL-2 receptor on resting T cells as well as the expression of MHC class II molecules. Apparently contradictory, IL-16 also has suppressive properties in so far that it is capable of inducing T cell anergy [66]. As was recently shown, IL-16 is significantly elevated in synovial fluids from patients with rheumatoid arthritis when compared to patients with other inflammatory or non-inflammatory joint diseases [67]. Furthermore, RA synovial fibroblasts have been identified as a major source of IL-16 within the synovium [67]. Therefore, it can be hypothesized that IL-16, produced by activated synovial fibroblasts, may attract $CD4^+$ T cells into the synovium and induce the expression of the IL-2 receptor on these T cells, thus accounting for the state of anergy found in synovial T cells. The reported reduction of Fas (CD95) expression on T cells and of subsequent apoptosis by IL-16 [68] might also point towards an increased life-span of these cells and contributes presumably to the accumulation of T cells within rheumatoid synovium, despite the low rate of proliferation. Taken together, the intriguing properties of IL-15 and IL-16 may help to explain the paradox between the abundance of T cells in the rheumatoid synovium and the lack of T cell derived cytokines in synovial fluid and tissue. Furthermore, in the absence of a clearly defined antigen, these non-antigen driven processes within the synovial membrane may offer a rationale for novel therapeutic approaches.

Attachment

Features such as synovial infiltration by inflammatory cells and up-regulation of cytokines and prostaglandins are shared by RA and several other joint diseases. However, the attachment and adhesion of synovial tissue to cartilage and bone appear to be unique in RA and are essential for localized delivery of matrix metalloproteins (MMPs) and cathepsins resulting in cartilage and joint destruction [1].

In this regard, important lessons have been learned from the above-mentioned MRL/lpr mouse model [17]. The initial stage of the disease was characterized by the proliferation of synovial cells with a "transformed" appearance as described by Fassbender for human rheumatoid arthritis [6]. Subsequently, these cells attached to cartilage and bone and aggressively invaded these tissues. Most significantly, inflammatory cells were absent during this initial stage of the disease and cartilage and bone erosions only occurred at the attachment site of "transformed" synovial lining cells [17].

Adhesion is mediated by various surface proteins. Three different families have now been characterized: selectins, integrins, and the Ig superfamily. Integrins contain at least 15 α and 8 β chains, which combine to form heterodimers [69]. Their ligands may be either cellular surface molecules or extracellular matrix proteins, and individual adhesion molecules may bind to more than one ligand. For example, CS-1, a spliced isoform of fibronectin, appears part of a bidirectional adhesion pathway operative in RA since it binds to the integrin VLA-4 (α4β1; CD49d/CD29) which also ligates with vascular cell adhesion molecule 1 (VCAM-1) [70]. The expression of VCAM-1 is upregulated in RA synovium [71]. Data by Koch et al., who reported that VCAM-1 is a strong inducer of angiogenesis [72], suggest that the activated synovial fibroblast overexpressing VCAM-1 might be responsible for neovascularization in RA synovium. The latter observation supports further the concept that T cell-independent pathways mediated by activated fibroblasts might contribute to angiogenesis in RA.

Most recently, osteopontin, an extracellular matrix protein that promotes cell attachment, could be demonstrated in synovial fibroblast-like cells [73]. In the same study, a stimulatory effect of osteopontin on the secretion of collagenase-1/ MMP-1 in articular chondrocytes was found. Hence it might be hypothesized that osteopontin mediates not only attachment of synovial cells to cartilage but also contributes to perichondrocytic matrix degradation [73].

Therefore, the role of adhesion molecules in RA is not restricted to the attachment of synovium to cartilage and bone, but includes also the recruitment of inflammatory cells and induction of cytokines and MMPs [69].

Matrix-degradation

Progressive joint destruction distinguishes RA from other inflammatory joint diseases and is mediated by the concerted action of various proteinases, the most prominent being MMPs [74] and cathepsins [75].

MMPs are characterized by a zinc molecule at the active site and include collagenase (MMP-1), stromelysin (MMP-3), gelatinases (MMP-2 and MMP-9) and membrane type MMPs (MT-MMP), which differ with respect to their substrate specificities. Whereas collagenase degrades collagen types I, II, III, VII, and X only when they are arranged in a triple helical structure, gelatinase can also cleave denatured collagen. Stromelysin is capable of activating collagenase as well as degrading proteoglycans. MMPs are secreted as inactive proenzymes and activated proteolytically by various enzymes such as trypsin, plasmin, and other proteases. Several reports have implicated collagenase [MMP-1) and stromelysin (MMP-3) in rheumatoid joint destruction [76, 77]. Both proteases are found to be elevated in synovial fluid of patients with RA as compared to OA and are released in large amounts from synovial fibroblast-like cells in culture [77, 78]. *In situ* studies revealed strong collagenase and stromelysin expression within rheumatoid synovium, both at the mRNA and protein level [76, 77, 79]. Synovial fibroblast-like cells within the lining layer or at the site of invasion have been identified as the major source for MMPs. This pattern of distribution is similar to that for proto-oncogenes and consistent with the notion that proto-oncogenes are involved in the activation of MMPs. For example, the proto-oncogene *fos* and the early growth response gene 1 (*egr-1*) have both been identified in collagenase-producing rheumatoid synovial fibroblasts [31].

The activity of MMPs is thought to be regulated by various mechanisms. Apart from being regulated at the transcriptional level, MMP activity is balanced by naturally-occuring tissue inhibitors of metalloproteinases (TIMP-1 and TIMP-2). These interact irreversibly with MMP-1 and MMP-3 and are synthesized and secreted by chondrocytes, synovial fibroblasts, and endothelial cells [78–80]. *In situ* hybridization studies demonstrated striking amounts of TIMP-1 mRNA in the synovial lining of patients with RA. However, it is the molecular relationship between MMPs and TIMP that are crucial for joint destruction, rather than the absolute levels of TIMP.

Of interest is that the degraded fibronectin also induces stromelysin and collagenase expression in synovial fibroblast-like cells [81]. Thus, the synthesis of matrix degrading enzymes in the inflamed joint is not only regulated by pro-inflammatory cytokines, but also by products of the destructive process itself in an amplifying fashion. Novel 3-dimensional *in vitro* models will allow further analysis of the distinct aspects of the destructive joint disease [82].

The fact that MMPs are inducible by cytokines such as IL-1 and TNFα and can be downregulated by anti-inflammatory cytokines such as IL-4 indicates a relationship between the action of synovial fibroblasts and macrophages during inflammatory and destructive processes in RA (Fig. 3). Supporting evidence is provided by data from an *in-vitro* model of human cartilage degradation [83] in which radiolabeled cartilage is used to measure the extent of degradation. In this model, macrophages accentuated cartilage degradation which could be inhibited by anti-IL-1, anti-IL-6, and anti-TNFα antibodies. Therefore, macrophage derived pro-inflammatory cytokines appear to amplify the destructive processes [5].

Recently, novel members of the MMP family have been characterized. Collagenase 3/ MMP-13 has been cloned from mammary carcinoma tissue and, subsequently, from osteoarthritic and rheumatoid synovial tissue [84, 85]. MMP-13 was reported to be expressed both at the mRNA [86] and protein levels [87] predominantly in the lining layer of rheumatoid synovium. Due to its localization, its substrate specifity for collagen type II, and its relative resistance to known MMP inhibitors, MMP-13 might play an important role in joint destruction.

Cathepsins are the other major group of proteases involved in joint destruction. They are classified by their catalytic mechanism and cleave cartilage types II, IX, and XI, as well as proteoglycans [75]. The cysteine proteases cathepsin B and L are upregulated in RA synovium [88]. In a similar fashion to MMPs, cathepsins are also activated by proto-oncogenes. It has been shown that transfection of fibroblasts with the ras proto-oncogene leads to cellular transformation and to the induction of cathepsin L [89]. This is supported by the *in vivo* finding of combined *ras* and cathepsin L expression, especially at sites of invasion [90]. Cathepsin K, a novel cysteine proteinase, has been suggested to play an important role in osteoclast-mediated bone resorption. Cathepsin K expression by RA synovial fibroblasts and macrophages has recently been reported. This occurs mainly at the site of synovial invasion into articular bone, suggesting a role in increased bone resorption in RA [91].

The majority of matrix-degrading enzymes are found to be expressed predominantly by activated synovial fibroblast-like cells at the site of invasion [8]. The co-expression of proto-oncogenes and some apoptosis-inhibiting molecules by these cells stresses the relationship between cellular activation, invasiveness, and destructive potential.

Therefore, inhibiting the action of MMPs and cathepsins appears a major target for the treatment of RA, namely the inhibition of joint destruction. Approaches *in vitro* and in animal models have included exogenous administration of the TIMP and synthetic peptides that inhibit MMPs [43]. Antibiotics such as tetracyclin and related compounds, which are inhibitors of MMPs, have been shown to be superior to placebo in controlled trials in RA [43]. In addition, using an animal model, fluoroketone-based inhibitors of cathepsins did not only inhibit cathepsin L and B activity, but also reduced joint destruction [92].

Based on the broad array of different MMPs and cathepsins, with different specificities towards components of the extracellular matrix, a combination of inhibitors may represent the required therapeutic approach.

Conclusions

Various T cell independent pathways have been elucidated. They include activation of synovial lining cells, attachment of RA synovium to articular cartilage and bone, and joint destruction by the combined action of various proteinases. Synovial fibroblast-like cells appear to be key players in these processes as they display an aggressive phenotype, mediate attachment of RA synovium to cartilage and bone, and release various matrix-degrading enzymes. The activated state of synovial fibroblast-like cells is further characterized by the production of chemokines and chemoattractant cytokines which modulate recruitment of inflammatory cells into RA synovium. Finally, increasing evidence implies an alteration of apoptotic pathways in RA. These data contribute to a comprehensive understanding of the pathogenic mechanisms in RA and, with regard to therapy [93], provide not only new possibilities but also indicate the necessity to interfere at different stages of the pathogenesis of RA. Based on the considerations of the molecular and cellular mechanisms of joint destruction in RA mentioned above, our laboratory is developing novel strategies to modulate the activation of synovial fibroblasts in RA using gene transfer techniques [94, 95, 96, 97].

References:

1 Gay S, Gay RE, Koopman WJ (1993) Molecular and cellular mechanisms of joint destruction in rheumatoid arthritis: two cellular mechanisms explain joint destruction? *Ann Rheum Dis* 52: S39–47

2 Weyand CM, Goronzy JJ (1997) Pathogenesis of rheumatoid arthritis. *Med Clin N Am* 81: 29–55

3 Kelly PMA, Bliss E, Morton JA, Burns J, McGee JOD (1988) Monoclonal antibody EBM/11: high cellular specifity for human macrophages. *J Clin Pathol* 41: 510–515

4 Höyhtyä M, Myllylä R, Piuva J, Kivirikko KI, Tryggvason K (1984) Monoclonal antibodies to human prolyl 4-hydroxylase. *Eur J Biochem* 141: 477–482

5 Burmester GR, Stuhlmüller B, Keyszer G, Kinne RW (1997) Review: Mononuclear phagocytes and rheumatoid synovitis: Mastermind or workhorse in arthritis? *Arthritis Rheum* 40: 5–18

6 Fassbender HG (1983) Histomorphological basis of articular cartilage destruction in rheumatoid arthritis. *Coll Relat Res* 3: 141–155

7 Firestein GS (1996) Invasive fibroblast-like synoviocytes in rheumatoid arthritis. Passive responders or transformed aggressors? *Arthritis Rheum* 39: 1781–1790

8 Müller-Ladner U, Gay RE, Gay S (1997) Structure and function of synoviocytes. In: Koopman WJ (ed): *Arthritis and Allied Conditions. A Textbook of Rheumatology* (13th edition). Williams and Wilkins, Baltimore, 243–253

9 Aicher WK, Heer AH, Trabandt A, Bridges SL Jr, Schroeder HW Jr, Stransky G, Gay RE, Eibel H, Peter HH, Siebenlist U et al (1994) Overexpression of zinc-finger transcription factor Z-255/Egr-1 in synoviocytes from rheumatoid arthritis patients. *J Immunol* 152: 5940–5948

10 Nykanen P, Bergroth V, Raunio P, Nordstrom D, Kottinen YT (1986) Phenotypic characterization of 3H-thymidine incorporating cells in rheumatoid arthritis synovial membrane. Rheumatol Int 6: 269–271

11 Mohr W, Hummler N, Peister B, Wessinghage D (1986) Proliferation of pannus tissue cells in rheumatoid arthritis. *Rheumatol Int* 6: 127–132

12 Petrow KP, Theis B, Eckard A, Karbowski A, Eysel P, Salzmann G, Gaumann A, Gay RE, Gay S, Klein C, et al (1997) Determination of proliferating cells at the sites of cartilage invasion in patients with rheumatoid arthritis (abstract). *Arthritis Rheum* 40 (suppl.): S251
13 Kinne RW, Palombo-Kinne E, Emmrich F (1995) Activation of synovial fibroblasts in rheumatoid arthritis. *Ann Rheum Dis* 54: 501–504
14 Matsumoto S, Müller-Ladner U, Gay RE, Nishioka K, Gay S (1996) Multistage apoptosis and Fas antigen expression of synovial fibroblasts derived from patients with rheumatoid arthritis. *J Rheumatol* 23: 1345–1352
15 Nakajima T, Aono H, Hasunuma T, Yamamoto K, Shirai T, Hirohata K, Nishioka K (1995) Apoptosis and functional Fas antigen in rheumatoid arthritis synoviocytes. *Arthritis Rheum* 38: 485–491
16 Firestein GS, Yeo M, Zvaifler N (1995) Apoptosis in rheumatoid arthritis synovium. *J Clin Invest* 96: 1631–1638
17 O'Sullivan FX, Fassbender HG, Gay S, Koopman WJ (1985) Etiopathogenesis of the rheumatoid arthritis-like disease in MRL/lpr mice. I. The histomorphologic basis of joint destruction. *Arthritis Rheum* 28: 529–536
18 Wu J, Zhou T, He J, Mountz JD (1993) Autoimmune disease in mice due to integration of an endogenous retrovirus in an apoptosis gene. *J Exp Med* 178: 461–468
19 Chu JL, Drappa J, Parnassa A, Elkon KB (1993) The defect in Fas mRNA expression in MRL/lpr mice is associated with insertion of the retrotransposon, ETn. *J Exp Med* 178: 723–730
20 Asahara H, Hasunuma T, Kobata T, Inoue H, Müller-Ladner U, Gay S, Sumida T, Nishioka K (1997) In situ expression of protooncogenes and Fas/Fas ligand in rheumatoid arthritis synovium. J Rheumatol 24: 430–435
21 Freiberg RA, Spencer DM, Choate KA, Duh HJ, Schreiber SL, Crabtree GR, Khavari PA (1997) Fas signal transduction triggers either proliferation or apoptosis in human fibroblasts. *J Invest Dermatol* 108: 215–219
22 Aicher WA, Peter HH, Eibel H (1996) Human synovial fibroblasts are resistant to Fas induced apoptosis (abstract). *Arthritis Rheum* 39 (suppl): S75
23 Zhang H, Yang Y, Horton JL, Samoilova EB, Judge TA, Turka LA, Wilson JM, Chen Y (1997) Amelioration of collagen-induced arthritis by CD95 (APO-1/Fas)-ligand gene transfer. *J Clin Invest* 100: 1951–1957
24 Franz JK, Hummel KM, Aicher WK, Müller-Ladner U, Gay RE, Gay S (1997) Sentrin, a novel anti-apoptotic molecule is strongly expressed in synovium of patients with rheumatoid arthritis (RA) (abstract). *Arthritis Rheum* 40 (suppl): S116
25 Okura T, Gong L, Kamitani T, Wada T, Okura I, Wie CF, Chang HM, Yeh ET (1996) Protection against Fas/APO-1- and tumor necrosis factor-mediated cell death by a novel protein, sentrin. *J Immunol* 157: 4277–4281
26 Firestein GS, Nguyen K, Aupperle KR, Yeo M, Boyle DL, Zvaifler NJ (1996) Apoptosis in rheumatoid arthritis. p53 overexpression in rheumatoid arthritis synovium. *Am J Pathol* 149: 2143–2151

27 Firestein GS, Echeverri F, Yeo M, Zvaifler NJ, Green DR (1997): Somatic mutations in the p53 tumor suppressor gene in rheumatoid arthritis synovium. *Proc Natl Acad Sci USA* 94:10895–10900
28 Migita K, Eguchi K, Ichinose Y, Kawabe Y, Tsukada T, Aoyagi T, Nagataki S (1997) Effects of rapamycin on apoptosis of rheumatoid synovial cells. *Clin Exp Immunol* 108: 199–203
29 Hui A, Kulkarni GV, Hunter WL, McCulloch CAG, Cruz TF (1997): Paclitaxel selectively induces mitotic arrest and apoptosis in proliferating bovine synoviocytes. *Arthritis Rheum* 40: 1073–1084
30 Fujisawa Y, Asahara H, Okamoto K, Aono H, Hasunuma T, Kobata T, Iwakura Y, Yonehara S, Sumida T, Nishioka K (1996) Therapeutic effect of the anti-fas antibody on arthritis in HTLV-1 tax transgenic mice. *J Clin Invest* 98: 271–278
31 Trabandt A, Aicher WK, Gay RE, Sukhatme VP, Fassbender HG, Gay S (1992) Spontaneous expression of immediately-early response genes c-fos and egr-1 in collagenase-producing rheumatoid synovial fibroblasts. *Rheumatol Int* 12: 53–59
32 Shiozawa S, Tanaka Y, Fujita T, Tokuisha T (1992) Destructive arthritis without lymphocyte infiltration in H2-c-fos transgenic mice. J Immunol 148: 3100–3104
33 Müller-Ladner U, Kriegsmann J, Gay RE, Gay S (1995) Oncogenes in rheumatoid synovium. *Rheum Dis Clin N Am* 21: 675–690
34 Lafyatis R, Remmers EF, Roberts AB, Yocum DE, Sporn MB, Wilder RL (1989) Anchorage-independent growth of synoviocytes from arthritic and normal joints: stimulation by exogenous platelet-derived growth factor and inhibition by transforming growth factor-b and retinoids. *J Clin Invest* 83: 1267–1276
35 Brinckerhoff CE, Harris ED (1981) Survival of rheumatoid synovium implanted into nude mice. *Am J Pathol* 103: 411–419
36 Geiler T, Kriegsmann J, Keyszer G, Gay RE, Gay S (1994) A new model for rheumatoid arthritis generated by engraftment of rheumatoid synovial tissue and normal human cartilage into SCID mice. *Arthritis Rheum* 37: 1664–1671
37 Müller-Ladner U, Kriegsmann J, Franklin BN, Matsumoto S, Geiler T, Gay RE, Gay S (1996) Synovial fibroblasts of patients with rheumatoid arthritis attach to and invade normal human cartilage when engrafted into SCID mice. *Am J Pathol* 49: 1607–1615
38 Müller-Ladner U, Kriegsmann J, Gay RE, Koopman WJ, Gay S, Chatham WW (1995) Progressive joint destruction in a HIV-infected patient with rheumatoid arthritis. *Arthritis Rheum* 38: 1328–1332
39 Fontana A, Hengartner H, Weber E, Fehr K, Grob PJ, Cohen G (1982) Interleukin-1 activity in the synovial fluid of patients with rheumatoid arthritis. *Rheumatol Int* 2: 49–53
40 Arend WP (1997) The pathophysiology and treatment of rheumatoid arthritis. *Arthritis Rheum* 40: 595–597
41 Firestein GS, Zvaifler N (1997) Anticytokine therapy in rheumatoid arthritis. *N Engl J Med* 337: 195–197
42 Mulherin D, Fitzgerald O, Bresnihan B (1996) Clinical improvement and radiological

deterioration in rheumatoid arthritis: Evidence that the pathogenesis of synovial inflammation and articular erosion may differ. *Br J Rheumatol* 35: 1263-1268

43 Moreland LW, Heck LW, Koopman WJ (1997) Biological agents for treating rheumatoid arthritis. *Arthritis Rheum* 40: 397–409

44 Kalden JR, Gay S (1994) Retroviruses and autoimmune rheumatic diseases. *Clin Exp Immunol* 98:1–5

45 Stransky G, Moreland LW, Gay RE, Gay S (1993) Virus-like particles (VLP) in synovial fluids from patients with rheumatoid arthritis. *Br J Rheumatol* 32: 1044–1048

46 Müller-Ladner U, Roberts CR, Gay RE, Gay S (1995) Messenger-RNA of a novel homolog of the transducin-like enhancer protein is detected by conserved retroviral sequences and present in rheumatoid arthritis (abstract). *Arthritis Rheum* 38 (suppl): S215

47 Haas C, Aicher WK, Dinkel A, Peter HH, Eibel H (1997) Characterization of SV40T antigen immortalized human synovial fibroblasts: Maintained expression patterns of EGR-1, HLA-DR and some surface receptors. *Rheumatol Int* 16: 241–247

48 Abe M, Tanaka Y, Saito K, Shirakawa F, Koyama Y, Goto S, Eto S (1997) Regulation of interleukin (IL)-1β gene transcription induced by IL-1β in rheumatoid synovial fibroblast-like cells, E11, transformed with simian virus 40 large T antigen. *J Rheumatol* 24: 420–429

49 Zhang HG, Blackburn WD Jr, Minghetti PP (1997) Characterization of a SV40-transformed rheumatoid synovial cell line which retains genotypic expression patterns: A model for evaluation of anti-arthritic agents. *In Vitro Cell Dev Biol Anim* 33: 37–41

50 Hasunuma T, Morimoto T, Hoa TTM, Müller-Ladner U, Aono H, Ogawa R, Gay S, Nishioka K (1997) Tenosynovial nodulosis in a patient infected with human T cell leukemia virus I. *Arthritis Rheum* 40: 578–582

51 Miossec P (1995) Pro- and antiinflammatory cytokine balance in rheumatoid arthritis. *Clin Exp Rheumatol* 13 (suppl 12): S13–16

52 Arend WP, Dayer JM (1995) Inhibition of the production and effects of interleukin-1 and tumor necrosis factor alpha in rheumatoid arthritis. Arthritis Rheum 38: 151–160

53 Van den Loo FA, Kuiper S, van Enckevort FH, Arntz OJ, van den Berg WB (1997) Interleukin-6 reduces cartilage destruction during experimental arthritis. A study in interleukin-6-deficient mice. *Am J Pathol* 151: 177–191

54 Kotake S, Schumacher HR, Yarboro CH, Arayssi TK, Pando JA, Kanik KS, Gourley MF, Klippel JH, Wilder RL (1997) *In vivo* gene expression of type 1 and type 2 cytokines in synovial tissues from patients in early stages of rheumatoid, reactive, and undifferentiated arthritis. *Proc Assoc Am Physicians* 109: 286–301

55 Faharat MN, Yanni G, Poston R, Panayi GS (1993) Cytokine expression in synovial membranes of patients with rheumatoid arthritis and osteoarthritis. *Ann Rheum Dis* 52: 870–875.

56 Simon K, Seipelt E, Sieper J (1994) Divergent T cell cytokine patterns in inflammatory arthritis. *Proc Natl Acad Sci USA* 91: 8562–8566

57 Firestein GS, Wu, Townsend K, Broide D, Alvaro-Gracia J, Glasebrook A, Zvaifler NJ

(1988) Cytokines in chronic inflammatory arthritis. I. Failure to detect T cell lymphokines (interleukin 2 and interleukin 3) and presence of macrophage colony-stimulating factor (CSF-1) and a novel mast cell growth factor in rheumatoid synovitis. *J Exp Med* 168: 1573–1586
58 Miossec P, Chomarat P, Dechanet J (1996) Bypassing the antigen to control rheumatoid arthritis. *Immunol Today* 17: 170–173
59 Robinson E, Keystone EC, Schall TJ, Gillett N, Fish EN (1995) Chemokine expression in rheumatoid arthritis (RA): evidence of RANTES and macrophage inflammatory protein (MIP)-1 production by synovial T cells. *Clin Exp Immunol* 101(3): 398–407
60 Al-Mughales J, Blyth TH, Hunter JA, Wilkinson PC (1996) The chemoattractant activity of rheumatoid synovial fluid for human lymphocytes is due to multiple cytokines. *Clin Exp Immunol* 106: 230–236
61 Seitz M, Dewald B, Gerber N, Baggiolini M (1991) Enhanced production of neutrophil-activating peptide-1/interleukin-8 in rheumatoid arthritis. *J Clin Invest* 87: 463–469
62 McInnes IB, Al-Mughales J, Field M, Leung BP, Huang FP, Dixon R, RD, Wilkinson PC, Liew FY (1996) The role of interleukin-15 in T-cell migration and activation in rheumatoid arthritis. *Nature Med* 3(2): 189–195
63 Panayi GS (1997) T-cell-dependent pathways in rheumatoid arthritis. *Curr Opin Rheumatol* 9: 236–240
64 Cruikshank WW, Center DM, Nisar N, Natke B, Theodore A, Kornfeld H (1994) Molecular and functional analysis of a lymphocyte chemoattractant factor: association of biological function with CD4 expression. *Proc Natl Acad Sci USA* 91: 5109–5113.
65 Center DM, Kornfeld H, Cruikshank WW (1996) Interleukin 16 and its function as a CD4 ligand. *Immunol Today* 17: 476–481
66 Cruikshank WW, Lim K, Theodore AC, Cook J, Fine G, Weller PF, Center DM (1996) IL-16 inhibition of CD3-dependent lymphocyte activation and proliferation. *J Immunol* 157: 5240–5248
67 Franz JK, Hummel KM, Kolb SA, Lahrtz F, Neidhart M, Aicher W, Gay R, Fontana A, Gay S (1997) Rheumatoid synovial fibroblasts (SF) express interleukin-16 – a potent chemoattractant factor for $CD4^+$ T cells (abstract). *Arthritis Rheum* 40 (suppl): S197
68 Baier M, Bannert N, Werner A, Lange K, Kurth R (1997) Molecular cloning, sequence, expression, and processing of the interleukin 16 precursor. *Proc Natl Acad Sci USA* 94: 5273–5277
69 Mojcik CF, Shevach EM (1997) Adhesion molecules. A rheumatologic perspective. *Arthritis Rheum* 40: 991–1004
70 Müller-Ladner U, Elices MJ, Kriegsmann JB, Strahl D, Gay RE, Firestein GS, Gay S (1997) Alternatively spliced CS-1 fibronectin isoform and its receptor VLA-4 in rheumatoid arthritis synovium. *J Rheumatol* 24:1873–1880
71 Kriegsmann J, Keyszer GM, Geiler T, Bräuer R, Gay RE, Gay S (1995) Expression of vascular cell adhesion molecule-1 mRNA and protein in rheumatoid synovium demonstrated by in situ hybridization and immunohistochemistry. *Lab Invest* 72: 209–213
72 Koch AE, Halloran MM, Haskell CJ, Shah MR, Polverini PJ (1995) Angiogenesis medi-

ated by soluble forms of E-selectin and vascular cell adhesion molecule-1. *Nature* 376: 517–519.

73 Petrow P, Franz JK, Müller-Ladner U, Hummel K, Gay RE, Prince CW, Gay S (1996) Expression of osteopontin mRNA in synovial tissue of patients with rheumatoid arthritis (RA) and osteoarthritis (OA) (abstract). *Arthritis Rheum* 39 (suppl): S36

74 Krane SM, Conca W, Stephenson ML, Amento EP, Goldring M (1990) Mechanisms of matrix degradation in rheumatoid arthritis. *Ann NY Acad Sci* 580: 340–354

75 Müller-Ladner U, Gay RE, Gay S (1996) Cysteine proteinases in arthritis and inflammation. *Perspectives in drug discovery and design.* ESCOM Science Publishers B.V., Leyden, 87–98

76 Gravallese EM, Darling JM, Ladd AL, Katz JN, Glimcher L (1991) *In situ* hybridization studies on stromelysin and collagenase mRNA expression in rheumatoid synovium. *Arthritis Rheum* 34: 1071–1084

77 Firestein GS, Paine M (1992) Expression of stromelysin and and TIMP in rheumatoid arthritis synovium. *Am J Pathol* 140: 1309–1314

78 Clark IM, Powell LK, Ramsey S, Hazelman BL, Cawston TE (1993) The measurement of collagenase, TIMP and collagenase-TIMP complex in synovial fluids from patients with osteoarthritis and rheumatoid arthritis. *Arthritis Rheum* 36: 372–380.

79 Okada Y, Gonoij Y, Nakanishi I, Nagase H, Hayakawa T (1990) Immunohistochemical demonstration of collagenase and tissue inhibitor of metalloproteinases (TIMP) in synovial lining cells of rheumatoid synovium. *Virch Arch B Cell Pathol* 59: 305–312

80 DiBattista JA, Pelletier J-P, Zafarullah M, Fujimoto N, Obata KíI, Martel-Pelletier J (1995) Coordinate regulation of matrix metalloproteases and tissue inhibitor of metalloproteinase expression in human synovial fibroblasts. *J Rheumatol* 22 (suppl 43): 123–128.

81 Werb Z, Tremble PM, Behrendtsen O, Crowley E, Damsky CH (1989) Signal transduction through the fibronectin receptor induces collagenase and stromelysin gene expression. *J Cell Biol* 109: 877–889

82 Schultz O, Keyszer G, Zacher J, Sittinger M, Burmester G (1997) Development of *in vitro* model systems for destructive joint diseases. Novel strategies for establishing inflammatory pannus. *Arthritis Rheum* 40: 1420–1428.

83 Scott BB, Weisbrot LM, Greenwood JD, Bogoch ER, Paige CJ, Keystone EC (1997) Rheumatoid arthritis synovial fibroblast and U937 macrophage/monocyte cell line interaction in cartilage degradation. *Arthritis Rheum* 40: 490–498

84 Mitchell PG, Magna HA, Reeves LM, Lopresti-Morrow LL, Yocum SA, Rosner PJ, Geoghegan KF, Hambor JE (1996) Cloning, expression, and type II collagenolytic activity of matrix metalloproteinase-13 from human osteoarthritic cartilage. *J Clin Invest* 97: 761–768

85 Wernicke D, Seyfert C, Hinzmann B, Gromnica-Ihle E (1995) Cloning of collagenase 3 from the synovial membrane and its expression in rheumatoid arthritis and osteoarthritis. *J Rheumatol* 23: 590–595

86 Petrow P, Hummel KM, Franz J, Kriegsmann J, Müller-Ladner U, Gay RE, Gay S (1997)

In situ-detection of MMP-13 mRNA in the synovial membrane and cartilage–pannus junction in rheumatoid arthritis (abstract). *Arthritis Rheum* 40 (suppl): S336

87 Lindy O, Konttinen YT, Sorsa T, Ding Y, Santavirta S, Ceponis A, López-Otín C (1997) Matrix metalloproteinase 13 (collagenase 3) in human rheumatoid synovium. *Arthritis Rheum* 40: 1391–1399

88 Keyszer GM, Heer AH, Kriegsmann J, Geiler T, Trabandt A, Keysser M, Gay RE, Gay S (1995) Comparative analysis of cathepsin L, cathepsin D, and collagenase messenger RNA expression in synovial tissues of patients with rheumatoid arthritis and osteoarthritis, by in situ hybridization. *Arthritis Rheum* 38: 976–984

89 Joseph L, Lapid S, Sukhatme VP (1987) The major ras induced protein in NIH 3T3 cells is cathepsin L. *Nucleic Acids Res* 15: 3186

90 Trabandt A, Aicher WK, Gay RE, Sukhatme VP, Nilson-Hamilton M, Hamilton RT, McGhee JR, Fassbender HG, Gay S (1990) Expression of the collagenolytic and ras-induced cysteine proteinase cathepsin L and proliferation-associated oncogenes in synovial cells of MRL/lpr mice and patients with rheumatoid arthritis. *Matrix* 10: 349–361

91 Hummel KM, Petrow PK, Jeisy E, Franz J, Gay RE, Brömme D, Gay S (1997) Cathepsin K mRNA is expressed in synovium of patients with rheumatoid arthritis (RA) at sites of bone destruction (abstract). *Arthritis Rheum* 40 (suppl): S250

92 Esser RE, Angelo RA, Murphey MD, Watts LM, Thornburg LP, Palmer JT, Talhouk JW, Smith RE (1994) Cysteine proteinase inhibitors decrease articular cartilage and bone destruction in chronic inflammatory arthritis. *Arthritis Rheum* 37: 236–247.

93 Hummel KM, Gay RE, Gay S (1997) Novel strategies for the therapy of RA. *Br J Rheumatol* 36: 265–267.

94 Müller-Ladner U, Roberts CR, Franklin BN, Gay RE, Robbins PD, Evans CH, Gay S (1997) Human IL-1Ra gene transfer into human synovial fibroblasts is chondroprotective. *J Immunol* 158: 3492–3498

95 Müller-Ladner U, Roberts CR, Franklin BN, Robbins PD, Gay RE, Evans CH, Gay S (1996) Gene transfer of the TNFα receptor p55 into human synovial fibroblasts and implantation into the SCID mouse (abstract). *Arthritis Rheum* 39 (suppl): S307

96 Müller-Ladner U, Franklin BN, Roberts CR, Robbins PD, Gay RE, Evans CH, Gay S (1996) Gene transfer of interleukin-10 into human synovial fibroblasts and implantation into the SCID mouse (abstract). *Arthritis Rheum* 39 (suppl): S160

97 Hummel KM, Petrow PK, Nawrath M, Müller-Ladner U, Neidhart M, Pavlovic J, Gay RE, Mölling K, Gay S (1997) Retroviral gene transfer of a c-raf dominant negative mutant does not inhibit synovial fibroblasts (SF) to invade cartilage in the SCID mouse model (abstract). *Arthritis Rheum* 40 (suppl): S120

Role of T cells in arthritis: Lessons from animal models

Wim B. van den Berg

Dept. of Rheumatology, University Hospital Nijmegen, NL-6500 HB Nijmegen, The Netherlands

Introduction

Rheumatoid arthritis (RA) is a systemic disease of unknown etiology, with the main manifestation being chronic inflammation in multiple joints. In many patients the arthritis is characterized by exacerbations and remissions. Current theories of the pathogenesis of the chronic arthritis include a sustained immune reaction directed at unknown exogenous agents that localize to the joints or articular autoantigens such as cartilage matrix molecules. In addition, chronicity might be linked to a deranged "tumor like" behaviour of the synovial tissue cells of RA patients, including macrophages and synovial fibroblasts. These cells show an aggressive phenotype and prolonged growth in culture, without an apparent need for further stimuli. It might be argued that the underlying trigger is co-isolated with the cells, still being present in the culture and hence creating a seemingly autonomous activation. In that sense, viruses may be likely candidates.

Models of chronic arthritis in experimental animals can mimic certain aspects of human RA. As such they may provide insight into pathogenetic pathways of chronic joint inflammation and can be used to study mechanisms of joint destruction, including cartilage and bone erosions. It is evident that chronic arthritis can be induced through T cell driven reactions to (auto)antigens in the joint and the first models were based on this principle. Lateron, it was shown that chronicity may also develop through direct activation of synovial cells by non-antigenic triggers, with limited involvement of T cells. Recent interest has focused on cytokine involvement in chronic joint inflammation and it has been shown that continued overexpression of tumor necrosis factor (TNF) and Interleukin (IL)-1 may lead to chronic arthritis and concomitant joint destruction in various animal species. In the absence of a proven T cel antigen in RA, clinical therapy is directed at the blocking of TNF and IL-1, as well as nonspecific suppression of T cell and macrophage function. Present research in animal models includes a continued search for novel putative antigens, detailed understanding of the regulation of T cell driven joint pathology, and novel pathways of induction of tolerance. In addition to antigen specific tolerisation, great

T Cells in Arthritis, edited by P. Miossec, W.B. van den Berg and G.S. Firestein

interest has emerged for the therapeutic application of socalled "bystander suppression"; this potentially enables suppression of an arthritis, driven by an unknown stimulus, through suppressive cytokines generated at the site by Th2 or Th3 reactions against joint specific stimuli.

The present chapter will address general mechanisms of arthritis in animal models, including both T cell and macrophage involvement. Special attention will be given to key elements of chronicity, the occurrence of arthritis in the absence of T cells, as well as the clear amplifying and modulatory role of T cells. It should be noted that animal models can only provide insight into mechanisms and the potential validity of therapeutic approaches, but it will on its own never solve the dilemma of whether human RA is more of a T cell or a macrophage disease.

Classic models of arthritis

Chronicity of joint inflammation can be understood in terms of the continuous presence of an arthritogenic stimulus. This can be exogenous in nature, such as bacteria or viruses, with a perpetual supply from the circulation and/or persistence in joint tissues. The potential relevance of such mechanisms is illustrated in the widely studied models of antigen-induced arthritis (AIA) and Streptococcal cell wall (SCW) arthritis [1–4]. In those models protein antigens are trapped in collagenous reservoirs of the joint, such as ligaments or cartilage (AIA), or partly undegradable cell wall fragments are retained in synovial tissue cells (SCW-A), providing persistent stimulation in the presence of T cell immunity. In addition, structures of the joint itself may function as a persistant antigen, the arthritis then being the result of an autoimmune attack (Tab. 1). In general, any component of the articular cartilage is a potential arthritogen, provided that tolerance against this stimulus can be broken and that sufficient amounts are accessible or released, by turnover in the joint, to sustain the autoimmune process. Well known examples are the models of collagen arthritis and proteoglycan arthritis [5, 6], in which heterologous collagen type II or enzymatically modified proteoglycans are used to facilitate the generation of cross-reactive autoimmunity. Recently, models have been developed along these principles [7–9] using Collagen type IX or XI, COMP (cartilage derived oligomeric protein) and HC GP39 (hyalin cartilage glycoprotein 39), all molecules that are normally expressed in cartilage. Before accepting any of these autoantigens as a true arthritogen in human RA, T cell responses have to be identified in reasonable numbers of patients and, more importantly, antigen specific immunomodulation must then alter the course of the disease. Interestingly, destructive forms of RA tend to decline at the moment that the cartilage is fully destroyed. Moreover, total joint replacement often results in total remission of the arthritis in that particular joint, without the need of concomitant synovectomy. These are arguments for a direct role of cartilage in an autoimmune pathogenesis of RA or an indirect, as yet uniden-

Table 1 - Common principles of chronicity in classic models of arthritis

Classic models of arthritis					
Model	**Immun.**	**Induction**	**Pers. Stim**	**Antibodies**	**T cell**
AIA	Ag/CFA	i.a. Ag	Ag	+	+
SCW	–	i.p. SCW	PG?	?	+
AA	CFA	–	PG?	?	+
CIA	CII/CFA	–	CII	++	+
Oil-arthritis	Oil	–	?	–	+
MRL-lpr/lpr	–	–	Fas-defect	–	?

Ag, antigen; CFA, Complete Freunds Adjuvant; CII, collagen type II, PG, proteoglycan; SCW, streptococcal cell walls; i.p., intraperitoneal; i.a., intraarticular.
Persistent stimulus relates to a defined antigen in the joint, when applicable.

tified, role of cartilage components in the maintenance of inflammatory processes in the joint.

Microbial components as arthritogenic triggers

The principle of cross-reactive autoimmunity may have physiological relevance when it is initiated by exogenous stimuli. Microbial components, including cell wall fragments from enteric organisms, have long been considered as potential arthritogenic agents and there is ample evidence that bacterial infections and developement of arthritis may somehow be related. Examples are reactive arthritis or arthritis associated with jejunal bypass surgery for obesity, the resulting blind loop in the gastrointestinal tract often showing bacterial overgrowth. Apart from their ability to induce arthritis by direct localization to joint tissues [10, 11], bacterial fragments can induce arthritis remotely, probably as a result of generation of a T cell reaction to bacterial epitopes cross-reacting with endogenous bacterial fragments continuously present in the synovial tissues or with cartilagenous autoantigens. In adjuvant arthritis (AA), the oldest classic model, the arthritis is induced by intradermal adminstration of Freund's complete adjuvant containing heat killed mycobacteria. The active component in the bacteria is the cell wall peptidoglycan, the disease can be induced with various bacteria and the strongest argument for an autoimmune process is the proper transfer of arthritis with T cells from diseased rats. Some T cell lines and clones showed to transfer arthritis, also recognized cartilage proteoglycan epitopes [12–14].

It is almost a matter of taste whether persistent microorganisms or autoantigens should be considered as different entities or that they both reflect integral parts of the body, needing tight regulation of tolerance. Both the classic autoimmune arthritides such as collagen and proteoglycan arthritis, as well as adjuvant arthritis, are genetically restricted and only inducible in particular strains of rats or mice. Tolerance against AA and SCW-A can be induced by pretreatment of the animals with bacterial heat shock proteins [13–16]. A bacterium specific pathogenesis is further supported by the resistance to AA and SCW-A in most conventionally bred Fisher and Wistar rats, whereas clear susceptibility is noted in germ-free animals of these strains [17, 18]. Colonization with bacteria before induction of arthritis prevented the susceptibility, suggesting that germ-free animals, lacking early contact with bacteria, are not tolerant.

A complicating but intriguing aspect of our current understanding of adjuvant arthritis is that not all adjuvant-active materials are derived from bacteria. Some mineral oils are adjuvant-active and can induce an arthritis indistinguishable from the classic adjuvant arthritis, still being T cell dependent and also showing strong strain dependency for particular rats or mice [19, 20]. It suggests that at least 2 mechanisms may underly chronicity in adjuvant disease, one related to cross-reactive autoimmune T cell reactions triggered by the response to bacterial antigens and a second one, based on nonspecific immunomodulation by bacterial components or oil preparations, resulting in unmasking of normally suppressed autoimmunity. The latter mechanism implies the potential involvement of a range of unidentified autoantigens.

The fact that cartilage destruction is minor in early adjuvant arthritis, unlike the situation in autoimmune collagen arthritis [21], makes it unlikely that cartilage autoantigens are a dominant element in AA. On the other hand, it should be noted that cartilage destruction in collagen and proteoglycan arthritis is linked to high levels of autoantibodies, creating immune complex depositions on the cartilage surface and directing the inflammatory process to that site. Such deposits are not noted in the AA and SCW-Arthritis. Another striking difference between the models is the fact that AA as well as oil induced arthritis produce a self-limiting arthritis, rendering animals recovering from arthritis resistant to reinduction, which is not the case in collagen arthritis.

Recent observations make it clear that bacteria are potent inducers of IL-12. This cytokine is shown to be a pivotal mediator in the generation of Th1 lymfocytes and the production of proinflammatory mediators from mature Th1 cells. It implies that any bacterial infection, by generation of IL-12, may shift balances of Th1/Th2 responses, and hence may unmask autoimmunity [22]. This principle has already been shown in other autoimmune diseases and it seems likely that similar events may occur in arthritis. IL-12 can greatly enhance susceptibility to collagen induced arthritis in mice, both during the early stages of the cross-reactive immunization process as well as at the onset of arthritis, whereas anti-IL-12 antibodies can prevent the onset [23, 24].

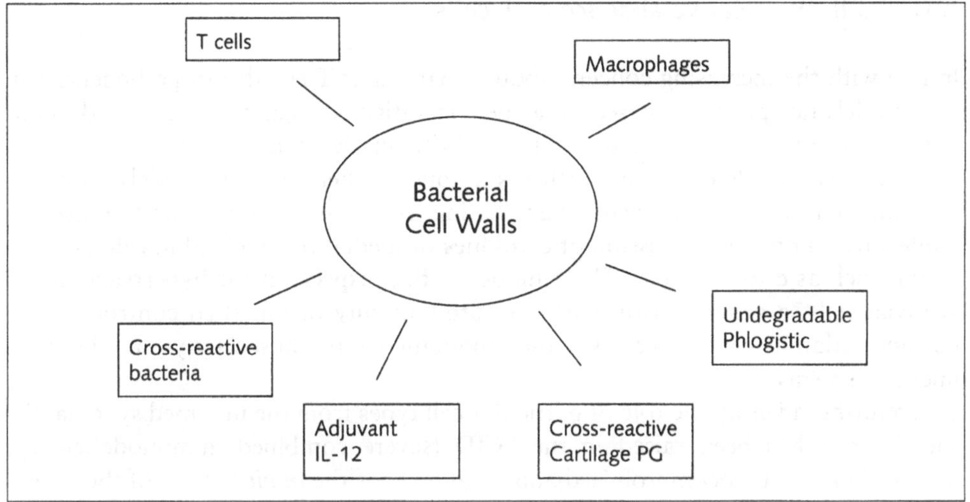

Figure 1
Determinants in the triggering of T cells and macrophages by bacterial components.

In conclusion, bacterial fragments can be involved in arthritis at various levels (Fig. 1). They may be phlogistic through direct macrophage activation, resulting in a chronic arthritis when the fragments are partly undegradable. Generation of T cell responses against such fragments may greatly enhance the inflammation. Adjuvant properties may further enhance this specific T cell reactivity, but may also unmask unrelated autoimmune responses. Finally, cross reactivity between bacterial epitopes and cartilage-specific epitopes may contribute to cartilage-specific autoimmunity. A critical issue in "bacterial" arthritis is of course the proper understanding as to why inflammation should occur in the joints. Both preferential localization in synovial tissues as well as cross reactive autoimmunity may be pivotal elements in this.

Interestingly, bacteria are potent inducers of TNF and in contrast to the limited role of TNF in the joint inflammation of AIA and CIA in the mouse, the joint swelling of arthritis induced with SCW (streptococcal cell walls) was highly TNF dependent [25–27]. Given the strong TNF dependence of human RA, the cytokine profile of bacterial arthritis seems in line with these clinical findings. As an aside, the cartilage destruction in SCW arthritis is IL-1 dependent and IL-1 production occurs independently of TNF, as noted in recent studies in SCW arthritis with anti-TNF antibodies or TNF soluble receptors [25]. The findings of TNF independent generation of IL-1 and cartilage destruction were confirmed in TNF knockout mice (unpub observ) and argue for dual inhibition of both TNF and IL-1 in RA patients to obtain full protection.

Arthritis in the relative absence of T cells

In line with the increasing concern about a particular T cell driven pathogenesis in RA, models not primarily based on a specific antigenic trigger have recieved major attention in recent years. These include arthritis models with various types of oils, spontaneous models displaying arthritis amongst other changes, models based on superantigens or viral antigens exacerbating established models, and transgenic models based on overexpression of cytokines or mediators involved in cellular activation such as c-fos or c-jun. These models reflect aspects of the hyperreactivity of synovial cells, a general disturbance of autoimmunity or impaired control of self-limiting inflammatory processes, either spontaneous or caused by yet unidentified microorganisms.

To further identify the role of particular cell types from the inflamed synovial tissue, interest has been raised in the SCID (severe combined immunodeficiency) mouse. This immunocompromised animal allows for the *in vivo* study of the potential of synovial cells to induce arthritic changes. Interesting approaches include the transfer of pieces of synovial tissue or selected cells from animal models or RA patients. Another intriguing design is the combination of cells or synovial tissue with engrafted cartilage as target tissue, to obtain further insight into the mechanisms of cartilage damage. It was convincingly demonstrated that RA synovial fibroblasts keep their transformed appearance and maintain cartilage invasive and destructive behaviour over prolonged periods of time, in the absence of T cells [28]. This nicely proves the direct destructive potential of such fibroblasts. On the other hand, *in vitro* activated T cells, originally isolated from inflamed joints of RA patients, can induce a severe destructive arthritis upon transfer to SCID mice [29]. The challenge yet remaining is to identify the relative contribution of particular cell types in the arthritic process in the presence of functional regulatory cells. The latter are absent in the SCID mouse when selected cell populations are transferred and this may result in over-interpretation of apparent arthritogenicity and destructive character.

Spontaneous arthritis is observed in the MRL-lpr/lpr mice [30]. These animals develop a severe autoimmune disease, mainly characterized by massive lymphadenopathy, arteritis, immune complex-mediated glomerulonephritis and chronic arthritis. The arthritis is characterized by synovial and mesenchymal cell hyperplasia, late T cell infiltration and cartilage damage, suggestive for a T cell independent onset. The synovial cells show a transformed appearance and cartilage invasive behaviour. A draw back for experimental studies is the mild severity and late onset, significant arthritis; routinely not observed before the age of 5 months. A viral cause has been suggested but not proven and it is now clear that these mice have a defect in Fas-mediated apoptosis. Expression can be enhanced by injection of Freund's complete adjuvant [31] or superantigen, the latter probably by induction of T cell anergy [32]. This acceleration is TNF-dependent since severity can be reduced with concomitant anti-TNF treatment [33].

The potential involvement of retroviral antigens in chronic arthritis was further underlined by the occurrence of arthritis after 2–3 months in mice transgenic for human T cell leukemia virus [34, 35]. The role of disturbed apoptosis in this viral model was demonstrated by the improved arthritis after anti-Fas antibody treatment [36]. Further evidence that overactivation of synovial cells might contribute to chronicity of arthritis has emerged from the construction of transgenic mice overexpressing c-fos. Plain overexpression of c-fos did not lead to arthritis. However, when classic T cell arthritis models were induced in these c-fos mice this yielded a more severe and more destructive arthritis. The latter was found for both antigen induced arthritis and autoimmune collagen arthritis [37]. Remarkably, the cellular infiltrate in these mice contained hardly any lymphocytes, yet marked cartilage destruction was found, stressing the effector role of mesynchemal cells in the damage. Intriguingly, c-fos overexpression enhances expression of the cartilage destructive enzymes stromelysin and collagenase, suggesting that the synovial cells then harbour sort of bombs, needing only minor activation by T cells to display a highly destructive character.

A final model to be described here is the transgenic mouse overexpressing TNF. These mice develop a chronic polyarthritis, with synovial hyperplasia, pannus formation, and cartilage destruction. The pattern illustrates that mere TNF is sufficient to trigger full expression of the whole arthritic process. Of interest, membrane bound TNF is sufficient to get full pathology, explaining the difficulty to demonstrate TNF in sufficient amounts in arthritic processes showing TNF dependence. Remarkably, arthritis could be blocked with anti-IL-1 Receptor antibodies, demonstrating that the effects of TNF are indirect [38–40]. Finally, similar arthritis could be induced by overexpression of TNF in recombination activation gene (RAG) mice lacking functional T cells [41]. This further underlines the fact that chronic, destructive arthritis can occur in the absence of T cells.

T cells and synovial cells in chronicity and joint destruction

None of the models discussed so far should be equated with specific forms of human RA, but the data may provide a general insight. The above examples in classic as well as more recent models illustrate that chronic arthritis may be the net result of various pathways, ranging from full T cell involvement in reactions against defined, persistant antigens in the joint to a total lack of T cell involvement in TNF and IL-1 overexpression systems (Fig. 2). In between, synergy of these systems seems highly likely. Examples are already given above, showing that preactivation/triggering of synovial cells by viruses or transgenic overexpression of downstream mediators in the cells, such as c-fos or c-jun, enhance the impact of a T cell driven arthritis. Similar amplification may occur in the arthritides directed against model protein antigens or bacterial fragments. Protein stimuli are in general hardly phlogistic on their

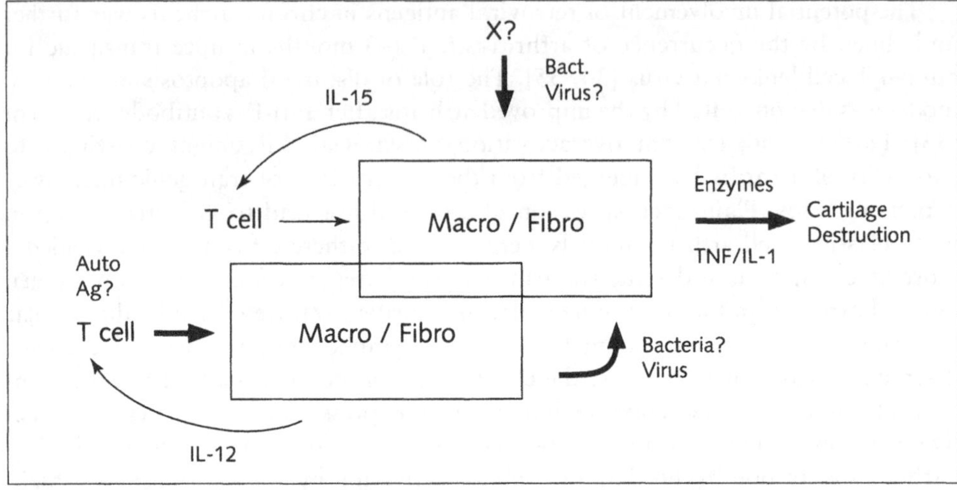

Figure 2
An activated synovial macrophage/fibroblast system needs minor or no further stimulation by T cells to cause cartilage destruction

own and can not trigger macrophages or fibroblasts to a significant extent. However, antibodies may amplify the system by generation of immune complexes which then are potent triggers of phagocytes. Such an amplifying role of antibodies has been demonstrated both in the antigen-induced arthritis and collagen arthritis. Expression of collagen arthritis is often low after a single immunization and can be markedly enhanced by a booster injection with collagen type II or passive administration of anti-CII antibodies [42]. Apart from this boosting of the onset, the T cells are more important, when compared to the antibodies, for proper chronicity. Low amounts of local antigen in joints is sufficient to sustain prolonged T cell activation, whereas much higher concentrations are needed to get prolonged arthritis with immune complexes.

A critical role for T cells in severity and chronicity has also been shown in arthritis induced by injection of streptococcal cell wall fragments into various strains of rats. When injected in Lewis or Fisher rats, both develop acute arthritis, linked to dissemination of cell wall fragments to the joints and local activation by uptake into synovial macrophages. However, the arthritis subsides in Fisher rats but becomes chronic in Lewis rats. Cogent evidence now exists that this chronic phase is dependent on T cells. The chronic phase is not inducible in nude Lewis rats. Moreover, Lewis rats mounted distinct SCW-specific T cell responses, whereas the resistant Fisher rats were unable to do so. The latter was linked to tolerance, since germ-free Fishers did mount SCW-specific T cell responses and showed chronic arthritis [1,

43, 44]. An important lesson from this is that macrophage-related joint inflammation is clear in the presence of large amounts of cell wall fragments, but at later stages, when the amount of retained fragments drops below a direct phlogistic treshold, chronicity is only seen when T cell reactivity becomes involved.

A few final remarks to be made on the involvement of T cells relate to the risk of overinterpretation of the relative paucity of T cell factors such as IL-2 or IFNγ in RA synovial tissue. It is clear from animal model studies that these factors are also scant in proven T cell dependent reactions and it must be underlined that histological analysis of chronic SCW arthritis also yields pictures dominated by macrophages and synovial fibroblasts, with scattered lymphocytes, yet the latter cells seem crucial in the chronicity. In addition, it must be mentioned that IL-15 is now found at a considerable concentration in RA joints and may represent a novel macrophage derived cytokine contributing to T cell activation [45, 46]. Studies to identify the trigger of IL-15 production and its role in animal models of arthritis are warranted. Finally, IL-17, a novel T cell derived cytokine with IL-1 like activity, can be found in distinct levels in RA synovia. Again, its role in models has yet to be examined.

Contribution of flare reactions to chronicity

In comparison to the chronic process of human RA, a general shortcoming of most models is the relatively short duration of the severe and rapidly destructive inflammation. In that respect, models based on repeated flares, with slower development of lesions, provide a valuable extension. Early studies in murine antigen induced arthritis made it clear that an arthritic joint containing retained antigen and bearing a chronic T cell infiltrate, displays a state of hyperreactivity against the retained antigen, contributing to chronicity. An early T cell infiltrate is rather nonspecific but may gain considerable specificity (enrichment of antigen-specific T cells) upon sustained stimulation by a retained antigen. Flares could then easily be induced in such joints with nanogram amounts of antigen, showing T cell dependence [47, 48] and a cartilage destructive character.

An important extension of the flare model was found by comparative dosing of IL-1 to naive joints and joints bearing a chronic inflitrate. The infiltrated joint was much more sensitive to IL-1 and the reactivity seemed to reside in the macrophage infiltrate [49].

In addition, flare reactions were studied using bacterial cell wall fragments. In line with earlier discussions it must be anticipated that flares with such fragments may be dualistic, rather high dosages causing direct activation of macrophages with concomitant cytokine release, low dosages only causing flares through T cells. As an aside, a correlation was found between susceptibility to flares and the level of IL-1 production by macrophages of particular rat strains [50]. With low dosages of SCW fragments reaching the arthritic joint, repeated flares could be induced in Lewis rats, mounting SCW-specific T cell hyperreactivity, but such flares were not noted in Fisher rats, in line with the inability to generate such T cell responses. Another crucial element of flares with bacterial fragments resides in the presence of considerable cross-reactivity between cell walls from different bacterial origins. Intriguingly, a strong correlation was noted between the capacity of heterologous cell walls to induce a flare of SCW arthritis in Lewis rats and to stimulate SCW-primed T cells of those animals *in vitro* [1, 44, 51]. Finally, such flares can also extend to cross-reactive autoantigens from the cartilage (Fig. 3). In conclusion, these principles open up a wide range of putative stimuli able to cause exacerbations, simultaneously complicating the search for the driving antigen in human RA.

Synovial macrophages as effector cells in arthritis

Macrophages in the synovial membrane might be pivotal cells when non-antigenic triggers are sustaining the arthritis but probably are major effector cells in T cell driven processes as well. In early stages of arthritis the synovial lining macrophages comprise a considerable portion of the synovial macrophages and apart from influx of monocytes a major event in early arthritis is the considerable thickening of the layer of synovial lining macrophages and fibroblasts. A strategy to selectively target macrophages at the cellular level is to make use of their phagocytic properties. When liposomes, containing the cytotoxic drug chlodronate, are given locally in the joint, these vesicles are almost selectively taken up by the lining macrophages, resulting in long-lasting elimination and depletion of these cells by an apoptotic process. This prevents unwanted damage to other cells or tissue upon treatment with toxic liposomes. Intriguingly, when arthritis is then induced in such a lining-macrophage-depleted joint, a considerable reduction of the arthritis is found when immune complexes are used as a trigger, but less so when the strong T cell dependent antigen induced arthritis (AIA) is elicited [52, 53]. Expression of collagen arthritis was also markedly reduced [54], probably confirming that immune complexes, in addition to T cells, are of major importance at the onset of this autoimmune arthritis. Interestingly, late treatment with chlodronate liposomes in established AIA markedly reduced the T cell mediated flare in such joints upon rechallenge with antigen [55]. Taken together, these are strong arguments that the lining macrophages are playing a pivotal role, not only in early arthritis, but also in exacerbations. Further analysis revealed that the lining cells were a major source of chemokines and IL-1 and TNF are pivotal intermediates in the production of chemokines by lining macrophages. Apart from direct neutralization of the key cytokines IL-1 and TNF, the targeting of the lining macrophages may offer an alternative therapeutic approach to modulating arthritis in the absence of proper knowledge of the driving arthritogen.

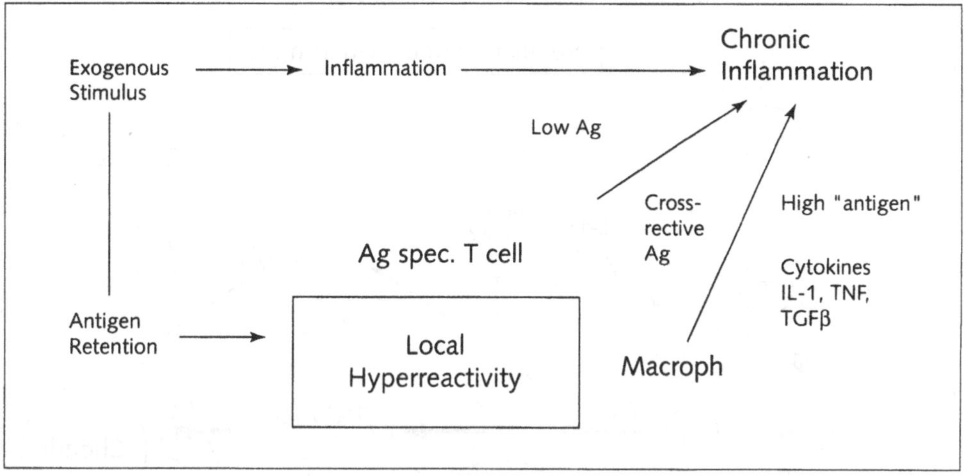

Figure 3
Local hyperreactivity plays a dominant role in propagation of chronic inflammation. This contains an antigen specific component and also a macrophage-driven pathway. Any insult causing cytokine release, such as TNFα or IL-1, may trigger exacerbations.

As outlined above, lining macrophages are important in directing cell influx. However, findings were less impressive when cartilage destruction was considered. Some reduction of cartilage proteoglycan loss was noted in immune complex arthritis in lining depleted joints, but no significant reduction was noted in AIA and CIA suggesting that local activation of synovial cells by T cell dependent mechanisms is already sufficient to trigger destruction, in the absence of a massive influx of monocytes. A more complete reduction of destruction was achieved when, apart from chlodronate-liposome treatment, the influx of monocytes was totally blocked with systemic treatment with anti-CR3 antibodies. The latter approach is efficient before onset of arthritis and suggests that under normal conditions infiltrating cells do amplify the destructive pathway. However, when applied to conditions of T cell mediated flares of smouldering arthritis cartilage destruction was still ongoing [52]. This indicates that sufficient synovial cell activation occurs upon triggering of T cells to sustain destruction, not necessarily needing further triggering or amplification by influx of monocytes.

Role of T cells in arthritis control

In spite of the ongoing debate on T cells or macrophages being dominant in the onset and propagation of arthritis, the overwhelming research efforts in understand-

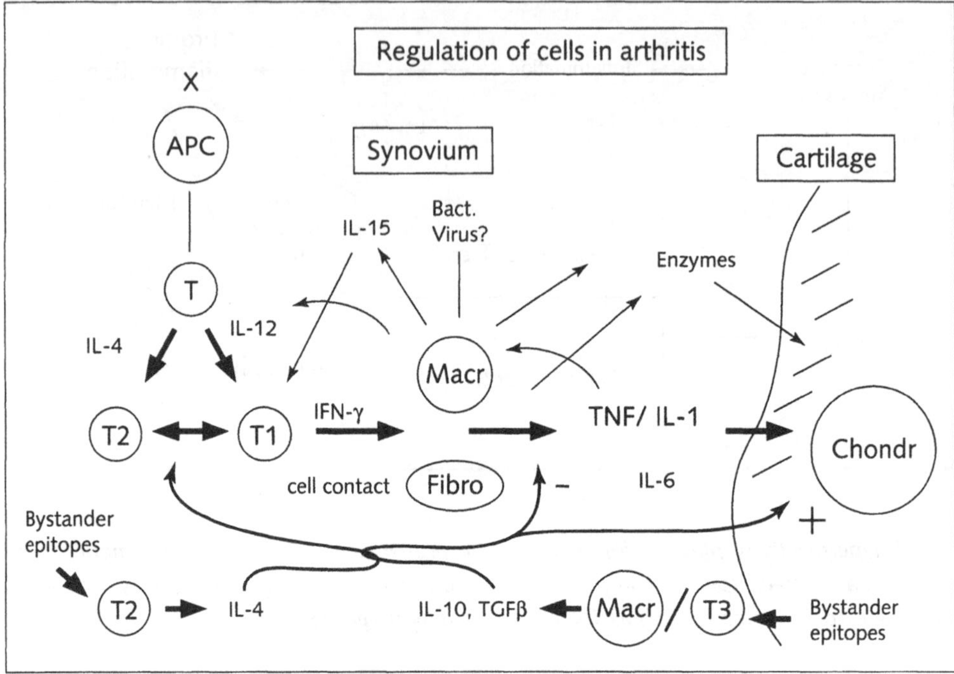

Figure 4
Cell and cytokine interplay in chronic joint inflammation

ing the regulation of T cell balances are of great benefit. In animal models of arthritis such as adjuvant arthritis or collagen arthritis it is well accepted that the disease severity is dependent on the balance of arthritic T cells and regulatory T cells [56–58] and there is old data that nonspecific T cell suppression in late collagen arthritis is making the arthritis worse [59], probably reflecting elimination of suppressive T cells. More recent studies suggest that arthritis induced by immunization with Collagen type II in Freunds complete adjuvant is driven by a mixture of Th1/Th2 cell responses and that suppression of arthritis can be achieved with T cells producing IL-4 or TGFβ [60, 61]. Accepted ways to promote suppressive subsets of T cells are antigen dosing at mucosal surfaces, through the oral or nasal route, and stimulation with modified antigens [62, 63]. An intriguing extension of antigen specific suppression of Th1 processes with cytokines produced at the site by Th2/Th3 cells is the concept of socalled "bystander suppression". Although Th2/Th3 responses are triggered by mucosal dosing with a specific antigen, the actual suppression is mediated by released cytokines and is therfore nonspecific. In that sense, tolerisation against a joint specific antigen can be used to suppress arthritogenic T cell responses against unknown antigens (Fig. 4). Efficacy of such an approach has been demonstrated for collagen type II in various arthritis models and heat shock proteins in oil induced arthritis [62, 64, 65]. In principle any cartilage epitope might be considered a joint specific bystander stimulus. The fact that IL-4 and TGFβ not only suppress Th1 reactions but are also potent suppressors of TNF and IL-1 production by macrophages does suggest that the principle is even applicable in non-immune arthritides, although it is conceivable that the dosages then have to be higher.

First studies in bystander suppression made use of collagen type II and although the data in animal models was encouraging, the clinical studies with oral dosing of CII in RA patients were disappointing [66, 67]. A major hurdle in application might be the fact that the suppressive subsets of T cells are generated at the mucosal sites and the draining lymph nodes, but display aberrant migration to synovial tissues. Th1 cells make use of specific P and E selectins to enter the joint [68] and Th2 cells have difficulty accumulating in joints. This might also explain the long recognized finding that Th2 cells are rather deficient in chronic synovial infiltrates. Alternative approaches using our knowledge of suppressive cytokines are to adminster recombinant IL-4 for prolonged periods of time or to use gene therapy to obtain prolonged expression. Approaches with IL-4 in arthritis have shown much better efficacy when combined with IL-10 [69]. An elegant extension of the gene therapy approach is the engeneering of T cell clones with controled cytokine production and desired migratory capacity. First experiments in this direction look promising [70, 71].

References

1 Van den Berg WB, van den Broek MF, van de Putte LBA, van Bruggen MCJ, van Lent PLEM (1991) Experimental arthritis: Importance of T cells and antigen mimicry in chronicity and treatment. In: Kresina TF (ed): *Monoclonal antibodies, cytokines, and arthritis*. Dekker, 237–252

2 Van den Berg WB, van der Kraan PM, van Beuningen HM (1998) Synovial mediators of cartilage damage and repair in OA. In: Brandt, KD, Doherty M, Lohmander LS (eds): *Oxford Textbook of Osteoarthritis*. Oxford University Press, Oxford, pp 157–167.

3 Van den Berg WB, van de Putte LBA, Zwarts WA, Joosten LAB (1984) Electrical charge of the antigen determines intraarticular antigen handling and chronicity of arthritis in mice. *J Clin Invest* 74: 1850–1859

4 Cromartie WL, Craddock JG, Schwab JH, Anderle SK, Yang CH (1977) Arthritis in rats after systemic injection of streptococcal cell walls. *J Exp Med* 146: 1485–1602

5 Trentham DE, Townes AS, Kang AH (1977) Autoimmunity to type II collagen: an experimental model of arthritis. *J Exp Med* 146: 857–868

6 Glant TT, Mikecz K, Arzoumanian A, Poole AR (1987) Proteoglycan-induced arthritis in Balb/C mice. Clinical features and histopathology. *Arthritis Rheum* 30: 201–212

7 Holmdahl R, Malmstrom V, Vuorio E (1993) Autoimmune recognition of cartilage collagens. *Ann Med* 25: 251–264

8 Cremer MA, Ye XJ, Terato K, Owens SW, Seyer JM, Kang AH (1994) Type XI collagen-induced arthritis in the Lewis rat. Characterization of cellular and humoral immune responses to native types XI, V, and II collagen and constituent α-chains. *J Immunol* 153: 824–832

9 Verheijden GFM, Rijnders AWM, Bos E, Coenen-de Roo CJJ, van Staveren CJ, Miltenburg AMM, Meijerink JH, Elewaut D, de Keyser F, Veys E, Boots AMH (1997) Human cartilage glycoprotein-39 as a candidate autoantigen in rheumatoid arthritis. *Arthritis Rheum* 40: 1115–1125

10 Stimpson SA, Brown RR, Anderle SK, Klapper DG, Clark RL, Cromartie WJ, Schwab JH (1986) Arthropathic properties of peptidoglycan-polysaccharide polymers from flora bacteria. *Infection and Immunity* 51: 240–249

11 Hazenberg MP, Klasen IS, Kool J, Ruseler-van Embden JGH, Severijnen AJ (1992) Are intestinal bacteria involved in the etiology of rheumatoid arthritis? *APMIS* 100: 1–9

12 Pearson CM (1956) Development of arthritis, periarthritis and periostitis in rats given adjuvants. *Proc Soc Exp Biol (NY)* 91: 95–101

13 Van Eden W, Hogervorst EJM, Henssen EJ, van der Zee R, van Embden JDA, Cohen IR (1989) A cartilage-mimicking T-cell epitope on a 65k mycobacterial heat-shock protein: Adjuvant arthritis as a model for human rheumatoid arthritis. *Curr Topics Microbiol Immunol* 145: 27–43

14 Holoshitz J, Naparstek Y, Ben-Num A, Cohen IR (1983) Lines of T lymphocytes induce or vaccinate against autoimmune arthritis. *Science* 219: 56-58

15 Van den Broek MF, Hogervorst EJM, van Bruggen MCJ, van Eden W, van der Zee R, van den Berg WB (1989) Protection against streptococcal cell wall-induced arthritis by pretreatment with the 65 kD mycobacterial heat shock protein. *J Exp Med* 170: 449–466

16 Van Eden W (1991) Heatshock proteins as immunogenic bacterial antigens with the potential to induce and regulate autoimmune arthritis. *Immunol Rev* 121: 5

17 Kohashi O, Kohashi Y, Takahashi T, Ozawa A, Shigematsu N (1986) Suppressive effect of Escherichia coli on adjuvant-induced arthritis in germ-free rats. *Arthritis Rheum* 29: 547–553

18 Van de Langerijt AGM, van Lent PLEM, Hermus ARMM, Sweep CGJ, Cools AR, van den Berg WB (1994) Susceptibility to adjuvant arthritis: relative importance of adrenal activity and bacterial flora. *Clin Exp Immunol* 97: 33–38

19 Kleinau S, Erlandsson H, Holmdahl R, Klareskog L (1991) Adjuvant oils induce arthritis in the DA rat. I. Characterization of the disease and evidence for an immunological involvement. *J Autoimmunity* 4: 871–880

20 Lorentzen JC, Klareskog L (1996) Susceptibility of DA rats to arthritis induced with adjuvant oil or rat collagen is determined by genes both within and outside the major histocompatibility complex. *Scand J Immunol* 44: 592–598

21 Van de Langerijt AGM, Huitinga I, Joosten LAB, Dijkstra CD, van Lent PLEM, van den Berg WB (1994) Role of β2 integrins in the recruitment of phagocytic cells in joint inflammation in the rat. *Clin Immunol Immunopathol* 73: 123–131

22 Segal BM, Shevach EM (1996) IL-12 unmasks latent autoimmune disease in resistant mice. J Exp Med 184: 771–775

23 Joosten LAB, Lubberts E, Helsen MMA, van den Berg WB (1997) Dual role of IL-12 in early and late stages of murine collagen type II arthritis. *J Immunol* 159: 4094–4102

24 Germann T, Szeliga J, Hess H, Störkel S, Podlaski F, Gately M, Schmitt E, Rüde E (1995) Administration of IL-12 in combination with type II collagen induces severe arthritis in DBA/1 mice. *Proc Natl Acad Sci USA* 92: 4823–4827

25 Kuiper S, Joosten LAB, Bendele AM, Edwards CK III, Arntz OJ, Helsen MMA, van de Loo FAJ, van den Berg WB (1998) Different roles of TNFα and IL-1 in murine streptococcal cell wall arthritis. *Cytokine; in press*

26 Van de Loo AAJ, Joosten LAB, van Lent PLEM, Arntz OJ, van den Berg WB (1995) Role of Interleukin-1, Tumor Necrosis Factor α and Interleukin-6 in cartilage proteoglycan metabolism and destruction. Effect of *in situ* cytokine blocking in murine antigen- and zymosan-induced arthritis. *Arthritis Rheum* 38: 164–172

27 Joosten LAB, Helsen MMA, van de Loo FAJ, van den Berg WB (1996) Anticytokine treatment of established type II collagen-induced arthritis in DBA/1 mice: a comparative study using anti-TNFα, anti-IL-1α/β, and IL-1ra. *Arthritis Rheum* 39: 797–809

28 Müller-Ladner U, Kriegsmann J, Franklin BN, Matsumoto S, Geiler T, Gay RE, Gay S (1996) Synovial fibroblasts of patients with rheumatoid arthritis attach to and invade normal human cartilage when engrafted into SCID mice. *Am J Pathol* 149: 1607–1615

29 Mima T, Saeki Y, Ohshima S, Nishimoto N, Matsushita M, Shimizu M, Kobayshi Y, Nomura T, Kishimoto T (1995) Transfer of rheumatoid arthritis into severe combined immunodeficent mice. The pathogenic implications of T cell populations oligoclonally expanding in the rheumatoid joints. *J Clin Invest* 96: 1746–1758

30 Koopman WJ, Gay S (1988) The MRL-lpr/lpr mouse. A model for the study of rheumatoid arthritis. *Scand J Rheumatol Suppl* 75: 284–289

31 Ratkay LG, Zhang L, Tonzetich J, Waterfield JD (1993) Complete Freund's Adjuvant induces an earlier and more severe arthritis in MRL-lpr mice. *J Immunol* 151: 5081–5087

32 Mountz JD, Zhou T, Long RE, Bluethmann HM, Koopman WJ, Edwards CK (1994) T cell influence on superantigen-induced arthritis in MRL-lpr/lpr mice. *Arthritis Rheum* 37: 113–124

33 Edwards CK, Zhou T, Zhang J, Baker TJ, Long RE, Borcherding DR, Bowlin TL, Bluethmann H, Mountz JD (1996) Inhibition of superantigen-induced proinflammatory cytokine production and inflammatory arthritis in MRL-lpr/lpr mice by a transcriptional inhibitor of TNFα. *J Immunol* 157: 1758–1772

34 Iwakura Y, Tosu M, Yoshida E, Takiguchi M, Sato K, Kitajima I, Nishioka K, Yamamoto K, Takeda T, Hatanaka M, Yamamoto H, Sekiguchi T (1991) Induction of inflammatory arthropathy resembling rheumatoid arthritis in mice transgenic for HTLV-I. *Science* 253: 1026–1028

35 Yamamoto H, Sekiguchi T, Itagaki K, Saijo S, Iwakura Y (1993) Inflammatory pol-

yarthritis in mice transgenic for human T cell leukemia virus type I. *Arthritis Rheum* 36: 1612–1620
36 Fujisawa K, Asahara H, Okamoto K, Aono H, Hasunuma T, Kobata T, Iwakra Y, Yonehara S, Sumida T, Nishioka K (1996) Therapeutic effect of the anti-Fas antibody on arthritis in HTLV-I fax transgenic mice. *J Clin Invest* 98: 271–278
37 Shiozawa S, Tanka Y, Fujita T, Tokuhisa T (1992) Destructive arthritis without lymphocyte infiltration in H2-c-fos transgenic mice. *J Immunol* 148: 3100–3104
38 Keffer J, Probert L, Cazlaris H, Georgopoulos S, Kaslaris E, Kioussis D, Kollias G (1991) Transgenic mice expressing human tumor necrosis factor: a predictive genetic model of arthritis. *EMBO J* 13: 4025–4031
39 Probert L, Plows D, Kontogeorgos G, Kollias G (1995) The type I interleukin receptor acts in series with TNF to induce arthritis in TNF-transgenic mice. *Eur J Immunol* 25: 1794–1798
40 Douni E, Akassoglou K, Alexopoulou L, Georgopoulos S, Haralambous S, Hill S, Kassiotis G, Kontoyiannis D, Pasparakis M, Plows D, Probert L, Kollias G (1996) Transgenic and knockout analyses of the role of TNF in immune regulation and disease pathogenesis. *J Inflammation* 47: 27–38
41 Georgopoulos S, Plows D, Kollias G (1996) Transmembrane TNF is sufficient to induce localized tissue toxicity and chronic inflammatory arthritis in transgenic mice. *J Inflammation* 46: 86–97
42 Joosten LAB, Helsen MMA, van den Berg WB (1994) Accelerated onset of collagen-induced arthritis by remote inflammation. *Clin Exp Immunol* 97: 204–211
43 Van den Broek MF, van Bruggen MCJ, van de Putte LBA, van den Berg WB (1988) T cell responses to streptococcal antigens in rats: relation to susceptibility to streptococcal cell wall-induced arthritis. *Cell Immunol* 116: 216–229
44 Van den Broek MF, van Bruggen MCJ, Stimpson SA, Severijnen AJ, van de Putte LBA, van den Berg WB (1990) Flare-up reaction of streptococcal cell wall-induced arthritis in Lewis and F344 rats: The role of T lymphocytes. *Clin Exp Immunol* 79: 297–306
45 McInnes LB, Leung BP, Sturrock RD, Field M, Liew FY (1997) IL-15 mediates T–cell dependent regulation of TNFα production in rheumatoid arthritis. *Nature Med* 3: 189– 195
46 Kouskoff V, Korganow AS, Duchatelle V, Degott C, Benoist C, Mathis D (1996) Organ-specific disease provoked by systemic autoimmunity. *Cell* 87: 811–822
47 Lens JW, van den Berg WB, van de Putte LBA, Berden JHM, Lems SPM (1984) Flare-up of antigen-induced arthritis in mice after challenge with intravenous antigen: effects of pretreatment with cobra venom factor and antilymphocyte serum. *Clin Exp Immunol* 57: 520–528
48 Van de Loo AAJ, Arntz OJ, Bakker AC, van Lent PLEM, MJM Jacobs, van den Berg WB (1995) Role of Interleukin-1 in antigen-induced exacerbations of murine arthritis. *Am J Pathol* 146: 239–249
49 Van de Loo AAJ, Arntz OJ, van den Berg WB (1992) Flare-up of experimental arthritis in mice with murine recombinant IL-1. *Clin Exp Immunol* 87: 196–202
50 Bristol LA, Durum SK, Eisenberg SP (1993) Differential regulation of group A strepto-

coccal peptidoglycan-polysaccharide (PG-APS)-stimulated macrophage production of IL-1 by rat strains susceptible and resistant to PG-APS-induced arthritis. *Cell Immunol* 149: 130–143

51 Van den Broek MF, van den Berg WB, van de Putte LBA, Severijnen AJ (1988) Streptococcal cell wall induced arthritis and flare-up reactions in mice induced by homologous and heterologous cell walls. *Am J Pathol* 133: 139–149

52 Van den Berg WB, van Lent PLEM (1996) Role of macrophages in chronic arthritis. *Immunobiol* 195: 614–623

53 Van Lent PLEM, van den Hoek AEM, van den Bersselaar LAM, Spanjaards MFR, van Rooijen N, Dijkstra CD, van de Putte LBA, van den Berg WB (1993) *In vivo* role of phagocytic synovial lining cells in onset of experimental arthritis. *Am J Pathol* 143: 1226–1237

54 Van Lent PLEM, Holthuysen AEM, van den Bersselaar LAM, van Rooijen N, Joosten LAB, van de Loo FAJ, van de Putte LBA, van den Berg WB (1996) Phagocytic lining cells determine local expression of inflammation in type II collagen-induced arthritis. *Arthritis Rheum* 39: 1545–1555

55 Van Lent PLEM, Holthuysen AEM, van den Bersselaar L, van Rooijen N, van de Putte LBA, van den Berg WB (1995) Role of macrophage-like synovial lining cells in localization and expression of experimental arthritis. *Scand J Rheumatol* 24 (Suppl 101): 83–89

56 Mauri C, Williams RO, Walmsley M, Feldmann M (1996) Relationship between Th/Th2 cytokine patterns and the arthritogenic response in collagen-induced arthritis. *Eur J Immunol* 26: 1511–1518

57 Chu CQ, Londei M (1996) Induction of Th2 cytokines and control of collagen-induced arthritis by nondepleting anti-CD4 Abs. *J Immunol* 157: 2685–2689

58 Doncardi A, Stasiuk LM, Fournier C, Abehsira-Amar O (1997) Conversion in vivo from an early dominant Th0/Th1 response to a Th2 phenotype during the development of collagen-induced arthritis. *Eur J Immunol* 27: 1451–1458

59 Maeda T, Saikawa I, Hotokebuchi T, Sugioka Y, Eto M, Murakami Y, Nomoto K (1994) Exacerbation of established collagen-induced arthritis in mice treated with an anti-T cell receptor antibody. *Arthritis Rheum* 37, 406–413

60 Myers LK, Seyer JM, Stuart JM, Kang AH (1997) Suppression of murine collagen-induced arthritis by nasal administration of collagen. Immunol 90: 161–164

61 Miossec P, van den Berg WB (1997) Th1/Th2 cytokine balance in arthritis. *Arthritis Rheum* 40; 2105–2115

62 Weiner HL (1997) Oral tolerance: Immune mechanisms and treatment of autoimmune diseases. *Immunol Today* 18: 335–343

63 Tian J, Atkinson MA, Clare Salzler M, Herschenfeld A, Forsthuber T, Lehmann PV, Laufman DL (1996) Nasal administration of glutamate decarboxylase (GAD65) peptides induces Th2 responses and prevents murine-dependent diabetes. *J Exp Med* 183: 1561–1567

64 Williams NA, Stasiuk LM, Nashar TO, Richards CM, Lang AK, Day MJ, Hirst TR

(1997) Prevention of autoimmune disease due to lymphocyte modulation by the B-subunit of Escherichia coli heat-labile enterotoxin. *Proc Natl Acad Sci USA* 94: 5290–5295
65 Prakken BJ, van der Zee R, Anderton SM, van Kooten PJS, Kuis W, van Eden W (1997) Peptide-induced nasal tolerance for a myobacterial heat shock protein 60 T cell epitope in rats suppresses both adjuvant arthritis and nonmicrobacterially induced experimental arthritis. *Proc Natl Acad Sci* USA 94: 3284–3289
66 Trentham DE, Dynesius–Trentham RA, Orav EJ, Combitchi D, Lorenzo C, Sewell KL, Hafler DA, Weiner HL (1993) Effects of oral administration of type II collagen on rheumatoid arthritis. *Science* 261: 1727–1730
67 Sieper J, Kary S, Sorensen H, Alten R, Eggens U, Huge W, Hiepe F, Kuhne F, Listing J, Ulbrich N, Braun J, Zink A, Mitchison NA (1996) Oral type II collagen treatment in early rheumatoid arthritis: a double-blind, placebo-controlled, randomized trial. *Arthritis Rheum* 39: 41–51
68 Austrup F, Vestweber D, Borges E, Lohning M, Brauer R, Herz U, Renz H, Hallmann R, Scheffold A, Radbruch A, Hamann A (1997) P- and E-selectin mediate recruitment of T-helper-1 but not T-helper-2 cells into inflamed tissues. *Nature* 385: 81–83
69 Joosten LAB, Lubberts E, Durez P, Helsen MMA, Jacobs MJM, Goldman M, van den Berg WB (1997) Role of IL-4 and IL-10 in murine collagen-induced arthritis. *Arthritis Rheum* 40: 249–259
70 Chernajovsky Y, Adams G, Triantaphyllopoulos K, Ledda MF, Podhajcer OL (1997) Pathogenic lymphoid cells engineered to express TGFβ1 ameliorate disease in a collagen-induced arthritis model. *Gene Therapy* 4: 553–559
71 Mathisen PM, Yu M, Johnson JM, Drazba JA, Tuohy VK (1997) Treatment of experimental autoimmune encephalomyelitis with genetically modified memory T cells. *J Exp Med* 186: 159–164.

The Th1/Th2 cytokine balance in arthritis

Pierre Miossec

Clinical Immunology Unit, Departments of Immunology and Rheumatology, Hôpital Edouard Herriot, F-69437 Lyon, France.

Introduction

The contribution of T cells to the pathogenesis of rheumatoid arthritis (RA) has been a matter of debate which is addressed in a number of reviews and chapters of this book [1–3]. The contribution of monocytes through the production of proinflammatory cytokines has been simpler to demonstrate [4]. Accordingly, Interleukin (IL)-1 and tumor necrosis factor (TNF)α have been selected as important therapeutic targets [5].

With respect to the production of T cell derived cytokines in RA, the low level of expression and production by RA synovium of T cell derived cytokines was first described for IL-2 and Interferon (IFN)γ, then extended to TNFβ and IL-4 [6–9]. The relative failure to detect these factors has been one reason to question the role of T cells. However, another way to look at the contribution of T cells in RA focuses on the analysis of their cytokine profile and the associated subsets of T cells. Indeed, such subsets have been associated with the development of different disease patterns in mouse and man. More importantly, the modulation of such cytokine profiles is now considered a therapeutic goal [10].

The Th1/Th2 cytokine balance from mouse to man:

In 1986, Mossmann and Coffman showed that mouse CD4 T cell clones could be classified into distinct subsets according to their cytokine pattern [11]. These studies established that Th1 clones produce IL-2 and IFNγ, whereas Th2 clones produce IL-4 and IL-5. Later, other cytokines were added and classified as Th1 (TNF-β) or as Th2 (IL-6, IL-10 and IL-13). Simultaneously a precursor (Tho) subset producing IL-4, IL-2 and IFNγ was described [12]. These precursor cells are themselves derived from virgin T cells (Thp) which secrete IL-2 following activation.

Regarding their function, Th1 cytokines favour T cell-mediated cellular immunity and cytotoxicity, delayed type hypersensitivity (DTH), and activation of mono-

T Cells in Arthritis, edited by P. Miossec, W.B. van den Berg and G.S. Firestein

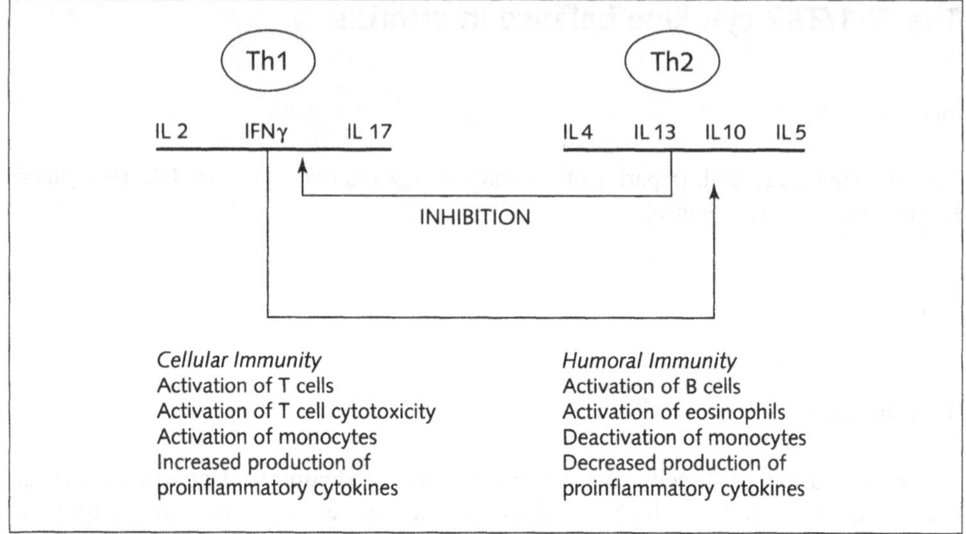

Figure 1
The Th1/Th2 cytokine balance and biological functions
A predominant Th1 profile is implicated in T cell-mediated immunity whereas a predominant Th2 profile is implicated in B cell-mediated immunity. The opposite effects on monocyte activation are the basis for the control of chronic inflammation. IL-17 has been added as a Th1 cytokine.

cytes leading to the production of proinflammatory cytokines. Conversely, Th2 cytokines favour B cell-mediated humoral immunity, induce IgE production with IL-4 and IL-13, activate eosinophils with IL-5, and deactivatation of monocytes leading to an anti-inflammatory cytokine pattern (Fig. 1). Observations in animal models indicated the contribution of Th1 cells to DTH and that of Th2 cells in allergy and some parasitic infections [12].

The same dichotomy was later applied to human T cells, first with T cell clones and later applied to various diseases [13, 14]. In the case of arthritis, T cell clones from the RA synovium site were found to produce large amounts of IFNγ, but not IL-4, leading to their classification as Th1 cells and RA as a Th1 condition [15, 16]. A similar conclusion was reached for autoimmune diabetes, thyroiditis, and multiple sclerosis (Fig. 2). Conversely, in allergic reactions, CD 4 T cells infiltrating the conjunctiva of patients with allergic conjunctivitis or allergen specific T cell clones obtained from atopic patients were essentially of the Th2 type [17]. Similarly, the contribution of IL-4 in scleroderma and of IL-10 in lupus led to the classification of these diseases as Th2 conditions [18–20].

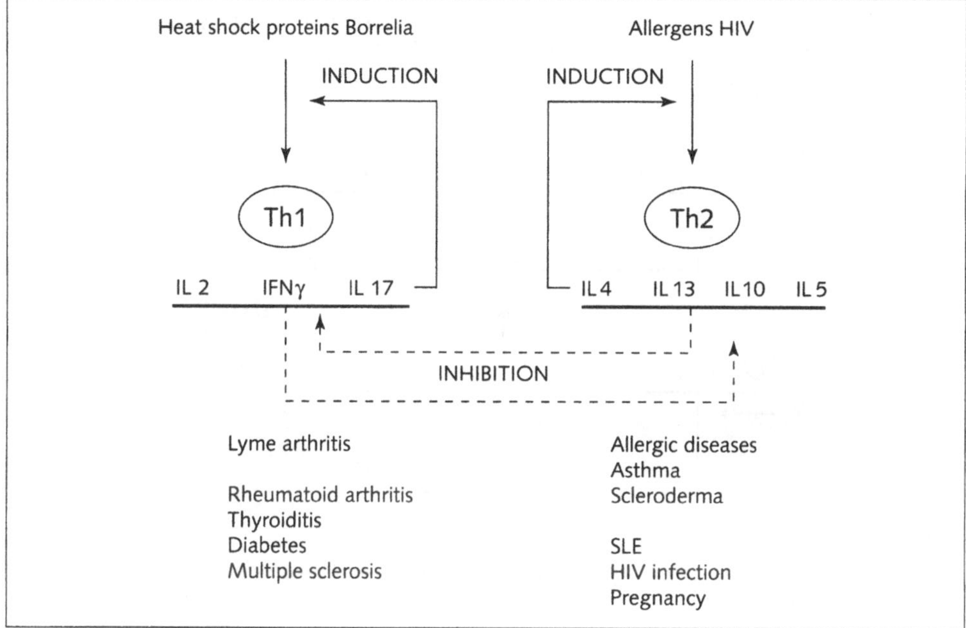

Figure 2
The Th1/Th2 cytokine balance and diseases
A predominant Th1 profile has been associated with rheumatoid arthritis, Lyme arthritis, multiple sclerosis, diabetes, and thyroiditis. Due to its effect on inflammation, IL-17 has been added as a Th1 cytokine. A Th2 profile with the predominant contribution of IL-4 and IL-5 has been associated with allergic diseases and scleroderma. The main contribution of IL-10, altough not predominantly of T cell origin, has been suggested in pregnancy, lupus, and early HIV infection.

Extension of the Th1/Th2 cytokine balance

Extension to other cell subsets

Further studies in mouse and man showed that T cell clones produce quite often a mixture of cytokines. In the case of RA, a large proportion of the heat shock protein (HSP) specific αβ CD 4 clones, producing large amounts of IFNγ, also released significant levels of IL-10 [16, 21]. In addition, some of these cytokines are produced by cells other than Th cells such as CD8 cytotoxic T cells, γδ T cells, and even by cells other than T cells [22]. IL-4 is produced also by mast cells, basophils, and eosinophils, whereas human IL-10 is produced by monocytes, B cells, and Th1 cells.

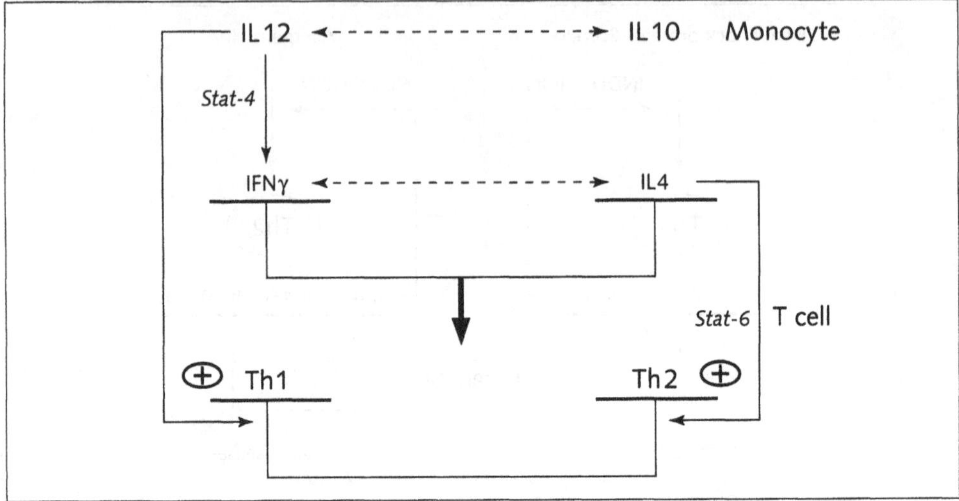

Figure 3
Control of the Th1/Th2 cytokine balance by monocyte and T-cell derived regulatory cytokines
IL-12 is the critical monocyte-derived cytokine which induces IFNγ production and a Th1 profile through the activation of Stat-4. IL-4 is the critical cytokine which induces a Th2 profile through the activation of Stat-6. Plain lines represent stimulatory effects; dotted lines represent inhibitory effects.

In RA synovium, IL-10 comes mainly from monocytes and not from T cells [23]. Thus, with respect to the relative amount of cytokine, IL-10 cannot be considered as a major T cell derived cytokine.

Recently a new Th3 subset has been defined for transforming growth factor (TGF)β producing T cells. However, TGFβ is largely a monocyte/mesenchymal cell-derived growth factor. Indeed the monocyte cytokine balance parallels the T cell cytokine balance. On the one hand, IL-12 produced by monocytes acts on T cells and NK cells inducing the production of IFNγ leading to a Th1 pattern. On the other hand, and in a symmetrical fashion, IL-10 produced by monocytes inhibits the production of IFNγ and thus counteracts the effect of IL-12 [10] (Fig. 3).

Cytokine specificity within the balance

Cytokines such as IL-4, IL-13 and IL-10 have been classified as Th2 cytokines. Although they share major functions, such as the inhibition of proinflammatory cytokine production by monocytes, they have a number of opposite effects on other targets [24–26]. For example, IL-10 induces full differentiation of plasma cells when B cells are in contact with synoviocytes, an effect which is strongly inhibited with IL-4 [27]. IL-4 and IL-13 share their antiinflammatory properties, but the effect of IL-4 on T cells appears more potent than that of IL-13. Furthermore, combination of the two cytokines results in an inhibitory effect as they compete for the same multi-chain receptor [28].

New members of the Th1/Th2 cytokine balance

New cytokines have been isolated and their classification is pending. Among them, IL-17 is of particular interest in inflammation. This cytokine is produced apparently only by CD 4 T cells and represents the human counterpart of mouse CTLA-8 [29]. IL-17 induces a proinflammatory pattern with the induction of IL-6, GM-CSF, and PGE2 production by mesenchymal cells, such as synoviocytes [29, 30]. Recent results indicate that IL-17 is actively produced by RA synovium. In addition, RA T cell clones producing IFNγ also produce IL-17. According to these characteristics, IL-17 can be classified as a type 1 cytokine. Furthermore, a combination of suboptimal concentrations of IL-17 with low levels of monocyte-derived cytokines strongly enhances cytokine production by synoviocytes. This pathway appears to represent an important component of the regulatory function of T cells in inducing an inflammatory pattern.

The kinetics of the Th1/Th2 cytokine balance

The dynamic pattern of the Th1/Th2 cytokine balance

The balance is regulated both positively and negatively. The stimulatory regulation implies that each Th cytokine subset induces its own production and favors the differentiation of naive T cells into the same subset. Thus IFNγ induces its own production and Th1 cell activation whereas IL-4 activates Th2 function.

Conversely, the inhibitory pathway implies that each subset can regulate the activities of the others. Both IL-4 and IL-10 are strong inhibitors of IFNγ production and IFNγ inhibits IL-10 production [31] (Fig. 1).

It is in the nature of the antigen to induce a particular T cell cytokine profile. Normal T cells produce Th1 cytokines in response to mycobacterial antigens and Th2 cytokines in response to allergens [14]. Furthermore, normal T cells cultured in the presence of either IFNγ or IL-4 gave rise to the development of either Th1 or Th2 clones respectively [32].

Recent results have shown that the identification of the inducing antigen is not mandatory for manipulating the balance. Human cord blood naive T cells activated by mitogens can be directed towards Th1 when cultured in the presence of IL-12 and anti-IL-4, and towards Th2 in the presence of IL-4 and anti-IL-12 [33]. These findings demonstrate the critical role of IL-12 and that of IL-4 in the switch to Th1 or Th2 respectively (Fig. 3). Such findings are of interest when considering their application to the treatment of disease where the cause is unknown.

It was expected that these cells would express specific subset markers. Indeed, a number of studies have suggested that this could be the case for markers such as CD27, CD30, and CD45 isoforms. However, additional studies have questioned their subset specificity. Regarding arthritis, blood CD4 $CD^{45RB\,Dim}$ CD^{27-} T cells have been characterized as the IL-4 producing subset [34]. Recent studies have indicated a good correlation between the Th1 pattern and the expression of the β2 chain of the IL-12 receptor and the Th2 pattern and the expression of the β chain of the IFNγ receptor [33, 34].

Molecules controlling the Th1/Th2 cytokine balance

Various molecules contribute to the control of Th1/Th2 development. The co-stimulatory molecules B7-1 (CD80) and B7-2 (CD86) expressed on antigen presenting cells act as a second signal and control the differentiation of the two major subsets [35]. Their ligands on T cells are CD28 and CTLA4 [36]. This second step of activation follows the first signal given by the interaction between the T cell receptor and the antigen MHC complex which confers T cell specificity. CD28 co-stimulation was found to promote the production of Th2 cytokines by mouse T cells through an IL-4 dependent mechanism [37].

Initial results in the mouse have indicated that activation of the B7-1 pathway stimulates the Th1 subset whereas B7-2 activation stimulates the Th2 subset. Conversely, blockage of B7-1 was able to control Th1 mediated diseases such as diabetes and encephalomyelitis [38, 39]. However results in other systems indicate the complexity of such regulation [40].

Applying these findings to man has proven to be even more difficult. The contribution of IL-4 appears to be critical. B7-2 stimulation controls specifically IL-4 production by naive T cells whereas both B7-1 and B7-2 can induce IL-4 production by memory T cells [41]. In the absence of the regulatory properties of IL-4, T cells remain sensitive to other regulatory cytokines such as IL-12 which induces IFNγ and a strong Th1 profile. At this stage, the presence or absence of IL-4 appears to represent the most critical factor in inducing the Th1/Th2 switch.

Signal transducer and activator of transcription (STAT) factors are critical in controling the intracellular signalling pathways of these cytokines. IL-12 acts through the activation of Stat-4. Indeed, inactivation of the STAT-4 gene in mouse leads to a defect in IL-12 production and Th1 functions combined with increased Th2 functions [42]. Conversely, STAT-6 is critical for the IL-4 and Th2 mediated events, as shown with Stat-6 knock-out mice [43, 44]. The transcription factor

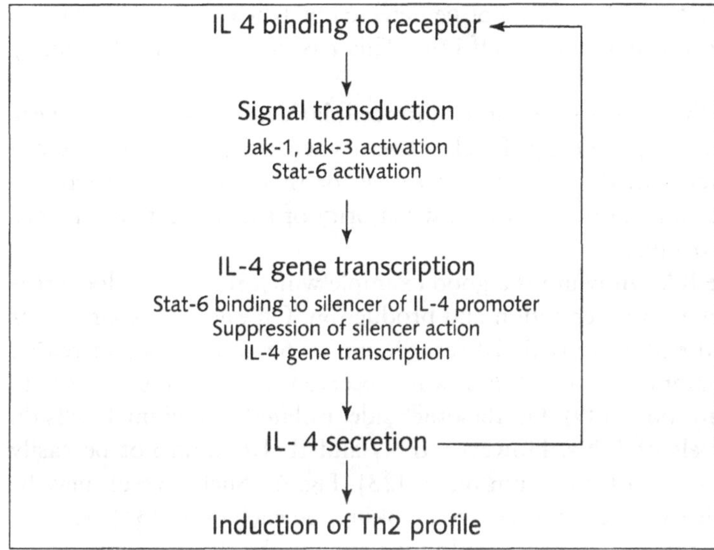

Figure 4
Control of IL-4 gene activation in the presence of IL-4
In the presence of IL-4 and upon its binding to a functional IL-4 receptor, receptor signal transduction is performed with the activation of the kinases Jak-1 and Jak-3. Phosphorylation activates Stat-6 transcription factor which enters the nucleus and binds to a silencer element which normally suppresses IL-4 transcription. Inhibition of the element's action leads to IL-4 gene transcription and IL-4 production [46]. Conversely, under the action of IL-12, the silencer is active and inhibits IL-4 production preventing the induction of a Th2 profile.

GATA-3 has been shown to be necessary and sufficient for Th2 pattern expression in mouse T cells [45]. STAT-6 activates IL-4 gene transcription by the inactivation of a silencer of the IL-4 promoter (Fig. 4) [46].

The Th1/Th2 cytokine balance in arthritis

Expression in the synovium

This simple classification has been more difficult to reconstitute when looking at the cytokines produced by the synovium itself. Findings on the levels of these T cell derived cytokines in RA have been contradictory and their specific detection difficult, despite the infiltration of the synovium by many T cells [6, 47]. Although contradictory results have been published, the expression of IL-2 and IFNγ mRNA by RA synovium was not detected even when using the most recent and sensitive methods [9]. IL-4 protein and mRNA could not be detected in synovial fluid, in synovium supernatants, or in the synovium itself [48]. This has been confirmed in many studies.

It should be noted that direct staining for intracellular cytokines showed a very low frequency of cytokine-producing T cells. Even when using Th1 or Th2 cell clones, only a few percent of the cells stain positive for IFNγ or IL-4 respectively. More importantly, the contribution of the vast majority of these negative cells has not been addressed in details.

The situation in the RA synovium is a good example which reflects the local regulation of cytokines on each other action and production. On one side, staining for IL-10 was positive and endogenous IL-10 was shown to be active since increased production of proinflammatory cytokines was observed in the presence of an inhibitory anti-IL-10 antibody [49]. On the other side, isolated synovium T cells do produce significant levels of IFNγ. However, IFNγ and IL-10 could not be easily detected in the supernatants of synovium pieces [23] (Fig. 4). Such a result may be explained by the inhibitory effect of these two cytokines on each other [31]. The relative ratio between the two components could then explain the flares observed during the disease course.

The Th1/Th2 cytokine balance and the search for the cause of RA

In Lyme arthritis, the histological aspect of the synovium is very similar to that seen in RA and antigen-specific T cell clones produce large amounts of IFNγ with no IL-4, as in RA [50]. Similarly, Th1 cells have been implicated in tuberculosis and some forms of leprosy [51, 52]. In the same line, T cells infected by the retrovirus HTLV-1 tend to produce an extended cytokine profile combining Th1 T cell and monocyte derived cytokines. Such profile could contribute to the rheumatoid-like clinical presentation observed both in man and in a transgenic mouse model for the Tax regulatory protein from HTLV-1 [53]. Such mechanism may apply to the pathogenesis of human diabetes with the contribution of a newly-identified endogenous retrovirus [54].

The Th1/Th2 cytokine balance and the chronicity of RA

Following initial stimulation of a few antigen-specific T cells, the tissue destruction appears to result from the contribution of a large infiltrate of bystander T cells. Increased migration of this polyclonal population results in the formation of the inflammatory lesion. Endothelial cell swelling, leading to the formation of high endothelium venules, is one of the earliest pathological findings. These changes are associated with an increased expression of adhesion molecules, leading to increased cell migration. In mouse arthritis, migration of Th1 cells rather than Th2 cells is facilitated through the use of the E and P selectins [55]. Thus, expression of such adhesion molecules may be sufficient to increase the migration of T cells in a non-antigen-specific fashion. Results in various animals models suggest that targeting the migration of inflammatory cells is of therapeutic interest. Indeed, targeting of intracellular adhesion molecule (ICAM)-1 has been applied to the treatment of RA [56]. To further refine such a concept, a more specific approach could be to block the migration of Th1, disease-inducing T cells, in favour of the protective Th2 cells [57].

Differences between systemic and synovial sites

Differences in migration patterns are associated with differences between systemic and synovial sites. During chronic inflammation, migration of proinflammatory cells is increased whereas that of protective cells is defective, leading to their relative accumulation in the blood stream [55]. In RA blood, a defect in IFNγ production has been reported [58]. Studies at the level of cytokine production have been limited because the production of IL-4 is difficult to detect. Results with a very sensitive IL-4 assay indicated that activated RA whole blood cells produced more IL-4 than controls with a higher IL-4/IFNγ ratio. Such findings are in line with the increased production in blood as well as in activated PBMC supernatants of sCD 23, the production of which is under the control of IL-4 [59]. These results obtained in blood are opposite to those found in RA synovium where a Th1 pattern is predominant. Similar differences have been found when comparing the response of monocytes from either blood or the synovial site with respect to these cytokines [60].

Acting on the Th1/Th2 cytokine balance to control RA

Administration of exogenous cytokines

Preclinical studies have been performed with synovium pieces and cell suspensions obtained after enzymatic digestion. Addition to synovium pieces of exogenous IL-4, IL-13, and to a lesser extent IL-10, strongly reduced the production of proinflammatory cytokines whereas that of IL-1Ra was enhanced [48, 49, 61]. Furthermore, addition of IL-4 to bone pieces reduced bone resorption through an apparent effect on osteoclast activity and survival [62]. Moreover, there is evidence that IL-4 has a direct protective effect against chondrocyte driven cartilage degradation [63] (Fig. 4) [64]. The regulatory role of IL-4, IL-13 and IL-10 has been convincingly demonstrated in most, but not all, animal models of arthritis. A better suppression was found with the combination of IL-4 and IL-10. These results in animal models are reviewed in the chapter by Wim van den Berg (this volume).

Combined together, such results provide the rationale for treatment [65]. The most simple approach is the administration of exogenous cytokines. However, their half-life is very short and such molecules will bind to specific receptors before reaching the inflammatory site. Local administration would not be difficult but will be limited by the number of affected joints. Preliminary phase I trials have started in RA using the systemic administration of IL-10 and IL-4.

Administration of cytokine by gene therapy has proven to be successful in arthritis animal models [66]. The precise local control of such genes, however, remains to be resolved. Another mean could be the *ex-vivo* stimulation of circulating lymphocytes with exogenous cytokines before injecting them back. Such a procedure has already been used with IL-2 to obtain lymphokine activated killer (LAK) cells in cancer treatment. *Ex-vivo* activation with Th2 cytokines can be a way of inducing the differentiation of uncommitted or Th1 cells into Th2 cells, provided that migration patterns are simultaneously modified.

Induction of the endogenous production of protective cytokines

The production of cytokines by T cells is under the control of numerous factors: the antigen structure: arthritogenic vs. tolerogenic epitopes, the mode of administration: systemic vs. oral, the nature of the antigen presenting cells: dendritic cells vs. B cells, and the cytokine and steroid environment: Th1 vs. Th2 [67].

Induction of a remission or cure of RA has been observed in a number of clinical conditions in the absence of an obvious action at the level of the cause [8]. These conditions are important to consider since it is tempting to reproduce such modulation. The most obvious situation is the remission of RA during pregnancy and the flare following delivery. In this situation, T cell mediated immunity, i.e. foetus rejection has to be down-regulated whereas the foetus has to be protected with maternal IgG [68]. These two components suggest the contribution of factors such as TGFβ and IL-10. Indeed, high expression of IL-10 at the placental interface has been observed in the mouse [69, 70]. More importantly, the improvement of RA appears to be directly related to the degree of maternal-paternal disparity, which results in increased foetus tolerance [71]. Similar observations have been made for the side-effects to slow-acting drugs [72] for early HIV infection [73] and allogeneic bone marrow transplantation [74] (Fig. 2). These conditions appear to be associated with a Th2 cytokine profile (Fig. 2) [7, 75].

Whatever the mechanism, such observations indicate that even long-standing inflammatory disease can improve without antigen-specific intervention. The next logical step is to reproduce these situations *in vitro* and *in vivo*. Although the clinical data from the first small trials with collagen type II dosing in RA patients looked promising [76], more extensive studies did not confirm efficacy [77] and we are yet at the beginning of exploring focused manipulation of local Th1/Th2/Th3 balances.

Interestingly, activated Th2/Th3 cells may protect individuals from Th1-dependent arthritis through antigen driven generation of IL-4, IL-10, or TGFβ. The principle of so-called bystander suppression through this set of cytokines provides a means to bypass the lack of information on particular autoantigens involved in the disease [78]. In particular, induction of bystander suppression by oral tolerance could represent a simple way to control inflammation.

It should be kept in mind that an excessive Th2 switch may be armful. Excess IL-4 and IL-13 could lead to allergy and asthma. Excess IL-10 could favor B cell/plasma cell activation with increased autoantibody production. Such events may contribute to some extra-articular manifestations such as rheumatoid vasculitis or lymphomas as seen during the course of RA.

Conclusion

Not knowing the cause of RA remains a major limitation in terms of its treatment. The concept of cytokine balance in arthritis is of interest since it may act in a cause independent fashion. Nevertheless this implies early treatment before destruction occurs in patients at high risk. In addition, recent findings suggest that the invasive pattern of RA synoviocytes is associated with, and may be the consequence of, irreversible somatic mutations [79]. If this was the case, then endogenous control of such proliferation may remain limited once a chronic stage has been reached. Combined together, these factors strongly point to the need for better early diagnosis and prognosis markers to ensure early treatment. In this situation, acting on the endogenous regulatory cytokine balance may represent a more natural way to prevent the consequences of chronic inflammation.

Acknowledgements
These studies performed in the laboratory of the author have been supported in part by grants from the Hospices Civils de Lyon, the Association de Recherche sur la Polyarthrite and from the European Union (Biomed-2 program contract BMH4-CT96-1698).

References

1 Firestein GS, Zvaifler NJ (1990) How important are T cells in chronic rheumatoid synovitis? *Arthritis Rheum* 33: 768–772
2 Panayi GS, Lanchbury JS, Kingsley GH (1992) The importance of the T cell in initiating and maintaining the chronic synovitis of rheumatoid arthritis. *Arthritis Rheum* 35: 729–735

3 Fox D (1997) The role of T cells in the immunopathogenesis of rheumatoid arthritis. *Arthritis Rheum* 40: 598–609

4 Arend WP, Dayer JM (1995) Inhibition of the production and effects of Interleukin-1 and Tumor Necrosis Factor α in rheumatoid arthritis. *Arthritis Rheum* 38: 151–160

5 Elliott MJ, Maini RN, Feldmann M, Kalden JR, Antoni C, Smolen JS, Leeb B, Breedveld FC, Macfarlane JD, Bijl H, Woody JN (1994) Randomised double-blind comparison of chimeric monoclonal antibody to tumour necrosis factor α (cA2) versus placebo in rheumatoid arthritis. *Lancet* 344: 1105–1110

6 Firestein GS, Alvaro-Gracia J, Maki R (1990) Quantitative analysis of cytokine gene expression in rheumatoid arthritis. *J Immunol* 144: 3347–3353

7 Miossec P (1993) Acting on the cytokine balance to control auto-immunity and chronic inflammation. *Eur Cytokine Netw* 4: 245–251

8 Miossec P, Chomarat P, Dechanet J (1996) Bypassing the antigen to control rheumatoid arthritis. *Immunol Today* 17: 170–173

9 Chen E, Keystone EC, Fish EN (1993) Restricted cytokine expression in rheumatoid arthritis. *Arthritis Rheum* 36: 901–910

10 Abbas AK, Murphy KM, Sher A (1996) Functional diversity of helper T lymphocytes. *Nature* 383: 787–793

11 Mosmann TR, Cherwinski H, Bond MW, Giedlin MA, Coffman RL (1986) Two types of murine helper T cell clone. I. Definition according to profiles of activities and secreted proteins. *J Immunol* 136: 2348–2357

12 Mosmann TR, Schumacher JH, Street NF, Budd R, O'Garra A, Fong TAT, Bond MW, Moore KWM, Sher A, Fiorentino DF (1991) Diversity of cytokine synthesis and function of mouse $CD4^+$ T cells. *Immunol Rev* 123: 209–229

13 Romagnani S (1991) Human T_H1 and T_H2 subsets: doubt no more. *Immunol Today* 12: 256–257

14 Del Prete GF, De Carli M, Mastromauro C, Biagiotti R, Macchia D, Falagiani P, Ricci M, Romagnani S (1991) Purified protein derivative of *Mycobacterium tuberculosis* and excretory-secretory antigen(s) of *Toxocara canis* expand *in vitro* human T cells with stable and opposite (type 1 T helper or type 2 T helper) profile of cytokine production. *J Clin Invest* 88: 346–350

15 Miltenburg AMM, Van Laar JM, De Kuiper R, Daha MR, Breedveld FC (1992) T cells cloned from human rheumatoid synovial membrane functionally represent the Th1 subset. *Scand J Immunol* 35: 603–610

16 Quayle AJ, Chomarat P, Miossec P, Kjeldsen-Kragh J, Førre O, Natvig JB (1993) Rheumatoid inflammatory T-cell clones express mostly Th1 but also Th2 and mixed (Th0-like) cytokine patterns. *Scand J Immunol* 38: 75–82

17 Maggi E, Biswas P, Del Prete G, Parronchi P, Macchia D, Simonelli C, Emmi L, De Carli M, Tiri A, Ricci M, Romagnani S (1991) Accumulation of Th-2-like helper T cells in the conjunctiva of patients with vernal conjunctivitis. *J Immunol* 146: 1169–1174

18 Salmon Ehr V, Serpier H, Nawrocki B, Gillery P, Clavel C, Kalis B, Birembaut P,

Maquart FX (1996) Expression of interleukin-4 in scleroderma skin specimens and scleroderma fibroblast cultures. Potential role in fibrosis. *Arch Dermatol* 132: 802–806

19 Hasegawa M, Fujimoto M, Kikuchi K, Takehara K (1997) Elevated serum levels of interleukin 4 (IL-4), IL-10, and IL-13 in patients with systemic sclerosis. *J Rheumatol* 24: 328–332

20 Llorente L, Zou W, Levy Y, Richaud-Patin Y, Wijdenes J, Alcocer-Varela J, Morel-Fourrier B, Brouet J-C, Arlacon-Segovia D, Galanaud P, Emilie D (1995) Role of interleukin 10 in the B lymphocyte hyperactivity and autoantibody production of human systemic lupus erythematosus. *J Exp Med* 181: 839–844

21 Mauri C, Williams RO, Walmsley M, Feldmann M (1996) Relationship between Th1/Th2 cytokine patterns and the arthritogenic response in collagen-induced arthritis. *Eur J Immunol* 26: 1511–1518

22 Chomarat P, Kjeldsen-Kragh J, Quayle AJ, Natvig JB, Miossec P (1994) Different cytokine production profiles of γδ T cell clones. Relation to inflammatory arthritis. *Eur J Immunol* 24: 2087–2091

23 Chomarat P, Banchereau J, Miossec P (1995) Differential effects of interleukins 10 and 4 on the production of interleukin-6 by blood and synovium monocytes in rheumatoid arthritis. *Arthritis Rheum* 38: 1046–1054

24 de Waal Malefyt R, Abrams J, Bennett B, Figdor CG, de Vries JE (1991) Interleukin 10 (IL-10) inhibits cytokine synthesis by human monocytes: an autoregulatory role of IL-10 produced by monocytes. *J Exp Med* 174: 1209–1220

25 de Waal Malefyt R, Figdor CG, de Vries JE (1993) Effects of interleukin 4 on monocyte functions: comparison to interleukin 13. *Res Immunol* 144: 629–633

26 Isomaki P, Luukkainen R, Toivanen P, Punnonen J (1996) The presence of interleukin-13 in rheumatoid synovium and its antiinflammatory effects on synovial fluid macrophages from patients with rheumatoid arthritis. *Arthritis Rheum* 39: 1693–1702

27 Dechanet J, Merville P, Durand I, Banchereau J, Miossec P (1995) The ability of synoviocytes to support terminal differentiation of activated B cells may explain plasma cell accumulation in rheumatoid synovium. *J Clin Invest* 95: 456–463

28 Zurawski SM, Chomarat P, Djossou, Bidaud C, McKenzie AN, Miossec P, Banchereau J, Zurawski G (1995) The primary binding subunit of the human interleukin-4 receptor is also a component of the interleukin-13 receptor. *J Biol Chem* 270: 13869–13878

29 Yao Z, Painter SL, Fanslow WC, Ulrich D, Macduff BM, Spriggs MK, Armitage RJ (1995) Human IL-17: A novel cytokine derived from T cells. *J Immunol* 155: 5483–5486

30 Fossiez F, Djossou O, Chomarat P, Flores-Romo L, Ait-Yahia S, Maat C, Pin JJ, Garrone P, Garcia E, Saeland S, Blanchard D, Gaillard C, Das Mahapatra B, Rouvier E, Golstein P, Banchereau J, Lebecque S (1996) T cell Interleukin-17 induces stromal cells to produce proinflammatory and hematopoietic cytokines. *J Exp Med* 183: 2593–2603

31 Chomarat P, Rissoan M-C, Banchereau J, Miossec P (1993) Interferon γ inhibits interleukin-10 production by monocytes. *J Exp Med* 177: 523–527

32 Maggi E, Parronchi P, Manetti R, Simonelli C, Piccinni M-P, Rugiu FS, De Carli M, Ricci

M, Romagnani S (1992) Reciprocal regulatory effects of IFN-γ and IL-4 on the *in vitro* development of human Th1 and Th2 clones. *J Immunol* 148: 2142–2147

33 Szabo SJ, Dighe AS, Gubler U, Murphy KM (1997) Regulation of the Interleukin-12R β2 subunit expression in developing T helper 1 and Th2 cells. *J Exp Med* 185: 817–824

34 Groux H, Sornasse T, Cottrez F, de Vries JE, Coffman RL, Roncarolo MG, Yssel H (1997) Induction of human T helper cell type 1 differentiation results in loss of IFN-gamma receptor beta-chain expression. *J Immunol* 158: 5627–5631

35 Gause WC, Urban JF, Linsley P, Lu P (1995) Role of B7 signaling in the differentiation of naive CD4+ T cells to effector interleukin-4-producing T helper cells. *Immunol Res* 14: 176–188

36 Lenschow DJ, Walunas TL, Bluestone JA (1996) CD28/B7 system of T cell costimulation. *Annu Rev Immunol* 14: 233–258

37 Rulifson IC, Sperling AI, Fields PE, Fitch FW, Bluestone JA (1997) CD28 costimulation promotes the production of Th2 cytokines. *J Immunol* 158: 658–665

38 Lenschow DJ, Ho SC, Sattar H, Rhee L, Gray G, Nabavi N, Herold KC, Bluestone JA (1995) Differential effects of anti-B7-1 and anti-B7-2 monoclonal antibody treatment on the development of diabetes in the nonobese diabetic mouse. *J Exp Med* 181: 1145– 1155

39 Khoury SJ, Akalin E, Chandraker A, Turka LA, Linsley PS, Sayegh MH, Hancock WW (1995) CD28-B7 costimulatory blockade by CTLA4Ig prevents actively induced experimental autoimmune encephalomyelitis and inhibits Th1 but spares Th2 cytokines in the central nervous system. *J Immunol* 155: 4521–4524

40 Natesan M, Razi Wolf Z, Reiser H (1996) Costimulation of IL-4 production by murine B7-1 and B7-2 molecules. *J Immunol* 156: 2783–2791

41 Freeman GJ, Boussiotis VA, Anumanthan A, Bernstein GM, Ke XY, Rennert PD, Gray GS, Gribben JG, Nadler LM (1995) B7-1 and B7-2 do not deliver identical costimulatory signals, since B7-2 but not B7-1 preferentially costimulates the initial production of IL-4. *Immunity* 2: 523–532

42 Thierfelder WE, van Deursen JM, Yamamoto K, Tripp RA, Sarawar SR, Carson RT, Sangster MY, Vignali DA, Doherty PC, Grosveld GC, Ihle JN (1996) Requirement for Stat4 in interleukin-12-mediated responses of natural killer and T cells. *Nature* 382: 171–174

43 Hou J, Schindler U, Henzel WJ, Ho TC, Brasseur M, McKnight SL (1994) An interleukin-4-induced transcription factor: IL-4 Stat. *Science* 265: 1701–1706

44 Takeda K, Tanaka T, Shi W, Matsumoto M, Minami M, Kashiwamura S, Nakanishi K, Yoshida N, Kishimoto T, Akira S (1996) Essential role of Stat6 in IL-4 signalling. *Nature* 380: 627–630

45 Zheng W-P, Flavell RA (1997) The transcription factor GATA-3 is necessary and sufficient for Th2 cytokine gene expression in CD4 T cells. *Cell* 89: 587–596

46 Kubo M, Ransom J, Webb D, Hashimoto Y, Tada T, Nakayama T (1997) T-cell subset-specific expression of the IL-4 gene is regulated by a silencer element and STAT6. *Embo J* 16: 4007–4020

47 Miossec P, Elhamiani M, Chichehian B, Dupuy d'Angeac A, Sany J, Hirn M (1990) Interleukin 2 (IL-2) inhibitor in rheumatoid synovial fluid: correlation with prognosis and soluble IL 2 receptor levels. *J Clin Immunol* 10: 115–120
48 Miossec P, Briolay J, Dechanet J, Wijdenes J, Martinez-Valdez H, Banchereau J (1992) Interleukin 4 inhibits *ex vivo* production of proinflammatory cytokines and immunoglobulins by rheumatoid synovitis. Arthritis Rheum 35: 874–883
49 Katsikis PD, Chu CQ, Brennan FM, Maini RN, Feldmann M (1994) Immunoregulatory role of interleukin 10 in rheumatoid arthritis. *J Exp Med* 179: 1517–1527
50 Yssel H, Shanafelt M-C, Soderberg C, Schneider PV, Anzola J, Peltz G (1991) Borrelia burgdorferi activates a T helper type 1-like T cell subset in lyme arthritis. *J Exp Med* 174: 593–601
51 Yamamura M, Uyemura K, Deans RJ, Weinberg K, Rea TH, Bloom BR, Modlin RL (1991) Defining protective responses to pathogens: Cytokine profiles in leprosy lesions. *Science* 254: 277–279
52 Haanen JBAG, de Waal Malefyt R, Res PCM, Kraakman EM, Ottenhoff THM, de Vries RRP, Spits H (1991) Selection of a human T helper type 1-like T cell subset by mycobacteria. *J Exp Med* 174: 583–592
53 Iwakura Y, Tosu M, Yoshida E (1991) Induction of inflammatory arthropathy resembling rheumatoid arthritis in mice transgenic for HTLV-1. *Science* 253: 1026–1028
54 Conrad B, Weissmahr RN, Boni J, Arcari R, Schupbach J, Mach B (1997) A human endogenous retroviral superantigen as candidate autoimmune gene in type I diabetes. *Cell* 90: 303–313
55 Austrup F, Vestweber D, Borges E, Lohning M, Brauer R, Herz U, Renz H, Hallmann R, Scheffold A, Radbruch A, Hamann A (1997) P- and E-selectin mediate recruitment of T-helper-1 but not T-helper-2 cells into inflammed tissues. *Nature* 385: 81–83
56 Kavanaugh AF, Davis LS, Nichols LA, Norris SH, Rothlein R, Scharschmidt LA, Lipsky PE (1994) Treatment of refractory rheumatoid arthritis with a monoclonal antibody to intercellular adhesion molecule 1. *Arthritis Rheum* 37: 992–999
57 Meeusen EN, Premier RR, Brandon MR (1996) Tissue-specific migration of lymphocytes: a key role for Th1 and Th2 cells? *Immunol Today* 17: 421–424
58 Al Janadi M, Al Dalaan A, Al Balla S, Raziuddin S (1996) $CD4^+$ T cell inducible immunoregulatory cytokine response in rheumatoid arthritis. *J Rheumatol* 23: 809–814
59 Chomarat P, Briolay J, Banchereau J, Miossec P (1993) Increased production of soluble CD23 in rheumatoid arthritis, and its regulation by interleukin-4. *Arthritis Rheum* 36: 234–242
60 Hart PH, Jones CA, Finlay Jones JJ (1995) Monocytes cultured in cytokine-defined environments differ from freshly isolated monocytes in their responses to IL-4 and IL-10. *J Leukoc Biol* 57: 909–918
61 Chomarat P, Vannier E, Dechanet J, Rissoan M-C, Banchereau J, Dinarello CA, Miossec P (1995) The balance of IL-1 receptor antagonist/IL-1β in rheumatoid synovium and its regulation by IL-4 and IL-10. *J Immunol* 154: 1432–1439

62 Miossec P, Chomarat P, Dechanet J, Moreau J-F, Roux J-P, Delmas P, Banchereau J (1994) Interleukin 4 inhibits bone resorption through an effect on osteoclasts and proinflammatory cytokines in an ex vivo model of bone resorption in rheumatoid arthritis. *Arthritis Rheum* 37: 1715–1722
63 Yeh LA, Augustine AJ, Lee P, Riviere LR, Sheldon A (1995) Interleukin-4, an inhibitor of cartilage breakdown in bovine articular cartilage explants. *J Rheumatol* 22: 1740–1746
64 Van Roon JAG, Van Roy J, Duits A, Lafeber F, Bijlsma JWJ (1995) Proinflammatory cytokine production and cartilage damage due to rheumatoid synovial T helper-1 activation is inhibited by interleukin-4. *Ann Rheum Dis* 54: 836–840
65 Rocken M, Racke M, Shevach EM (1996) IL-4-induced immune deviation as antigen-specific therapy for inflammatory autoimmune disease. *Immunol Today* 17: 225–231
66 Bessis N, Boissier MC, Ferrara P, Blankenstein T, Fradelizi D, Fournier C (1996) Attenuation of collagen-induced arthritis in mice by treatment with vector cells engineered to secrete interleukin-13. *Eur J Immunol* 26: 2399–2403
67 Daynes RA, Araneo BA, Dowell TA, Huang K, Dudley D (1990) Regulation of murine lymphokine production in vivo. III. The lymphoid tissue microenvironment exerts regulatory influences over T helper cell function. *J Exp Med* 171: 979–996
68 Formby B (1995) Immunologic response in pregnancy: Its role in endocrine disorders of pregnancy and influence on the course of maternal autoimmune diseases. *Endocrinol Metab Clin North Am* 24: 187–205
69 Wegmann TG, Lin H, Guilbert L, Mosmann TR (1993) Bidirectional cytokine interactions in the maternal-fetal relationship: is successful pregnancy a Th2 phenomenon? *Immunol Today* 14: 353–356
70 Raghupathy R (1997) Maternal anti-placental cell-mediated reactivity and spontaneous abortions. *Am J Reprod Immunol* 37: 478–484
71 Nelson JL, Hughes KA, Smith AG, Nisperos BB, Branchaud AM, Hansen JA (1993) Maternal-fetal disparity in HLA class II alloantigens and the pregnancy-induced amelioration of rheumatoid arthritis. *New Engl J Med* 329: 466–471
72 Arasil TK, Tuncer S, Tosun M (1991) Sustained remission of rheumatoid arthritis following hypersensitivity reaction. *Arthritis Rheum* 34: 789–790
73 Calabrese LH, Wilke WS, Perkins AD, Tubbs RR (1989) Rheumatoid arthritis complicated by infection with the human immunodeficiency virus and the development of Sjögren's syndrome. *Arthritis Rheum* 32: 1453–1457
74 Marmont AM (1994) Immune ablation followed by allogeneic or autologous bone marrow transplantation: a new treatment for severe autoimmune disease? *Stem Cells* 12: 125–135
75 Meyaard L, Hovenkamp E, Keet IP, Hooibrink B, de Jong IH, Otto SA, Miedema F (1996) Single cell analysis of IL-4 and IFN-gamma production by T cells from HIV-infected individuals: decreased IFN-gamma in the presence of preserved IL-4 production. *J Immunol* 157: 2712–2718
76 Trentham DE, Dynesius-Trentham RA, Orav EJ, Combitchi D, Lorenzo C, Sewell KL,

Hafler DA, Weiner HL (1993) Effects of oral administration of type II collagen on rheumatoid arthritis. *Science* 261: 1727–1730

77 Sieper J, Kary S, Sorensen H, Alten R, Eggens U, Huge W, Hiepe F, Kuhne F, Listing J, Ulbrich N, Braun J, Zink A, Mitchison NA (1996) Oral type II collagen treatment in early rheumatoid arthritis. A double-blind, placebo-controlled, randomized trial. *Arthritis Rheum* 39: 41–51

78 Prakken BJ, van der Zee R, Anderton SM, van Kooten P, Kuis W, van Eden W (1997) Peptide-induced nasal tolerance for a mycobacterial heat shock protein 60 T-cell epitope in rats supresses both adjuvant arthritis and nonmicrobially induced experimental arthritis. *Proc Natl Acad Sci USA* 94: 3284–3289

79 Firestein GS, Echeverri F, Yeo M, Zvaifler NJ, Green DR (1997) Somatic mutations in the p53 tumor suppressor gene in rheumatoid arthritis synovium. *Proc Natl Acad Sci USA* 94: 10895–10900

Interactions between T cell plasma membranes and monocytes

Danielle Burger and Jean-Michel Dayer

Division of Immunology and Allergy, Hans Wilsdorf Laboratory, University Hospital, 24 rue Micheli-du-Crest, CH-1211 Geneva 14, Switzerland

Introduction

In chronic inflammation that leads to tissue destruction and fibrosis immunocompetent cells migrate through the vascular endothelium to the target tissue. Interactions between lymphocytes of different subsets and monocyte-macrophages result in the production of cytokines such as interleukin (IL)-1 and tumor necrosis factor (TNF)-α. In rheumatoid arthritis (RA), these cytokines induce connective tissue cells (e.g. fibroblasts, type B synovial cells) to produce large amounts of matrix-metalloproteinases (MMPs) which degrade the extracellular matrix (ECM) components (e.g. collagens and proteoglycans). Simultaneously, counter-regulatory mechanisms (cytokine inhibitors, anti-inflammatory cytokines, and protease inhibitors) set in as an attempt to block inflammation and tissue destruction. Shortly after the inflammatory process, attempts at repair take place to restore the integrity of the tissue. In pathologic conditions such as rheumatoid arthritis (RA), this attempt mostly results in non-functional tissue (fibrosis). These processes have been extensively reviewed by us [1–3] and others [4–6]. The present chapter aims at reviewing the role of direct contact between T lymphocytes and monocyte-macrophages in the above processes.

Relationship between cytokines and metalloproteinases

Inflammation involves the influx into the target tissue of migratory cells such as T and B lymphocytes, polymorphonuclear neutrophils, mastocytes and mononuclear phagocytes. Like in all processes involving cell migration and proliferation, the influx of inflammatory cells in the target tissue is associated with remodeling of the extracellular matrix. In normal biological processes, tissue remodeling consists of the controlled breakdown and neosynthesis of extracellular matrix elements, requiring the action, limited in time and space, of extracellular proteases such as plasminogen activators and matrix metalloproteinases (MMPs). The expression of these proteas-

T Cells in Arthritis, edited by P. Miossec, W.B. van den Berg and G.S. Firestein

es and their inhibitors is controlled by soluble extracellular factors such as cytokines [7–10]. In chronic inflammatory diseases, the production of cytokines by infiltrating and resident tissue cells escapes regulatory mechanisms, and induces tissue destruction either directly or indirectly through the activation of immune and inflammatory cells, e.g. by inducing them to produce inflammatory cytokines and proteases.

Cytokines such as TNF-α and IL-1 are implicated in the pathogenesis of RA. Indeed, *in vitro* studies on synovial tissue from RA patients suggest that the effects of TNF-α are amplified due to its potential to induce other pro-inflammatory cytokines, like IL-1 and granulocyte-macrophage colony-stimulating factor (GM-CSF) [5, 11]. A major function of both monocytes and macrophages is to release various cytokines including IL-1 and TNF-α which participate in the induction of MMP secretion on mononuclear phagocytes and fibroblast-like cells (i.e. synoviocytes) [12, 13]. It is therefore likely that mononuclear phagocytes in addition to fibroblasts occupy a pivotal position in the control of extracellular matrix turnover, being capable of mediating joint destruction in RA directly by generating their own MMPs and also indirectly by releasing cytokines which in turn induce synoviocyte MMP production. This activity is reflected at the systemic level, since stromelysin-1 (MMP-3) and tissue inhibitor of metalloproteinase (TIMP)-1 have been found in the serum and synovial fluid from RA patients where MMP-3 levels seem to correlate with disease activity [14–16].

Cell-cell contact

T cell and macrophage infiltration in synovial tissue

T lymphocytes are likely to play a pivotal role in the pathogenesis of chronic inflammatory diseases. In RA, T lymphocytes that display a mature helper phenotype (i.e. $CD3^+CD4^+$) are the main infiltrating cells in the pannus, ranging from 16% of total cells in “transitional areas” to 75% in “lymphocyte-rich areas” [17–20]. T lymphocyte extravasation occurs at the level of high endothelial venules [20]. Although the majority of T lymphocytes transmigrate through the endothelium in a nonactivated state, they become activated in the synovium as they move further away from blood vessels.

In the perivascular space, activated T lymphocytes bind to matrix proteins and fibroblasts [21, 22]. Tissue destruction takes place in areas where T lymphocytes are in close contact with monocytes, hinting at novel cell surface-mediated mechanisms potentiating inflammation. The T cell population in inflamed synovial tissue predominantly belongs to the Th1 subset [23]. Of special interest, these T cells show a very marked staining for the chemokine receptors CCR5 and CXCR3, and are only occasionally positive for CCR3 [24]. It appears that CCR5 is highly expressed on Th1 cells and rarely present in Th2 cells, whereas CCR3 is found in Th2 cells but not in Th1 cells. CXCR3 is highly expressed in both T cell subsets [24, 25]. MIP-1β appears to be a selective ligand for CCR5 [26, 27], eotaxin for CCR3 [28–30], and IP10 for CXCR3 [31].

Recently it was shown that transgenic mice expressing T cell-targeted membrane-associated mutant human TNF-α displayed proliferative synovitis and chronic inflammatory arthritis, suggesting that at least part of the pathogenic activities of T cells *in vivo* may be assigned to the expression of the membrane-associated form of TNF-α by T lymphocytes [32, 33]. However, the role of macrophage-derived cells is also crucial. The increased depth of lining cell layer is a result of accumulation of type A macrophage-derived lining cells, with local proliferation of type B fibroblast-like synoviocytes. Macrophages express mostly CD68 in the synovial lining and CD14 and CD68 in the sublining. A positive correlation was established between CD14 cells counts of both lining and sublining CD68 cells, and articular destruction [31]. Together these observations suggest that both T cells and macrophages are important and that contact of T cells with macrophages or other cells in the pannus might be involved in RA pathogenesis.

T cell signaling of monocyte-macrophages by direct cell-cell contact

The activation of effector cells mediated by T lymphocytes has been abundantly documented by the induction of B cell proliferation and antibody secretion, which require both direct cell-cell contact and soluble signals. Indeed, in the absence of antigen, B cells can be activated by direct contact with activated T cells [34, 35]. The simultaneous activation of both T and B cells involves numerous "cross-talk" signaling molecules that trigger a cascade of timed signals resulting in the induction of effector functions in both cell types.

Most studies relating to monocyte-macrophage activation have focused on the role of exogenous soluble factors such as lipopolysaccharides (LPS) and other bacterial or endogenous products such as IFNγ and CSFs, and to some extent TNF-α and IL-1 [36, 37]. Cytokines like TNF-α and IL-1 [38] potently stimulate nearby fibroblast-like cells to release MMPs [12, 13, 39–41] and prostaglandin E_2 (PGE_2), but have a very limited capacity for inducing monocyte-macrophages to produce MMPs [42]. It appears that most of the soluble cytokines mainly have an anti-inflammatory effect on monocyte-macrophage functions. Considering that cells from the monocytic lineage have been considered "professional" antigen-presenting cells (APC), it is amazing that while a tremendous number of studies has been devoted to APC signaling of T cells very few attempts have been made to address the question of T cell signaling of monocyte-macrophages in the context of direct cell-cell contact.

Some years ago it was observed that the expression of membrane-associated IL-1 (IL-1α) in mouse macrophages was mediated by both soluble factors and direct contact with T cells [43]. The contact between T cells and macrophages and its effect on IL-1 induction was observed with both Th1 and Th2 cells in the absence of lymphokine release [44]. We also observed that direct contact with stimulated T cells potently activated monocyte-macrophage functions [45, 46]. The production of IL-1β by human monocytes also required direct contact with anti-CD3-stimulated T cells [47]. Other observations have shown that the induction of mouse macrophage effector functions mediated by T lymphocytes in cocultures of living cells required signals delivered simultaneously by cell-cell contact and IFNγ [48–50]. However, fixed, stimulated T cells induced TNF-α production in murine macrophages in the absence of IFNγ [51]. Furthermore, isolated plasma membranes from both stimulated Th1 and Th2 cells were able to induce nitric oxide production by mouse IFNγ-primed macrophages [52], establishing that direct contact with stimulated T cells was a potent mechanism in inducing monocyte-macrophage effector functions.

Activation of human monocytes and monocytic cells by direct contact with stimulated T cells

In our attempts to elucidate the pathogenic mechanisms underlying connective tissue destruction and repair, typified by RA, we observed that IL-1 and TNF-α (mainly produced by monocyte-macrophages) are the principal cytokines stimulating the production of MMPs on fibroblasts/synovial cells. We subsequently described their antagonists: IL-1Ra and TNF-sR which counteract the pro-inflammatory, destructive properties of the two cytokines [53–57]. We further analyzed the mechanisms of regulation ruling the balance between agonistic and antagonistic cytokines. Furthermore, having measured cytokines and their inhibitors in patients, we concluded that our *in vitro* results were relevant to inflammatory diseases, particularly RA [1, 58, 59]. However, the factors or mechanisms inducing high levels of IL-1 and TNF-α on human monocyte-macrophages remained unclear. Indeed, many soluble lymphokines (IL-4, IL-10, IL-13) display inhibitory activity, whereas IFNγ is a weak activator.

We therefore hypothesized that soluble products of T lymphocytes were predominantly inhibitors of inflammation, whereas direct contact through cell surface activating factors on T cells had mainly an activating effect, in accordance with histological observations demonstrating that most of the destruction occurs at sites where inflammatory cells are in direct contact, adjacent to the ECM. This hypothesis was confirmed by our recent results emphasizing that cell-cell contact between stimulated T lymphocytes and surrounding cells is likely to be a potent and preferential process involved in these pathological mechanisms (Fig. 1).

The use of double-chamber culture systems has led to the seminal observation that in the presence of the T lymphocyte activator phytohemagglutinin (PHA) the coculture of viable T lymphocytes and freshly isolated blood monocytes in the same

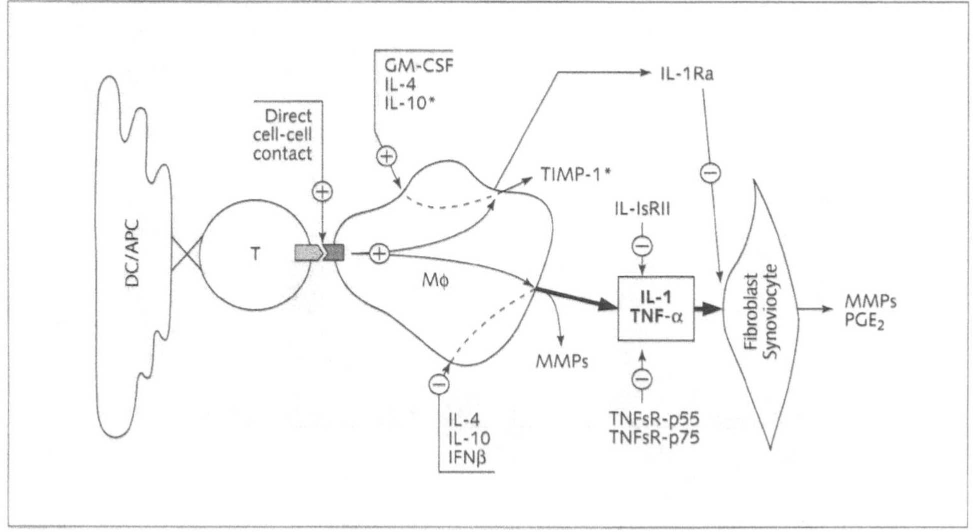

Figure 1
Scheme of the activation cascade from T lymphocytes to monocyte-macrophages and fibroblasts/synoviocytes
T lymphocytes are stimulated through the T cell receptor by putative antigen(s) presented by antigen presenting cells (APC; dendritic cells, DC). Stimulated T lymphocytes express cell surface factors which in turn activate monocyte-macrophages (MΦ). The activation of monocyte-macrophages is modulated by cytokines such as GM-CSF, IL-4. and IL-10 that up-regulate IL-1Ra production, but only IL-10 up-regulates TIMP-1 production (*), whereas IL-4, IL-10 and IFN-β [85] down-regulate the production of MMPs, IL-1, and TNF-α. IL-1 and TNF-α, whose respective activities are regulated by specific inhibitors (i.e. IL-1Ra, IL-1 soluble receptor II (IL-1sRII) and TNF soluble receptors (TNFsR) p55 and p75), trigger fibroblast-like synoviocytes to produce MMPs and PGE2 that in turn promote tissue destruction and the release of the mineral phase, respectively.

compartment resulted in a massive production of IL-1β and TNF-α by mononuclear phagocytes (Fig. 2). This was not observed when cells were physically separated by a permeable membrane. Thus the evidence was obtained that cell-cell contact with stimulated T lymphocytes activates monocytes. Subsequently, we determined that: (i) direct cell-cell contact with membranes of stimulated T cells is sufficient to transduce the activating signal; and (ii) cell-surface glycoproteins on stimulated T lymphocytes are involved in target cell activation [45, 46].

Our working hypothesis was that cell-cell contact between T lymphocytes and monocyte-macrophages represented an important mechanism for potentiating inflammation and tissue destruction. We confirmed the accuracy of this hypothesis

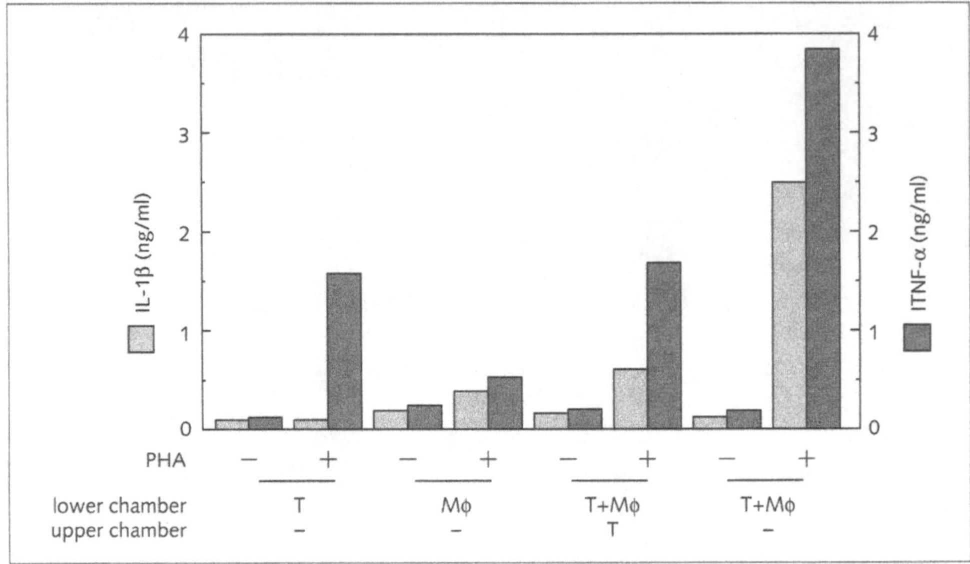

Figure 2
Induction of IL-1β and TNF-α production by monocytes upon contact with stimulated T lymphocytes
Freshly isolated T lymphocytes (T) and monocytes (MΦ) were cultured in a two-chamber cell culture system. Monocytes were induced to produce IL-1β and TNF-α only when they were cultured in the same chamber as stimulated T lymphocytes.

[45, 46, 60-63], demonstrating that cell-cell contact between stimulated T lymphocytes and monocyte-macrophages appears to be a preferential biological mechanism not only for the massive up-regulation of the inflammatory cytokines IL-1 and TNF-α but also for the induction of MMPs. Membranes of T cells stimulated with lectins and phorbol esters induce the production of pro-inflammatory cytokines (e.g. TNF-α, IL-1β, IL-8), cytokine inhibitors (IL-1Ra, TNF-sR), MMPs (MMP-1, MMP-9), and their inhibitor TIMP-1 by monocytes or the monocytic cell line THP-1 (Fig. 3) [45, 46, 60, 62].

Depending on T cell type and T cell stimulus, direct cell-cell contact with stimulated T cells can induce the unbalanced production of pro-inflammatory cytokines and their inhibitors as well as of MMPs and TIMP-1

Synovial tissue T cell clones stimulated by the immobilized anti-CD3 antibody OKT3 induced the production of MMP-1, but not TIMP-1, by THP-1 cells [61],

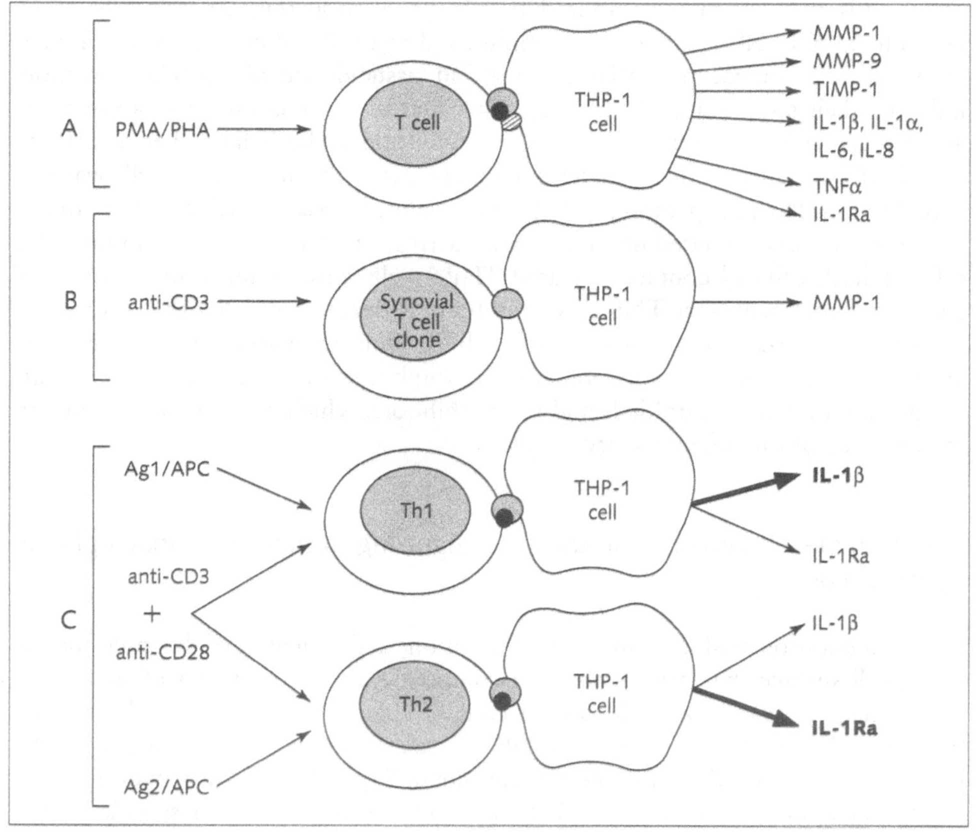

Figure 3
Depending on the stimulus and cell type, stimulated T cells induced the production of various products in monocyte-macrophages or monocytic cells
(A) When stimulated by PHA and PMA, T cells of any type induced the production of the indicated cytokines, MMPs and inhibitors; (B) Synovial T cell clones stimulated by immobilized anti-CD3 antibodies only induced the monocytic-production of MMP-1; (C) Th1 and Th2 clones stimulated by their respective antigen (Ag1 = PPD and Ag2 = tetanus toxoid) or anti-CD3 and anti-CD28 differentially induced the production of IL-1β and IL-1Ra. Th1 cells preferentially induced IL-1β production while Th2 cells preferentially induced IL-1Ra production.

resulting in an imbalance between the enzyme and its inhibitor. Similarly, Th1 T cell clones generated with purified protein derivative (PPD) as an antigen (Ag1) after stimulation with OKT3 and anti-CD28 or specific antigens preferentially induced IL-1β production in THP-1 cells, whereas Th2 clones generated with tetanus toxoid as an antigen (Ag2) mainly induced IL-1Ra production (Fig. 3) [63]. Therefore, depending on T cell type and T cell stimulus, direct cell-cell contact with stimulated T cells can induce pro-inflammatory and tissue-destructive products without inducing their specific inhibitors, suggesting that this mechanism may account for any imbalance arising under pathological conditions. The balance between IL-1β and IL-1Ra production by monocytes upon contact with stimulated T cells was regulated by Ser/Thr phosphatase(s) [64]. The balance between TNF-α and its soluble receptor was also regulated upon monocyte activation by contact with stimulated T cells. Indeed, cell-cell contact-activated THP-1 cells express membrane-associated protease(s) that neutralize TNF-α activity both by degrading the latter cytokine and by cleaving its receptors at the cell surface [65]. Thus, the triggering of these mechanisms by direct contact with stimulated T lymphocytes may differentially regulate the pro-inflammatory cytokines and their inhibitors, which balance dictates in part the outcome of the inflammatory process.

Surface molecules involved in the T cell signaling of monocyte-macrophages by direct contact

A crucial question arising from these observations is the identity of the molecules on the T cell surface that are involved in contact-dependent signaling of monocyte-macrophage activation as well as their counter-ligands. The use of cytokine inhibitors has shown that activation of fibroblasts, synoviocytes and microvascular endothelial cells by stimulated peripheral blood T lymphocytes was mainly due to membrane-associated TNFα and IL-1α [66, 67]. However, neither soluble TNF-α receptor nor IL-1Ra inhibited T cell-signaling of the monocytic cell line THP-1. Furthermore, neutralizing antibodies to TNF-α, IL-1, IL-2, IFN-γ and GM-CSF all failed to affect monocyte activation by membranes from stimulated T cells [45, 46, 60].

Besides membrane-associated cytokines, other surface molecules were assessed for their ability to activate monocyte-macrophages upon contact with stimulated T cells, e.g. lymphocyte function associated antigen (LFA)-1/ICAM-1, CD2/LFA3, and CD40/CD40L. It was demonstrated that CD40/CD40L was involved in the contact activation of both human and mouse monocyte-macrophages by T lymphocytes stimulated for 6 h [68, 69]. Furthermore, peripheral blood T lymphocytes isolated from CD40L-knockout mice and stimulated for 6 h were not able to induce monocyte activation. However, when stimulated for 24 h T lymphocytes isolated from both CD40L-knockout and wild type mice triggered monocyte activation, although to a lower extent [70].

In our system, human T lymphocytes which were stimulated for 48 h expressed a high capacity to induce cytokines and MMPs in monocyte-macrophages. Furthermore, the most effective human T cell line in inducing signaling of monocytes by direct contact was the human lymphocytic cell line HUT-78 [71] which does not express CD40L mRNA in resting or activating conditions [72]. Finally, the THP-1 cells we generally use as monocytic target cells do not express CD40 (C. Chizzolini, unpublished results). This suggests that CD40/CD40L might be involved in contact-activation of monocyte-macrophages by T lymphocytes stimulated for short periods of time. This does not apply to T lymphocytes stimulated for long periods since the latter cells do not express CD40L any longer [73].

A recent study showed that functional CD40L was expressed by synovial fluid T lymphocytes of RA patients. Although in synovial tissue immuno-histochemical analysis demonstrated CD40L expression in infiltrating cells of the vascular/perivascular area [74], no staining was observed in infiltrating cells which migrated farther. These results suggest that CD40L might be involved in the extravasation of T lymphocytes in the pannus through the vascular endothelium [75]. They also imply that cell surface factors other than CD40L were involved in T lymphocyte contact-signaling of monocytes. Other studies have shown that cytokine production was induced in monocytes by soluble CD23 [76, 77]. In monocytes, the counter-ligands of CD23 are CD11b/CD18 and CD11c/CD18 rather than CD21 [78]. Our studies and others have shown that LFA-1 (CD11a/CD18) and CD69 play a role in the activation of human monocytic cells by stimulated T cells [45, 79]. The latter data were recently confirmed in a study showing that IL-15 induced synovial T cells from RA patients to activate the production of TNF-α by macrophages. This effect was inhibited by antibodies to CD69, LFA-1, and ICAM-1 [80]. Thus it is possible that some already-identified surface molecules are involved in T cell signaling of monocyte-macrophages. However, inhibitors (e.g. antibodies) of these molecules fail to abolish monocyte activation altogether, suggesting that the required factor(s) for T cell signaling of human monocytes by direct contact remain(s) to be identified.

Subcellular fractionation showed that the activation factors are located in the plasma membranes of stimulated T cells. In addition to peripheral blood T lymphocytes, contact-activation factors were expressed by T cell lines JURKAT and HUT-78 [46], and by all 88 T cell clones expanded from a single healthy blood donor, although to varying extents [62]. This demonstrates that all stimulated T cells can express surface factors which activate monocyte-macrophages. Interestingly, the products that are induced in the target cell differ depending on the nature of the stimulating agent and the time of stimulation of T lymphocytes. This could imply that several contact-activation factors, likely to be acting synergistically, are expressed on the surface of stimulated T lymphocytes.

In our studies, antibodies to known cell surface antigens (CD2, CD11a, CD11b, CD11c, CD14, CD18, CD23, CD29, CD40, CD40L, CD54, CD69, CTLA4, CD95, CD95L) or membrane-associated cytokines (IFNγ, IL-2, GM-CSF, IL-1, TNF-α, LT), and cytokine inhibitors (IL-1Ra, TNF-soluble receptors) failed to abolish the activity of contact-activation factors in monocytes and THP-1 cells [45, 46, 60, and unpublished data by J.-M. Dayer, D. Burger]. Only antibodies to CD11a, CD11b, CD11c, and CD69 partially inhibited the activity of contact-activation factors [45, 46]. In addition, unstimulated HUT-78 cells expressing CD69, CD11a and TNF-α constitutively at their surface did not induce any contact-signaling in THP-1 cells, whereas PHA/PMA-stimulated HUT-78 cells, whose expression of CD69 and CD11a remained unchanged as compared to unstimulated HUT-78 cells, potently activated THP-1 cells (Fig. 4). Metabolic inhibitors such as cycloheximide and tunicamycin inhibited the expression of contact-activation factors on stimulated T cells demonstrating that contact-activation factors were glycoproteins [45, 46, 62]. Inhibitors of N-linked oligosaccharide processing [81] such as Swainsonine and N-methyldeoxynojirimycin did not inhibit the activity of contact-activation factors, implying that N-linked oligosaccharides may not be involved in T cell signaling of THP-1 cells.

Activation of human dermal fibroblasts, synoviocytes and endothelial cells by membranes of stimulated T cells

During advanced chronic inflammation, stimulated T-lymphocytes can potentially contact various cells, other than mononuclear phagocytes, that are involved in the pathogenic mechanisms. Such target cell types include interstitial fibroblasts such as synoviocytes and endothelial cells. We observed that contact with stimulated T lymphocytes potently affected dermal fibroblasts, synoviocytes and endothelial cells. Indeed, upon contact with membranes of stimulated T lymphocytes dermal fibroblasts and synoviocytes produce large amounts of MMP-1 and PGE_2 in the absence of TIMP-1 [82]. In addition, membranes of stimulated T lymphocytes induced the expression of cell adhesion molecules (ICAM-1, VCAM-1 and E-selectin) and the production of cytokines (IL-6 and IL-8) in microvascular endothelial cells [66].

The surface factors involved in contact activation of either microvascular endothelial cells [66, 83, 84] or fibroblasts and synoviocytes [82] have been identified as membrane-associated cytokines, mainly TNF-α and IL-1α. These cytokines are not involved in the activation of the monocyte-macrophages by T cell membranes (see above). It is therefore intriguing that T lymphocytes developed different cell-signaling systems adapted to the different target cells.

Conclusion

Our current experimental results strongly suggest that, by direct cell-cell contact, membranes of stimulated T lymphocytes attracted by specific chemokines, potentiate the inflammatory response. They do this by favouring the extravasation of cells

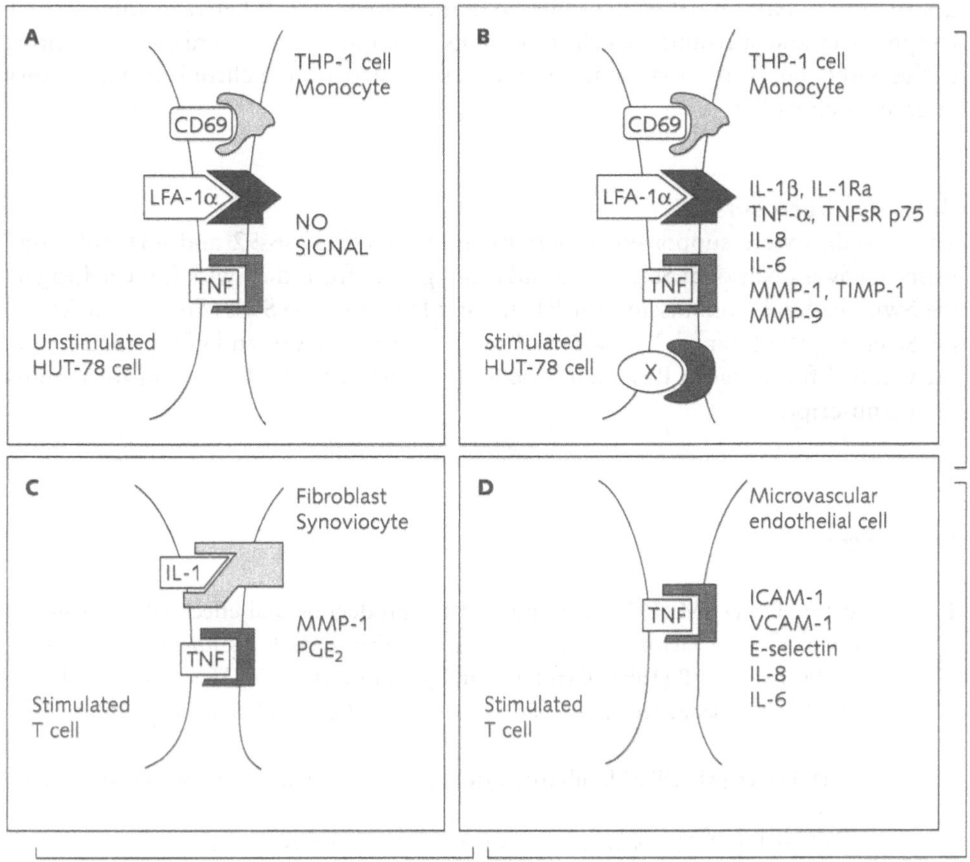

Figure 4
Different T cell surface molecules are involved in the signaling of the different target cells Although CD69, CD11a, and TNF-α are expressed by unstimulated HUT-78 cells they are not able to induce THP-1 cell activation (A), suggesting the necessity for other unidentified factor(s) (B). Fibroblasts and synoviocytes are activated by membrane-associated TNF-α and IL-1 (C), while microvascular endothelial cells are mainly activated by membrane-associated TNF-α (D).

from the immune system into the target tissue through the endothelium [66, 83], and by activating the production of pro-inflammatory cytokines and MMPs at inflammatory sites, i.e. by stimulating monocytes and fibroblast-like cells. This mechanism (cell-cell contact with stimulated T lymphocytes) induces an unbalanced production of MMPs and TIMP-1 *in vitro* and may, by analogy, favour tissue destruction *in vivo*. We thus hypothesize that cell-cell contact between stimulated T lymphocytes and surrounding cells represents an important mechanism contributing to the pathogenesis of inflammation and tissue destruction in chronic inflammatory diseases such as RA.

Acknowledgements
These studies were supported in part by grants #31-33786-92 and #31-50930-97 from the Swiss National Science Foundation, grants from the Swiss Cancer League, the Swiss Federal Commission for Rheumatic Diseases, the Swiss Society for Multiple Sclerosis, the Biomed 2 program of the European Union, and grant #3524 from the Council for Tobacco Research. The authors thank Dr. C. Chizzolini for reading the manuscript.

References

1 Arend WP, Dayer JM (1995) Inhibition of the production and effects of interleukin-1 and tumor necrosis factor alpha in rheumatoid arthritis. *Arthritis Rheum* 38: 151–160
2 Dayer JM, Arend WP (1997) Cytokines and growth factors. In: WN Kelley, EDJ Harris, S Ruddy, CS Sledge (eds): *Textbook of Rheumatology*. W.B. Saunders, Philadelphia, 267–286
3 Burger D, Dayer JM (1995) Inhibitory cytokines and cytokine inhibitors. *Neurology* 45: S39–S43
4 Harris ED (ed) (1997) *Rheumatoid Arthritis*. W.B. Saunders, Philadelphia
5 Feldmann M, Brennan FM, Maini RN (1996) Role of cytokines in rheumatoid arthritis. *Annu Rev Immunol* 14: 397–440
6 Smolen JS, Tohidastakrad M, Gal A, Kunaver M, Eberl G, Zenz P, Falus A, Steiner G (1996) The role of T-lymphocytes and cytokines in rheumatoid arthritis. *Scand J Rheumatol* 25: 1–4
7 Opdenakker G, van Damme J (1992) Cytokines and proteases in invasive processes: molecular similarities between inflammation and cancer. *Cytokine* 4: 251–258
8 Mauviel A (1993) Cytokine regulation of metalloproteinase gene expression. *J Cell Biochem* 53: 288–295
9 Ries C, Petrides PE (1995) Cytokine regulation of matrix metalloproteinase activity and its regulatory dysfunction in disease. *Biol Chem Hoppe Seyler* 376: 345–355
10 Birkedal-Hansen H (1995) Proteolytic remodeling of extracellular matrix. *Curr Opin Cell Biol* 7: 728–735
11 Unemori EN, Amento EP (1995) Role of cytokines in rheumatoid arthritis. In: BB Aggarwal, RK Puri (eds): *Human Cytokines: Their Role in Disease and Therapy*. Blackwell Science, Inc. Boston, 217–236

12 Busiek DF, Ross FP, McDonnell S, Murphy G, Matrisian LM, Welgus HG (1992) The matrix metalloprotease matrilysin (PUMP) is expressed in developing human mononuclear phagocytes. *J Biol Chem* 267: 9087–9092

13 Welgus HG, Campbell EJ, Cury JD, Eisen AZ, Senior RM, Wilhelm SM, Goldberg GI (1990) Neutral metalloproteinases produced by human mononuclear phagocytes. Enzyme profile, regulation, and expression during cellular development. *J Clin Invest* 86: 1496–1502

14 Yoshihara Y, Obata K, Fujimoto N, Yamashita K, Hayakawa T, Shimmei M (1995) Increased levels of stromelysin-1 and tissue inhibitor of metalloproteinases-1 in sera from patients with rheumatoid arthritis. *Arthritis Rheum* 38: 969–975

15 Ishiguro N, Ito T, Obata K, Fijimoto N, Iwata H (1996) Determination of stromelysin-1, 72 and 92 kDa type IV collagenase, tissue inhibitor of metalloproteinase-1 (TIMP-1), and TIMP-2 in synovial fluid and serum from patients with rheumatoid arthritis. *J Rheumatol* 23: 1599–1604

16 Manicourt DH, Fujimoto N, Obata K, Thonar EJ (1995) Levels of circulating collagenase, stromelysin-1, and tissue inhibitor of matrix metalloproteinases 1 in patients with rheumatoid arthritis. Relationship to serum levels of antigenic keratan sulfate and systemic parameters of inflammation. *Arthritis Rheum* 38: 1031–1039

17 Kurosaka M, Ziff M (1983) Immunoelectron microscopic study of the distribution of T cell subsets in rheumatoid synovium. *J Exp Med* 158: 1191–1210

18 Quayle A, Kjeldsen Kragh J, Forre O, Waalen K, Sioud M, Kalvenes C, Natvig JB (1989) Immunoregulatory T cell subsets and T cell activation in rheumatoid arthritis. A need for analysis on the clonal and molecular level. *Springer Semin Immunopathol* 11: 273–287

19 Tak PP, Smeets TJM, Daha MR, Kluin PM, Meijers KAE, Brand R, Meinders AE, Breedveld FC (1997) Analysis of the synovial cell infiltrate in early rheumatoid synovial tissue in relation to local disease activity. *Arthritis Rheum* 40: 217–225

20 Davis LS, Geppert TD, Meek K, Oppenheimer-Marks N, Lipsky PE (1997) Immune and inflammatory responses. In: WN Kelley, EDJ Harris, S Ruddy, CS Sledge (eds): *Textbook of Rheumatology*. W.B. Saunders, Philadelphia, 95–127

21 Harris ED (1997) T lymphocytes. In: ED Harris (ed): *Rheumatoid Arthritis*. W.B. Saunders, Philadelphia, 52–73

22 Harris ED (1997) Rheumatoid synovium: complex, and more than the sum of its parts. In: ED Harris (ed): *Rheumatoid Arthritis*. W.B. Saunders, Philadelphia, 126–149

23 Dolhain RJEM, Vanderheiden AN, Terhaar NT, Breedveld FC, Miltenburg AMM (1996) Shift toward T lymphocytes with a T helper 1 cytokine-secretion profile in the joints of patients with rheumatoid arthritis. *Arthritis Rheum* 39: 1961–1969

24 Loetscher P, Chizzolini C, Uguccioni M, Dayer JM, Baggiolini M, Moser B (1998) CCR5 is characteristic of Th1 lymphocytes. *Nature* 391: 344–345

25 Sallusto F, Mackay CR, Lanzavecchia A (1997) Selective expression of the eotaxin receptor CCR3 by human T helper 2 cells. *Science* 277: 2005–2007

26 Samson M, Labbe O, Mollereau C, Vassart G, Parmentier M (1996) Molecular cloning

and functional expression of a new human CC-chemokine receptor gene. *Biochemistry* 35: 3362–3367

27 Raport CJ, Gosling J, Schweickart VL, Gray PW, Charo IF (1996) Molecular cloning and functional characterization of a novel human CC chemokine receptor (CCR5) for RANTES, MIP-1beta, and MIP-1alpha. *J Biol Chem* 271: 17161–17166

28 Daugherty BL, Siciliano SJ, DeMartino JA, Malkowitz L, Sirotina A, Springer MS (1996) Cloning, expression, and characterization of the human eosinophil eotaxin receptor. *J Exp Med* 183: 2349–2354

29 Ponath PD, Qin S, Post TW, Wang J, Wu L, Gerard NP, Newman W, Gerard C, Mackay CR (1996) Molecular cloning and characterization of a human eotaxin receptor expressed selectively on eosinophils [see comments]. *J Exp Med* 183: 2437–2448

30 Combadiere C, Ahuja SK, Murphy PM (1995) Cloning and functional expression of a human eosinophil CC chemokine receptor. *J Biol Chem* 270: 16491–16494

31 Mulherin D, Fitzgerald O, Bresnihan B (1996) Synovial tissue macrophage populations and articular damage in rheumatoid arthritis. *Arthritis Rheum* 39: 115–124

32 Georgopoulos S, Plows D, Kollias G (1996) Transmembrane TNF is sufficient to induce localized tissue toxicity and chronic inflammatory arthritis in transgenic mice. *J Inflamm* 46: 86–97

33 Probert L, Akassoglou K, Alexopoulou L, Douni E, Haralambous S, Hill S, Kassiotis G, Kontoyiannis D, Pasparakis M, Plows D, et al (1996) Dissection of the pathologies induced by transmembrane and wild-type tumor necrosis factor in transgenic mice. *J Leukoc Biol* 59: 518–525

34 Parker DC (1993) T cell-dependent B cell activation. Annu Rev Immunol 11: 331–60

35 Clark EA, Ledbetter JA (1994) How B and T cells talk to each other. *Nature* 367: 425–428

36 Bevilacqua MP, Butcher E, Furie B, Gallatin M, Gimbrone M, Harlan J, Kishimoto K, Lasky L, McEver R, et al (1991) Selectins: a family of adhesion receptors. *Cell* 67: 233

37 Zhang J, Fujimoto N, Iwata K, Sakai T, Okada Y, Hayakawa T (1993) A one-step sandwich enzyme immunoassay for human matrix metalloproteinase 1 (interstitial collagenase) using monoclonal antibodies. *Clin Chim Acta* 219: 1–14

38 Zvaifler NJ (1995) Macrophages and the synovial lining. *Scand J Rheumatol Suppl* 101: 67–75

39 Cury JD, Campbell EJ, Lazarus CJ, Albin IJ, Welgus HG (1988) Selective upregulation of human alveolar macrophage collagenase production by lipopolysaccharide and comparison to collagenase production in fibroblasts. *J Immunol* 141: 4306–4312

40 Dayer JM, Beutler B, Cerami A (1985) Cachectin/tumor necrosis factor stimulates collagenase and prostaglandin E2 production by human synovial cells and dermal fibroblasts. *J Exp Med* 162: 2163–2168

41 Dayer JM, De Rochemonteix B, Burrus B, Demczuk S, Dinarello CA (1986) Human recombinant interleukin 1 stimulates collagenase and prostaglandin E2 production by human synovial cells. *J Clin Invest* 77: 645–648

42 Lacraz S, Nicod L, Galve-de Rochemonteix B, Baumberger C, Dayer JM, Welgus HG (1992) Suppression of metalloproteinase biosynthesis in human alveolar macrophages by interleukin-4. *J Clin Invest* 90: 382–388
43 Weaver CT, Unanue ER (1986) T cell induction of membrane IL-1 on macrophages. *J Immunol* 137: 3868–3873
44 Weaver CT, Duncan LM, Unanue ER (1989) T cell induction of macrophage IL-1 during antigen presentation: characterization of a lymphokine mediator and comparison of Th1 and Th2 subsets. *J Immunol* 142: 3469–3476
45 Vey E, Zhang JH, Dayer JM (1992) IFN-gamma and 1, 25(OH)2D3 induce on THP-1 cells distinct patterns of cell surface antigen expression, cytokine production, and responsiveness to contact with activated T cells. *J Immunol* 149: 2040–2046
46 Isler P, Vey E, Zhang JH, Dayer JM (1993) Cell surface glycoproteins expressed on activated human T-cells induce production of interleukin-1 beta by monocytic cells: a possible role of CD69. *Eur Cytokine Netw* 4: 15–23
47 Landis CB, Friedman ML, Fisher RI, Ellis TM (1991) Induction of human monocyte IL-1 mRNA and secretion during anti-CD3 mitogenesis requires two distinct T cell-derived signals. *J Immunol* 146: 128–135
48 Stout RD, Bottomly K (1989) Antigen-specific activation of effector macrophages by IFN-gamma producing (Th1) T cell clones: failure of IL-4-producing (Th2) T cell clones to activate effector function in macrophages. *J Immunol* 142: 760–765
49 Sypek JP, Wyler DJ (1991) Antileishmanial defense in macrophages triggered by tumor necrosis factor expressed on CD4+ T lymphocyte plasma membrane. *J Exp Med* 174: 755–759
50 Sypek JP, Matzilevich MM, Wyler DJ (1991) Th2 lymphocyte clone can activate macrophage antileishmanial defense by a lymphokine-independent mechanism in vitro and can augment parasite attribution *in vivo*. *Cell Immunol* 133: 178–186
51 Suttles J, Miller RW, Tao X, Stout RD (1994) T cells which do not express membrane tumor necrosis factor-alpha activate macrophage effector function by cell contact-dependent signaling of macrophage tumor necrosis factor-alpha production. *Eur J Immunol* 24: 1736–1742
52 Tao X, Stout R (1993) T cell-mediated cognate signaling of nitric oxide production by macrophages. Requirements for macrophage activation by plasma membranes isolated from T cells. *Eur J Immunol* 23: 2916–2921
53 Balavoine JF, De Rochemonteix B, Williamson K, Seckinger P, Cruchaud A, Dayer JM (1986) Prostaglandin E2 and collagenase production by fibroblasts and synovial cells is regulated by urine-derived human interleukin 1 and inhibitor(s). *J Clin Invest* 78: 1120–1124
54 Seckinger P, Williamson K, Balavoine JF, Mach B, Mazzei G, Shaw A, Dayer JM (1987) A urine inhibitor of interleukin 1 activity affects both interleukin 1 alpha and 1 beta but not tumor necrosis factor alpha. *J Immunol* 139: 1541–1545
55 Seckinger P, Lowenthal JW, Williamson K, Dayer JM, MacDonald HR (1987) A urine

inhibitor of interleukin 1 activity that blocks ligand binding. *J Immunol* 139: 1546–1549
56 Seckinger P, Isaaz S, Dayer JM (1988) A human inhibitor of tumor necrosis factor a. *J Exp Med* 167: 1511–1516
57 Seckinger P, Isaaz S, Dayer JM (1989) Purification and biologic characterization of a specific tumor necrosis factor alpha inhibitor. *J Biol Chem* 264: 11966–11973
58 Dayer JM, Goldring SR, Robinson DR, Krane SM (1980) Cell-cell interactions and collagenase production. In: DE Woolley, JM Evanson (eds): *Collagenase in Normal and Pathological Connective Tissues*. John Wiley & Sons Ltd, New York, 83–104
59 Dayer JM, Demczuk S (1984) Cytokines and other mediators in rheumatoid arthritis. *Springer Semin Immunopathol* 7: 387–413
60 Lacraz S, Isler P, Vey E, Welgus HG, Dayer JM (1994) Direct contact between T lymphocytes and monocytes is a major pathway for induction of metalloproteinase expression. *J Biol Chem* 269: 22027–22033
61 Miltenburg AMM, Lacraz S, Welgus HG, Dayer JM (1995) Immobilized anti-CD3 antibody activates T cell clones to induce the production of interstitial collagenase, but not tissue inhibitor of metalloproteinases, in monocytic THP-1 cells and dermal fibroblasts. *J Immunol* 154: 2655–2667
62 Li JM, Isler P, Dayer JM, Burger D (1995) Contact-dependent stimulation of monocytic cells and neutrophils by stimulated human T-cell clones. *Immunology* 84: 571–576
63 Chizzolini C, Chicheportiche R, Burger D, Dayer JM (1997) Human Th1 cells preferentially induce interleukin (IL)-1 beta while Th2 cells induce IL-1 receptor antagonist production upon cell/cell contact with monocytes. *Eur J Immunol* 27: 171–177
64 Vey E, Dayer JM, Burger D (1997) Direct contact with stimulated T cells induces the expression of IL-1 beta and IL-1 receptor antagonist in human monocytes. Involvement of serine/threonine phosphatases in differential regulation. *Cytokine* 9: 480–487
65 Vey E, Burger D, Dayer JM (1996) Expression and cleavage of tumor necrosis factor-alpha and tumor necrosis factor receptors by human monocytic cell lines upon direct contact with stimulated T cells. *Eur J Immunol* 26: 2404–2409
66 Lou J, Dayer JM, Grau GE, Burger D (1996) Direct cell/cell contact with stimulated T lymphocytes induces the expression of cell adhesion molecules and cytokines by human brain microvascular endothelial cells. *Eur J Immunol* 26: 3107–3113
67 Burger D, Rezzonico R, Modoux C, Welgus HG, Dayer JM (1996) Direct contact with stimulated T lymphocytes induces an imbalance between metalloproteinase and TIMP-1 production by human fibroblasts. *Eur Cytokine Netw* 7: 561
68 Malik N, Greenfield BW, Wahl AF, Kiener PA (1996) Activation of human monocytes through CD40 induces matrix metalloproteinases. *J Immunol* 156: 3952–3960
69 Wagner DH, Stout RD, Suttles J (1994) Role of the CD40-CD40 ligand interaction in CD4(+) T cell contact-dependent activation of monocyte interleukin-1 synthesis. *Eur J Immunol* 24: 3148–3154
70 Stout RD, Suttles J, Xu J, Grewal IS, Flavell RA (1996) Impaired T cell-mediated macrophage activation in CD40 ligand-deficient mice. *J Immunol* 156: 8–11

71 Gazbar AF, Carney DN, Bunn PA, Russel EK, Jaffe ES, Schechter GP, Guccion JG (1990) Mitogen requirements for the *in vitro* propagation of cutaneous T-cell lymphomas. *J Biol Chem* 55: 409–417
72 Gauchat J-F, Aubry J-P, Mazzei G, Life P, Jomotte T, Elson G, Bonnefoy J-Y (1993) Human CD40-ligand: molecular cloning, cellular distribution and regulation of expression by factors controlling IgE production. *FEBS Lett* 315: 259–266
73 Roy M, Waldschmidt T, Aruffo A, Ledbetter JA, Noelle RJ (1993) The regulation of the expression of gp39, the CD40 ligand, on normal and cloned CD4+ T cells. *J Immunol* 151: 2497–2510
74 MacDonnald KPA, Nishioka Y, Lipsky PE, Thomas R (1997) Functional CD40 ligand is expressed by T cells in rheumatoid arthritis. *J Clin Invest* 100: 2404–2414
75 Yellin MJ, Brett J, Baum D, Matsushima A, Szabolcs M, Stern D, Chess L (1995) Functional interactions of T cells with endothelial cells: the role of CD40L-CD40-mediated signals. *J Exp Med* 182: 1857–1864
76 Armant M, Rubio M, Delespesse G, Sarfati M (1995) Soluble CD23 directly activates monocytes to contribute to the antigen-independent stimulation of resting T cells. *J Immunol* 155: 4868–4875
77 Armant M, Ishihara H, Rubio M, Delespesse G, Sarfati M (1994) Regulation of cytokine production by soluble CD23: costimulation of interferon gamma secretion and triggering of tumor necrosis factor alpha release. *J Exp Med* 180: 1005–1011
78 Le Coanet-Henchoz S, Gauchat JF, Aubry JP, Graber P, Life P, Paul-Eugene N, Ferrua B, Corbi AL, Dugas B, Plater-Zyberk C, et al (1995) CD23 regulates monocyte activation through a novel interaction with the adhesion molecules CD11b-CD18 and CD11c-CD18. *Immunity* 3: 119–125
79 Manié S, Kubar J, Limouse M, Ferrua B, Ticchioni M, Breittmayer JP, Peyron JF, Schaffar L, Rossi B (1993) CD3-stimulated Jurkat T-cells mediate IL-1b production in monocytic THP-1 cells: role of LFA-1 molecule and participation of CD69 T-cell antigen. *Eur Cytokine Netw* 4: 7–13
80 McInnes IB, Leung BP, Sturrock RD, Field M, Liew FY (1997) Interleukin-15 mediates T cell-dependent regulation of tumor necrosis factor-alpha production in rheumatoid arthritis. *Nature Med* 3: 189–195
81 Elbein AD (1991) Glycosidase inhibitors: Inhibitors of N-linked oligosaccharide processing. *FASEB J* 5: 3055–3063
82 Burger D, Rezzonico R, Li JM, Modoux C, Welgus HG, Dayer JM (1998) Direct contact of human synoviocytes and fibroblasts with stimulated T lymphocytes induces the production of interstitial collagenase (MMP-1) but not of tissue inhibitor of metalloproteinases-1 (TIMP-1): involvement of membrane-associated cytokines and possible relevance to rheumatoid arthritis. *Arthritis Rheum*; *in press*
83 Burger D, Lou J, Dayer JM, Grau GE (1997) Both soluble and membrane-associated TNF activate brain microvascular endothelium: relevance to multiple sclerosis. *Mol Psychiatr* 2: 113–116
84 Lou J, Ythier A, Burger D, Zheng L, Juillard P, Lucas R, Dayer JM, Grau GE (1997)

Modulation of soluble and membrane-bound TNF-induced phenotypic and functional changes of human brain microvascular endothelial cells by recombinant TNF binding protein I. *J Neuroimmunol* 77: 107–115

85 Coclet-Ninin J, Dayer JM, Burger D (1997) Interferon-beta not only inhibits interleukin-1 beta and tumor necrosis factor-alpha but stimulates interleukin-1 receptor antagonist production in human peripheral blood mononuclear cells. *Eur Cytokine Netw* 8: 345–349

Adhesion molecules in arthritis: Control of T cell migration into the synovium

Nancy Oppenheimer-Marks and Peter E. Lipsky

Rheumatic Diseases Division of The Department of Internal Medicine, The University of Texas Southwestern Medical School, 5323 Harry Hines Blvd., Dallas, TX 75235-3577, USA

Introduction

Rheumatoid arthritis (RA) is a chronic inflammatory condition that affects approximately 0.8% of the world population [1, 2]. Although there are frequent systemic manifestations of inflammation, the primary physiological events occur within the synovial tissue lining of diarthrodial joints. In spite of intense investigation, the cause of RA and the precise pathophysiological events remain uncertain. Much attention has focused on T lymphocytes and the role they play in the pathogenesis of RA. Along with functional analyses of T cell populations, the mechanisms by which T cells enter rheumatoid synovium has been the focus of considerable investigation. A number of studies have demonstrated an essential role for cell surface adhesion receptors in T cell migration, although the specific receptors employed by T cells and their counterreceptors on endothelial cells have not been completely delineated. Postcapillary venules appear to be the site of T cell entry into the synovium, although this conclusion is based more on analogy to other tissue sites rather than direct experimental verification in the synovium.

The role of T cells in RA

In 1975, van Boxel and associates were the first to note that the rheumatoid synovium was heavily infiltrated with T lymphocytes [3]. This finding was rapidly confirmed by many other groups, who demonstrated that synovial tissue contained aggregates of $CD4^+$ T cells with an activated phenotype [4–6]. The observation that rheumatoid synovial tissue was heavily infiltrated with T cells, along with the findings that RA was associated with particular alleles of the class II major histocompatibility complex (MHC) [7], refocused thinking about the immunopathology of RA from the possibility that it was largely an immune complex-mediated disease to the probability that the disease involved activation of $CD4^+$ T cells, presumably responding to arthritogenic antigens.

T Cells in Arthritis, edited by P. Miossec, W.B. van den Berg and G.S. Firestein

Cytokines are thought to play an essential role in the immunopathogenesis of synovial inflammation, as well as the initiation of damage to cartilage and bone [8–10]. It was reasoned that if T cells were playing a central role in rheumatoid inflammation, they would be likely to produce large amounts of cytokines. However, initial studies quantitating the amount of T cell-derived cytokines, such as interferon (IFN)γ and interleukin (IL)-2, in rheumatoid inflammation indicated that they were found in small amounts and were much less abundantly produced than cytokines derived from macrophages and synovial fibroblasts [11, 12]. More recent studies using more sensitive techniques of immunohistology and quantitative PCR amplification of cytokine mRNAs have clearly shown the presence of T cell derived cytokines in rheumatoid synovitis [13–18]. The most prominent cytokine appears to be IFNγ that may be produced by as much as two to ten percent of synovial membrane $CD4^+$ T cells in RA [15]. The number of cytokine producing $CD4^+$ T cells in the rheumatoid synovium is comparable to that found in other chronic inflammatory diseases [19].

Despite perturbation of their function [20–22], synovial T cells exhibit an activated phenotype as gauged by expression of a variety of activation markers and upregulation of a number of functional activities [23–32]. For example, synovial $CD4^+$ T cells have a markedly enhanced capacity to provide help for B lymphocytes [22]. Part of this activity relates to the constitutive expression of the tumor necrosis factor (TNF) receptor family member CD40 ligand/CD154 that is essential for contact dependent activation of B cells and macrophages by T cells [33]. By virtue of the upregulation of CD40 ligand/CD154, synovial $CD4^+$ T cells not only can directly induce immunoglobulin production by B cells, but can also upregulate cytokine production by myeloid cells in a contact dependent manner [33]. These findings are consistent with the conclusion that synovial $CD4^+$ T cells provide both membrane signals and cytokines responsible for the inflammation characteristic of rheumatoid synovitis.

It has also become apparent that synovial $CD4^+$ T cells are markedly enriched in a subpopulation of highly differentiated memory T cells characterized by the phenotype, CD45RBdim, $CD27^-$ [24]. These cells have the capability of producing cytokines rapidly after stimulation, providing intense help for B cells and co-stimulating macrophage activation, but limited capability for proliferation [34]. Thus, when compared to a similar population of peripheral CD4+ memory T cells, functional capabilities of synovial $CD4^+$ T cells are reasonably intact. However, they appear to be markedly biased toward production of the pro-inflammatory cytokine, IFNγ, and markedly diminished in the capacity to produce the anti-inflammatory cytokine, IL-4 [13, 15, 17, 18, 35]. Unapposed production of IFNγ by differentiated $CD4^+$ effector cells appears to facilitate the ongoing inflammation in the synovium characteristic of RA.

Rheumatoid synovial tissue vasculature

The vascular endothelium plays a critical role in regulating the infiltration of specific subsets of memory CD4+ T cells into synovial tissue [23, 24]. It is apparent that such tissue specific migration is independent of the specificity of the antigen receptor expressed by individual T cells. The endothelium plays an active role in recruiting specific subsets of T cells as evidenced by the finding that specific subsets of memory T cells exhibited enhanced transendothelial migration *in vitro*, whereas in the absence of endothelial cells no selective migration of memory T cells was observed [36].

The vasculature of rheumatoid synovium is heterogeneous with regard to vessel size. During the progression of RA, neovascularization occurs throughout the tissue. T cell migration into tissue seems to occur at postcapillary venules, which are comprised of a single layer of endothelial cells supported by an underlying basement membrane. These vessels have been shown to be the sites of adhesion for peripheral blood mononuclear cells [37, 38]. During the course of RA, changes occur in many of the endothelial cells of the postcapillary venules, presumably in response to cytokines and other factors in the local mileau. The phenotype and functional characteristics of the endothelium tend to be altered, and the capacity of endothelial cells to mediate the transendothelial migration of T cells may be enhanced [39]. In this regard, postcapillary venules undergo a phenotypic change, developing the appearance of high endothelial venules (HEV) which are specialized postcapillary venules of lymphoid tissue. This change presumably represents a response to immunological activity and lymphocyte trafficking in the tissue [40–43]. The HEV of rheumatoid synovium and those of secondary lymphoid organs are different, however, in that the former support the migration of memory T cells, whereas the latter specifically promote the transendothelial migration of naive T cells [44]. This presumably relates to differences in the display of adhesion molecules and production of chemokines by HEV at these sites. Postcapillary venules of rheumatoid synovium in patients with active, untreated disease exhibit an HEV-like morphology, especially in regions near lymphocyte aggregates, whereas tissue samples from patients whose disease had been modified by treatment exhibited relatively flatter endothelium [42, 43, 45]. Only when lymphocyte aggregates were observed were tall HEV present, suggesting that in these instances, the morphological change may have developed in response to the local immunological activity. Moreover, trafficking into the tissue may be more restricted and confined to areas of lymphoid aggregates. HEV-like morphology and activity seems to develop in response to the trafficking of cells into the tissue and their subsequent production of cytokines. HEV-like blood vessels were found to develop in sites of delayed type hypersensitivity reactions in the skin of primates in response to exposure to proinflammatory cytokines. Concomitant stimulation with TNFα and IFNγ induced the appearance of HEV as well as the adhesion and extravasation of inflammatory cells [46]. In contrast, other studies have shown that HEV are not necessary for transendothelial migration of T cells, since migration similarly occurred through flat endothelium, although the transit time was considerably longer [47]. HEV, therefore, may provide an advantage over flat endothelium, due to optimal presentation of adhesion receptors to migrating cells, but may not be a requirement for migration and may, in fact, develop in response to the activity of T cells in the tissue after migration.

Adhesion receptor expression in rheumatoid synovium

Endothelial cells of rheumatoid synovium express a variety of adhesion receptors that bind T cells [48]. This is most likely a direct result of the activities of proinflammatory cytokines, such as IFNγ, IL-1-β and TNF-α, that are elaborated within the tissue, and which among their other activities, induce or upregulate the expression of adhesion receptors by endothelial cells. Thus, several reports have indicated that the endothelial cells of rheumatoid synovium express intercellular adhesion molecule-1 (ICAM-1; CD54), vascular cell adhesion molecule-1 (VCAM-1; CD106), E-selectin (CD62E), and P-selectin (CD62P) [49–52]. With the exception of P-selectin and ICAM-1, which seem to be expressed by endothelial cells of nearly all blood vessels of synovial tissue, there tends to be a wide variation in expression of the other adhesion molecules by endothelial cells. The reasons for this are not entirely certain, but they may be related to cytokine exposure of the endothelium, as well as the nature of the detection system used, and whether or not ligand was bound to the receptors and prevented recognition of the anti-receptor monoclonal antibodies. In addition, synovial tissue endothelial cells express inter-endothelial cell adhesion molecules, including platelet endothelial cell adhesion molecule (PECAM-1; CD31), as well as cadherins and a recently identified molecule, vascular adhesion protein-1 (VAP-1) [53–55]. The function of the former molecules are largely related to maintaining endothelial intgerity, although they may also play a role in regulating cellular traffic, whereas the function of the latter molecule involves mediating sialic acid-dependent, lymphocyte binding to endothelial cells [56].

To maintain their integrity, endothelial cells also interact with components of their basement membrane. Prominent among the molecules that mediate adhesion are members of the integrin family, including β1 (CD29) integrins, CD49d, CD49e, and CD49f. Both CD49dCD29 (α4β1, very late antigen-4 [VLA-4]) and CD49eCD29 (α5β1, VLA-5) mediate binding to fibronectin whereas CD49fCD29 (α6β1, VLA-6) interacts with laminin. In addition, collagen binding integrins are expressed by vascular endothelial cells, including CD49bCD29 (α2β1, VLA-2). αV, which associates with several β chains including β1, β3, and β5, has multiple specificities, the most prominent of which are vitronectin and fibronectin [57]. All of these receptors are expressed by endothelial cells. As new blood vessels develop in synovial tissue, their activity has been suggested to increase. For example, synovial tissue produces a number of endothelial growth factors, including vascular endothelial growth factor and basic-fibroblast growth factor. Among their actions is stimulation of expression of $\alpha V\beta 3$ and $\alpha V\beta 5$, which are important in mediating endothelial cell adhesion to vitronectin in the extracellular matrix, as well as inducing extracellular matrix-degrading enzymes [57].

T cells in synovial tissue similarly express a number of adhesion receptors. Among the receptors are those that mediate cell-cell adhesion, including leukocyte function-associated antigen-1 (LFA-1, CD11aCD18), VLA-4, and CD44, and those that bind extracellular matrix molecules, including CD26 and VLA-4 [26, 30]. In addition, RA synovial T cells also may be VLA-1^+ or VLA-2^+, suggestive of an activated phenotype, since they are expressed only after several rounds of proliferation [25]. Both adhesion receptors primarily mediate cell binding to collagen.

Cells require an activation signal before their integrin receptors become competent to bind their ligand [58]. This has been demonstrated for LFA-1 on T cells freshly isolated from peripheral blood of normal individuals. In contrast, a subset of circulating T cells from RA patients expresses LFA-1 in a ligand-binding-competent form and, therefore, these cells can directly bind to their counterreceptors without additional stimulation [31]. Expression of a ligand-binding-competent form of LFA-1 may be a feature related to an overall increased activation state of circulating T cells in RA patients, and may contribute to their increased accumulation within rheumatoid synovium by mediating their transendothelial migration into the tissue. Subsets of synovial tissue and fluid T cells also express activated VLA-4 as evidenced by their ability to bind to fibronectin-coated substrates [28, 59]. The data indicate that subsets of circulating T cells as well as those found at inflammatory sites in RA express activated integrins that can facilitate their entry into synovial tissue.

Adhesion receptor mediated infiltration of T cells into rheumatoid synovium

To access synovial tissue, T cells are selectively recruited by the vascular endothelial cells to migrate through postcapillary venules. This involves the concerted activities of specific cell surface adhesion receptors, as well as the functional activity of particular subsets of T cells and endothelial cells. Both T cells and endothelial cells possess multiple cell surface adhesion receptors which could facilitate T cell extravasation. The multi-step process of transendothelial migration involves initial contact of T cells with endothelial cell surfaces, the induction or activation of specific cell surface adhesion receptors to mediate stable, firm binding of T cells to the endothelium, and then a weakening of the attachments such that bound T cells transmigrate through the endothelial layer. Each of these steps is an adhesion receptor mediated process that involves specific receptor-counterreceptor pairs. The repertoire of adhesion receptors that may be involved in T cell binding to endothelial cells may be relatively large, whereas few receptors may be capable of mediating transendothelial migration. Central to the process of T cell extravasation is the intrinsic migratory capacity of T cells that facilitates T cell movement through the endothelial layer in a pathway directed by specific adhesion molecules.

Table 1 lists the adhesion receptors that are likely to facilitate the infiltration of T cells into sites of chronic inflammation. Adhesion receptors that are members of the immunoglobulin, selectin, and integrin superfamilies mediate much of the adhesive interactions that occur during the infiltration of leukocytes into sites of inflammation [48]. Additional adhesion receptors that are not members of these superfamilies, such as CD44, also play a role in T cell extravasation [48, 60]. At inflammatory sites, the expression of many receptors on endothelial cells is regulated by the actions of proinflammatory cytokines [39]. Each endothelial receptor binds at least one counterreceptor expressed by T cells, some of which are also functionally regulated by activation stimuli. For example, reagents, such as phorbol esters, which activate protein kinase C, as well as engagement of the T cell receptor/CD3 complex, induce changes in LFA-1 and VLA-4 activity without necessarily affecting their expression, such that the receptors become competent to bind their counterreceptors [61]. Additionally, ligation of CD31 on a subset of T cells leads to the functional activation of VLA-4 [62]. Moreover, cytokines that are produced in the rheumatoid synvoium, such as IL-15, can directly activate the binding capability of T cell-expressed LFA-1 and VLA-4 [63]. In contrast to this, there are adhesion receptors, such as L-selectin (CD62L), CD2 and CD44, that do not require an activation step to be able to bind their counterreceptors. Not only does the binding of adhesion receptors to specific counterreceptors facilitate adhesion and transendothelial migration, but ligation of adhesion receptors is also likely to deliver intracellular signals as well. Thus, adhesion receptors such as LFA-1 and VLA-4 deliver co-stimulatory signals to inflammatory cells when they are engaged by their counterreceptors, ICAM-1 and VCAM-1, or the extracellular matrix molecule fibronectin, respectively [64–69].

Several studies involving patients with RA have been carried out to examine the affect of agents that block cytokine or adhesion molecule activities. In one study, administration of a monoclonal antibody against ICAM-1 to RA patients with active disease had a marked modifying effect on disease activity [70]. Among its effects, the anti-ICAM-1 mAb caused a marked lymphocytosis and suppression of the patient's delayed type hypersensitivity response to recall antigen, implying that lymphocyte trafficking into tissues was altered. In another study, administration of an anti-TNFα mAb to patients with RA decreased the levels of adhesion receptors in the tissue and in the circulation [71]. Taken together, these studies support the role of adhesion receptors in lymphocyte trafficking in RA as well as that of proinflammatory cytokines modulating adhesion receptor expression and thereby facilitating entry of T cells into the rheumatoid synovium.

Table 1 - Adhesion receptors mediating T cell interactions with endothelial cells in chronic inflammation

T cell adhesion receptor	Endothelial cell counterreceptor
Receptors potentially mediating binding during early phase of acute inflammation[1]:	
CD2	LFA-3 (CD58), CD59, CD48
CD31	CD31, heparin, αVβ3
CD44	?
VLA-4 (CD49d/CD29)	VCAM-1, CS-1 fibronectin
L-selectin (CD62L)	GlyCAM-1, charged oligosaccharides
CLA	E-selectin (CD62E)
PSGL-1	P-selectin (CD62P)
?[2]	?
Receptors potentially mediating binding during late phase of acute and developing chronic inflammation:	
*[3]	*
LFA-1 (CD11a/CD18)	ICAM-1, ICAM-2
Receptors potentially mediating transendothelial migration:	
LFA-1 (CD11a/CD18)	ICAM-1
CD44	hyaluronan[4]

1 *All of the receptors listed are constitutively active. Although all have not been empirically tested, they potentially could mediate T cell-endothelial cell interactions at inflammatory sites.*
2 *As yet unidentified receptors also may mediate interactions.*
3 *All constitutively active receptors could continue contributing to T cell-endothelial cell binding while higher affinity interactions are developing.*
4 *To become competent for binding hyaluronan, CD44 requires an activation signal*

Our understanding of the steps of lymphocyte extravasation has evolved from studies examining this phenomenon in neutrophils. Normally, neutrophils roll along the surface of the endothelium [72, 73]. At sites of acute inflammation, where E-selectin and P-selectin are expressed by endothelial cells, this process has been shown to be mediated by either of these molecules binding to neutrophil L-selectin

[74]. This type of adhesive interaction is not stable and by itself does not lead to the transendothelial migration of neutrophils. Rather, stable interactions occur as a result of the formation of additional adhesions between integrins on neutrophils and ICAM-1 on endothelial cells. This stabilized binding and transendothelial migration of neutrophils occurs as a response of neutrophils to the activities of inflammatory mediators. Thus, leukotrienes, complement components, and chemokines such as IL-8, activate neutrophils and among the induced cellular changes is an increased activity of integrins leading to increased adhesiveness [75, 76]. In this series of events, L-selectin expression is down-regulated by cleavage from the surface of neutrophils. Concomitantly there is an increased expression and activation of Mac-1 which, by binding to ICAM-1, strengthens neutrophil interactions with endothelial cells. These mediators most likely also activate LFA-1 on neutrophils since both LFA-1 and Mac-1 have been suggested to mediate the transendothelial migration of neutrophils [77, 78]. CD31 also has been suggested to play a role in the transendothelial migration of neutrophils [79].

The precise mechanisms involved in the establishment of stabilized lymphocyte binding to endothelial cells have not been as clearly delineated. There is redundancy in the number of receptor-counterreceptor pairs that are capable of supporting lymphocyte adhesion to endothelial cells. L-selectin, which does not require an activation step, has been reported to mediate lymphocyte binding to TNF-α activated endothelial cells in addition to binding GlyCAM-1, a mucin-like adhesion molecule expressed by peripheral lymph node endothelial cells [80, 81]. Thus, the ligation of L-selectin may initiate intracellular signaling events that lead to stabilized T cell-endothelial cell binding. Normally, LFA-1 undergoes a conformational change for high affinity binding to its counterreceptor. This does not involve increased expression of LFA-1 by lymphocytes, but relates to conformational changes in its structure. LFA-1 mediates lymphocyte adhesion to endothelial cells, as does VLA-4, although all of the binding cannot be accounted for by the activities of these two molecules. LFA-1 functions during adhesion of resting or activated T cells to unstimulated endothelial cells by binding to both ICAM-1 and ICAM-2 [48]. VLA-4 mediates T cell adhesion to cytokine-activated endothelium by binding VCAM-1 [48]. Unlike LFA-1, multiple activation states for VLA-4 have been identified [82]. This may explain the findings that VLA-4 mediates lymphocyte binding to VCAM-1 under conditions of shear flow *in vitro* [83, 84]. Based upon these reports, suggestions have been made that VLA-4/VCAM-1 interactions occur before those of LFA-1/ICAM-1, anchoring the cells during the development of increased adhesiveness. Both E-selectin and P-selectin, which are expressed by activated endothelial cells, also appear to be involved in lymphocyte binding [48]. A subset of memory T cells adheres to E-selectin, and for many of these T cells this is mediated by cutaneous lymphocyte antigen (CLA) [85]. In addition, LFA-1 was recently shown to bind to E-selectin through its carbohydrate moieties [86]. The nature of the lymphocyte counterreceptor that binds P-selectin is most likely related to P-selectin glycoprotein ligand-1 (PSGL), a mucin-like transmembrane protein expressed by neutrophils and T cells, and which contains sialylated forms of blood group antigens, Lewis X and Lewis A [87]. All members of the selectin family specifically recognize these oligosaccharides [48]. CLA on T cells is also a ligand for P-selectin, becoming so by post-translational modification of PSGL-1 [88].

Unlike the process of T cell-endothelial cell binding, there are limited numbers of adhesion receptors that have been identified to mediate the transendothelial migration of lymphocytes. To date, the receptor pair LFA-1/ICAM-1, the homing receptor CD44, and CD31 have been implicated in the transendothelial migration of lymphocytes [48, 60]. Monoclonal antibody (MAb) blocking experiments conducted *in vitro* have demonstrated that the transendothelial migration of T cells bound to endothelial cells is inhibited by anti-LFA-1 or anti-ICAM-1 mAb, but not by mAb against VLA-4, VCAM-1, LFA-3 or E-selectin. Thus, although a number of adhesion receptors mediate initial adhesive events between T cells and endothelial cells, they do not necessarily serve a similar function during transendothelial migration.

Under conditions whereby both T cells and endothelial cells have been exposed to activation stimuli, part of the transendothelial migration of the activated lymphocytes is mediated by CD44 [60]. CD44 is not related to the integrin, immunoglobulin or selectin superfamilies. Rather, CD44 is more closely related to proteoglycan link protein. It has a number of different ligand specificities, hyaluronan and collagen, and it also has been reported to bind a receptor expressed by mucosal tissue endothelial cells. It is likely, therefore, that both lymphocyte-endothelial cell binding and transendothelial migration utilize a multiplicity of receptors. This redundancy may be necessary for a succession of adhesive interactions between lymphocytes and the endothelium that facilitate lymphocyte entry into tissue.

The nature of the initial interactions formed between lymphocytes and endothelial cells at sites of inflammation remains a matter of debate. At delayed times in an acute inflammatory response and during chronic inflammation, the forces of blood flow are not a major impediment to lymphocyte migration, as they may be during the initial phases of an acute inflammatory response, since blood flow is markedly diminished. The requirement for constitutively active adhesion receptors to tether the cells to the endothelium therefore is likely to be decreased. In addition, memory $CD4^+$ T cells that express a diminished density of L-selectin comprise the major peripheral blood migratory population at sites of inflammation [23, 24]. It is likely, however, that during the early acute phase of inflammation, receptors such as L-selectin may be important. For example, other migratory T cell subsets, such as $\gamma\delta TCR^+$ T cells, are L-selectin$^+$ [89]. In the scheme of things, L-selectin may mediate initial interactions of $\gamma\delta TCR^+$ T cells with the endothelium in the absence of marked inflammation, when blood flow is intact, and cells require adhesion to resist the shear force of the blood flow. Subsequent stabilization by integrin adhesion receptors may facilitate transendothelial migration of $\gamma\delta TCR^+$ T cells into tissue. As a result of their appearance in tissue and activation, phenotypic and functional changes may be induced in the endothelium resulting in decreased blood flow, enhanced adhesion molecule expression, and/or the elaboration of soluble mediators. Such conditions may allow migration competent αβTCR+ memory T cells to extravasate into, and accumulate within, the inflamed tissue and fluid compartments, therefore propagating the inflammatory process.

Cytokines and chemokines

Recently, knowledge of a group of low molecular weight (6–10 kDa) soluble mediators, referred to as chemokines, has increased enormously. Currently, there are more than thirty known chemokines which are related by primary structure, particularly by conservation of a 4 cysteine motif [90]. Based on the spacing of the cysteines, chemokines can be classified into two groups, C-X-C (also called α) and C-C (also called β), depending on whether the first two cysteines are adjacent or are separated by an intervening amino acid residue. Most recently, two other groups, C and CXXXC, have been identified [91, 92]. Table 2 lists chemokines that may impact T cell migration into and within chronically inflamed tissues. In general, members of the CXC group, such as IL-8, induce neutrophil migration, whereas the CC and C group members induce the migration of lymphocytes, monocytes, eosinophils, and mast cells. Reports, however, have suggested a role for IL-8 in lymphocyte migration since a subset of T cells express mRNA for the IL-8 receptors [90].

Chemokines are not expressed in most resting cells, but are rapidly upregulated on activation, when chemokine mRNA increases markedly. Secretion of chemokines usually occurs as a result of exposure of the cells to pro-inflammatory cytokines, such as IL-1, TNFα or IFNγ [90, 93]. Chemokines mediate their activity by binding cell surface receptors that are members of the rhodopsin superfamily of seven transmembrane spanning G-protein linked molecules [94]. Chemokine receptors (CR) may be specific for only one individual chemokine, or they may bind multiple types of molecules. For example, the receptor CCR-1 binds most of the CC chemokines, but none of the CXC chemokines, and CCR-2 exclusively binds IL-8. Many chemokines are present in synovial fluid, and may play an important role in facilitating the migration of cells into the tissue as well as directing their traffick in the interstitium. IL-8 is present in synovial fluid, and is produced by a variety of cell types, including synovial tissue macrophages, endothelial cells, fibroblasts, keratinocytes, and T cells [95]. Regulated on activation normal T cell expressed and secreted (RANTES) appears to be produced by antigen or mitogen-activated T lymphocytes [96]. On the other hand, macrophage inflammatory protein (MIP)-1α, MIP-1β, and monocyte chemotactic protein (MCP)-1 are produced by many cell types including B and T lymphocytes [97–99]. Chemokines also are involved in angiogenesis. Whether or not a CXC chemokine contains the structural motif glut-

Table 2 - Chemokines affecting T cell migration into and within chronically inflamed tissues

Chemokine	Chemokine receptor
CXC (α) chemokines:	
Interleukin-8 (IL-8)	CXCR1, 2, DARC[1]
Interferon-inducible protein (IP-10)	CXCR3
Stromal cell derived factor (SDF)-1	CXCR4
CC (β) chemokines:	
Monocyte chemotactic protein (MCP)-1, 2, 3, 4	CCR-1, 2, 3, 4, DARC[2]
Macrophage inflammatory protein (MIP)-1α	CCR-1, 3, 4
MIP-1β	CCR-1, 3, 5
Regulated on activation normal T cell expressed and secreted (RANTES)	CCR-1, 3, 4, 5, DARC
C chemokine:	
lymphotactin	?

1 DARC, duffy antigen receptor complex, a non-signal transducing receptor that binds many chemokines.

2 receptors for MCP-1 are CCR2 and CCR4; MCP-2, CCR1, CCR2; MCP-3, CCR1, CCR2, CCR3; MCP-4, CCR2, CCR3.

amine-leucine-arginine (ELR) will determine if it inhibits or stimulates angiogenesis. For example, IP-10 and platelet factor-4 contain ELR and inhibit angiogenesis, whereas IL-8 and growth related oncogene (GRO)-α do not have ELR and they promote angiogenesis [100, 101]. It is important to consider, therefore, that the local concentrations of these molecules in inflamed tissue may be important in regulating both T cell migration and angiogenesis.

A number of the chemokines have been reported to facilitate transendothelial migration of T cells by stimulating integrin mediated interactions with endothelial cells [102]. Recently, the cytokine IL-15 was identified in synovial tissue and synovial fluid, and was also shown to be chemotactic for T cells [103, 104]. Other studies have confirmed this observation and additionally have shown that IL-15 stimulates the transendothelial migration of T cells [63]. Moreover, it was found that IL-15 is chemokinetic and not chemotactic, that it is produced by endothelial cells, and that endothelial cell-derived IL-15 stimulates transendothelial migration of T cells *in vitro*. In addition, a combination of TNFα and IFNγ induces the appearance of IL-15 on endothelial cell surfaces. In an *in vivo* model in which RA synovial tissue

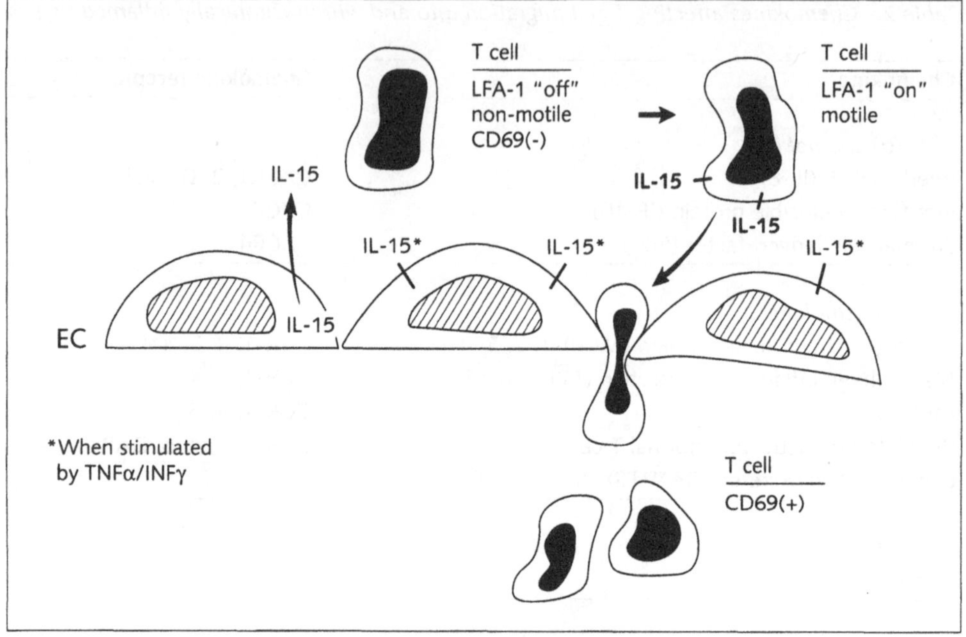

Figure 1
Model of IL-15-stimulated transendothelial migration of T cells
Depicted is the role of IL-15 in transendothelial migration. Similar events may also occur in response to chemokines that promote the transendothelial migration of T cells.

is engrafted into the severe combined immunodeficient (SCID) mouse, IL-15 was shown to dramatically increase T cell infiltration into the synovial tissue grafts [63]. IL-15 also was found to activate the binding capability of LFA-1, and to stimulate T cell motility, which could contribute to the local migration of T cells into inflammatory sites (Fig. 1). Finally, in addition to stimulating high affinity binding between LFA-1 on T cells and ICAM-1 on endothelium, IL-15 also activates migrating T cells to express the early activation marker, CD69. The activity of IL-15 may, therefore, contribute to the initial activation of $CD4^+$ T cells in rheumatoid synovium, as has been described previously [23, 24, 27].

Concluding remarks

T cell extravasation into rheumatoid synovial tissue is a critical aspect of rheumatoid inflammation. Adhesion receptors play central roles in the pathogenesis of RA by mediating T cell interactions with the endothelium and with the extracellular matrix, as well as by delivery of co-stimulatory signals to the cells. Soluble chemokines and cytokines emerging from tissue profoundly influence adhesion receptor mediated T cell trafficking into and within the synovium, and thus control the organization and compartmentalization of the various cell populations within the tissue. Future approaches to modulate adhesion receptor and chemokine/cytokine activities will have a profound impact on the development of therapeutics to control rheumatoid inflammation.

References

1 Lipsky PE (1997) Rheumatoid Arthritis. In: AS Fauci, E Braunwald, KJ Isselbacher, JD Wilson, JB Martin, DL Kasper, SL Hauser and DL Longo (eds): *Harrison's Principles of Internal Medicine*, 14th edition. New York: McGraw Hill, 1880–1888
2 Harris ED (ed) (1997) *Reumatoid Arthritis*. Philadelphia: W.B. Saunders
3 Van Boxel JA, Paget SA (1975) Predominantly T cell infiltrate in rheumatoid synovial membranes. *N Engl J Med* 293: 517–520
4 Janossy G, Panay GS, Duke O, Bofill M, Poulter LW, Goldstein G (1981) Rheumatoid arthritis: a disease of T lymphocyte/macrophage immunoregulation. Lancet 2: 839–842
5 Kurosaka M, Ziff M (1983) Immunoelectron microscopic study of the distribution of T cell subsets in rheumatoid synovium. *J Exp Med* 158: 1191–210
6 Cush JJ, Lipsky PE (1988) Phenotypic analysis of synovial tissue and peripheral blood lymphocytes isolated from patients with rheumatoid arthritis. *Arthritis Rheum* 31: 1230–1238
7 Stastny P (1978) Association of the B-cell alloantigen DRw4 with rheumatoid arthritis. *N Engl J Med* 298: 869–871
8 Lipsky PE, Davis LS, Cush JJ, Oppenheimer-Marks N (1989) The role of cytokines in the pathogenesis of rheumatoid arthritis. *Springer Semin Immunopathol* 11: 123–162
9 Feldmann M, Brennan FM, Maini RN (1996) Role of cytokines in rheumatoid arthritis. *Ann Rev Immunol* 14: 397–440
10 Koch AE, Kunkel SL, Strieter RM (1995): Cytokines in rheumatoid arthritis. *J Invest Med* 43: 28–38
11 Firestein GS, Xu WD, Townsend K, Broide D, Alvaro-Gracia J, Glasebrook A, Zvaifler NJ (1988) Cytokines in chronic inflammatory arthritis. I. Failure to detect T cell lymphokines (IL-2 and IL-3) and presence of macrophage colony-stimulating factor (CSF-1) and a novel mast cell growth factor in rheumatoid synovitis. *J Exp Med* 168: 1573–1586
12 Firestein GS, AlvaroGarcia JM, Maki R (1990) Quantitative analysis of cytokine gene expression in rheumatoid arthritis. *J Immunol* 144: 3347–3353
13 Simon AK, Seipelt E, Sieper J (1994) Divergent T-cell cytokine patterns in inflammatory arthritis. *Proc Natl Acad Sci USA* 91: 8562–8566

14 Brennan FM, Field M, Chu CQ, Feldmann M, Maini RN (1991) Cytokine expression in rheumatoid arthritis. *Brit J Rheumatol* 30: (suppl 1): 76–80

15 Dolhain RJEM, van der Heiden AN, ter Haar NT, Breedveld FC, Miltenburg AMM (1997) Shift toward T lymphocytes with a T helper 1 cytokine-secretion profile in the joints of patients with rheumatoid arthritis. *Arthritis Rheum* 39: 1961–1969

16 Isomäki P, Luukkainen R, Toivanen P, Punnonen J (1996) The presence of interleukin-13 in rheumatoid synovium and its antiinflammatory effects on synovial fluid macrophages from patients with rheumatoid arthritis. *Arthritis Rheum* 39: 1693–1702

17 Kotake S, Schumacher Jr HR, Yarboro CH, Arayssi TK, Pando JA, Kanik KS, Gourley MF, Klippel JH, Wilder RL (1997) *In vivo* gene expression of type 1 and type 2 cytokines in synovial tissues from patients with early stages of rheumatoid, reactive, and undifferentiated arthritis. *Proc Assn Amer Phy* 109: 286–301

18 Bucht A, Larsson P, Weisbrot L, Thorne C, Pisa P, Smedegard G, Keystone EC, Grönberg (1996) Expression of interferon-gamma (IFN-), IL-10, IL-12 and transforming growth factor-beta (TGF-) mRNA in synovial fluid cells from patients in the early and late phases of rheumatoid arthritis (RA). *Clin Exp Immunol* 103: 357–367

19 Wagner AD, Bjornsson J, Bartley GB, Goronzy JJ, Weyand CM (1996) Interferon gamma producing T cells in giant cell vasculitis represent a minority of tissue infiltrating cells and are located distant from the site of pathology. *Amer J Pathol* 148: 1925–1933

20 Maurice MM, Nakamura J, van der Voort EAM, van Vliet AI, Staal FJT, Tak PP, Breedveld FC, Verweij CL (1997) Evidence for the role of an altered redox state in hyporesponsiveness of synovial T cells in rheumatoid arthritis. *J Immunol* 158: 1458–1465

21 Maurice MM, Lankester AC, Bezemer AC, Geertsma MF, Tak PP, Breedveld FC, van Lier RAW Verweij CL (1997) Defective TCR-medicated signaling in synovial T cells in rheumatoid arthritis. *J Immunol* 159: 2973–2978

22 Thomas R, McIlraith M, Davis L, Lipsky PE (1992) Rheumatoid synovium is enriched in CD45RBdim memory T cells that are potent helpers for B cell differentiation. *Arthritis Rheum* 35: 1455–1465

23 Cush JJ, Lipsky PE (1988) Phenotypic analysis of synovial tissue and peripheral blood lymphocytes isolated from patients with rheumatoid arthritis. *Arthritis Rheum* 31: 1230–1238

24 Kohem CL, Brezinschek RI, Wisbey H, Tortorella C, Lipsky PE, Oppenheimer-Marks N (1996) Enrichment of differentiated $CD45RB^{dim}$, CD27-memory T cells in the peripheral blood, synovial fluid, and synovial tissue of patients with rheumatoid arthritis. *Arthritis Rheum* 39: 844–854

25 Hemler ME, Glass D, Coblyn JS, Jacobson JG (1986) Very late activation antigens on rheumatoid synovial T lymphocytes. Association with stages of T cell activation. *J Clin Invest* 78: 696–702

26 Takahashi H, Söderström K, Nilsson E, Kiessling R, Patarroyo M (1992) Integrins and

other adhesion molecules on lymphocytes from synovial fluid and peripheral blood of rheumatoid arthritis patients. *Eur J Immunol* 22: 2879–2885
27 Afeltra A, Galeazzi M, Ferri GM, Amoroso A, De Pita O, Porzio F, Bonomo L (1993) Expression of CD69 antigen on synovial fluid T cells in patients with thrumatoid arthritis and chronic synovitis. *Ann Rheum Dis* 52: 457–460
28 Laffon A, Garcia Vicuna R, Humbria A, Postigo AA, Corbi AL, de Landazuri MO, Sanchez Madrid F (1991) Upregulated expression and function of VLA-4 fibronectin receptors on human activated T cells in rheumatoid arthritis. *J Clin Invest* 88: 546–552
29 Sfikakis PP, Zografou A, Viglis V, Iniotaki-Theodoraki A, Piskontaki I, Tsokos GC, Sfikakis P Choremi-Papadopoulou H (1995) CD28 expression on T cell subsets in vivo and CD28-mediated T cell response in vitro in patients with rheumatoid arthritis. *Arthritis Rheum* 38: 649–644
30 Kelleher D, Murphy A, Hall Nicola, Omary MB, Kearns G, Long A Casey EB (1995) Expression of CD44 on rheumatoid synovial fluid lymphocytes. *Ann Rheum Dis* 54: 566–570
31 Yokota A, Murata N, Saiki O, Shimizu M, Springer TA Kishimoto T (1995) High avidity state of leukocyte function-associated antigen-1 on rheumatoid synovial fluid T lymphocytes. *J Immunol* 155: 4118–4124
32 Isomäki P, Aversa G, Cocks BG, Luukkainen R, Saario R, Toivanen P, de Vries JE Punnonen J (1997) Increased expression of signaling lymphocytic activation molecule in patients with rheumatoid arthritis and its role in the regulation of cytokine production in rheumatoid synovium. *J Immunol* 159: 2986–2993
33 MacDonald KPA, Nishioka Y, Lipsky PE, Thomas R (1997) Functional CD40 ligand is expressed by T cells in rheumatoid arthritis. *J Clin Invest* 100: 2404–2414
34 Tortorella C, Schulze-Koops H, Thomas R, Splawski JB, Davis LS, Picker LJ, Lipsky PE (1995) Expression of CD45RB and CD27 identifies subsets of CD4+ memory T cells with different capacities to induce B cell differentiation. *J Immunol* 155: 149–162
35 Schulze-Koops H, Lipsky PE, Kavanaugh AF, Davis LS (1995) Elevated Th1 or Th0-like cytokine mRNA in peripheral circulation of patients with rheumatoid arthritis. Modulation by treatment with anti-ICAM-1 correlates with clinical benefit. *J Immunol* 155: 5029–5037
36 Brezinschek RI, Lipsky PE, Galea P, Vita R, Oppenheimer-Marks N (1995) Phenotypic characterization of CD4+ T cells that exhibit a transendothelial migratory capacity. *J Immunol* 154: 3062–3077
37 Jalkanen S, Steere AC, Fox RI, Butcher EC (1986) A distinct endothelial cell recognition system that controls lymphocyte traffic into inflamed synovium. *Science* 233: 556–558
38 Oppenheimer-Marks N, Ziff M (1986) Binding of normal human mononuclear cells to blood vessels in rheumatoid arthritis synovial membrane. *Arthritis Rheum* 29: 789–792
39 Kavanaugh AF, Oppenheimer-Marks N (1992) The role of the endothelium in the pathogenesis of vasculitis. In: EC LeRoy (ed): *Systemic Vasculitis: The Biological Basis* New York: Marcel Dekker, Inc 27–48

40 Freemont AJ (1987) Molecules controlling lymphocyte-endothelial interactions in lymph nodes are produced in vessels in inflamed synovium. *Ann Rheum Dis* 4: 924–928

41 Freemont AJ, Jones CJP, Bromley M, Andrews P (1983) Changes in vascular endothelium related to lymphocyte collections in diseased synovia. *Arthritis Rheum* 26: 1427–1433

42 Iguchi T, Ziff M (1986) Electron microscopic study of rheumatoid synovial vasculature. *J Clin Invest* 77: 355–361

43 Yanni G, Whelan, A, Feighery, C, Fitzgerald, O, Bresnihan, B (1993) Morphometric analysis of synovial membrane blood vessels in rheumatoid arthritis: Associations with the immunohistologic features, synovial fluid, cytokine levels and the clinical course. *J Rheum* 20: 634–638

44 Picker LJ, Siegelman MH (1993) Lymphoid tissues and organs. In: Paul, WE (ed): *Fundamental Immunology* 3rd edn. New York: Raven Press. 145–197

45. Ziff M, Iguchi T (1987) Electron microscopic study of rheumatoid synovial vasculature: Intimate relationship between tall endothelium and lymphoid aggregation. *Int. J. Tissue Reactions* 9: 273–276

46. Munro JM, Pober JS, Cotran RS (1989) Tumor necrosis factor and interferon- induce distinct patterns of endothelial activation and associated leukocyte accumulation in skin of Papio Anubis. *Am J Path* 135: 121–133

47 Fossum S, Smith ME, Ford WL (1983). The recirculation of T and B lymphocytes in the athymic, nude rat. Scand. J. Immunol. 17: 551–557

48 Oppenheimer-Marks N, Lipsky, PE (1994) Transendothelial migration of T cells in chronic inflammation. *The Immunologist* 2: 58–64

49 Hale LP, Martin ME, McCollum DE, Nunley JA, Springer TA, Singer KH, Haynes BF (1989) Immunohistologic analysis of the distribution of cell adhesion molecules within the inflammatory synovial microenvironment. *Arthritis Rheum* 32: 22–30

50 Koch A, Burrows JC, Haines GK, Carlos TM, Harlan JM, Leibovich SJ (1991) Immunolocalization of endothelial and leukocyte adhesion molecules in human rheumatoid and osteoarthritic synovial tissue. *Lab Invest* 64, 313–320

51 Tak PP, Thurkow EW, Daha MR, Kluin PM, Smeets TJ, Meinders AE, Breedveld FC (1995) Expression of adhesion molecules in early rheumatoid synovial tissue. *Clin Immunol Immunopathol* 77: 236–242

52 Grober JS, Bowen BL, Ebling H, Athey B, Thompson CB, Fox DA, Stoolman LM (1993) Monocyte-endothelial adhesion in chronic rheumatoid arthritis. *In situ* detection of selectin and integrin dependent interactions. *J Clin Invest* 91, 2609–2619

53 Yousseff PP, Triantafillou S, Parker A, Coleman M, Roberts-Thomson PJ, Ahern MJ, Smith MD (1997) Variability in cytokine and cell adhesion molecule staining in arthroscopic synovial biopsies: quantification using color video image analysis. *J Rheumatol* 24: 2291–2298

54 Geiger B, Ayalon O (1992) *Cadherins Annu Rev Cell Biol* 8: 307–332

55 Salmi M, Kalimo K, Jalkanen S (1993) Induction and function of vascular adhesion protein-1 at sites of inflammation. *J Exp Med* 178: 2255–2260

56 Salmi M, Jalkanen S (1996) Human vascular adhesion protein 1 (VAP-1) is a unique sialoglycoprotein that mediates carbohydrate-dependent binding of lymphocytes to endothelial cells. *J Exp med* 183: 569–579
57 Friedlander M, Brooks PC, Schaffer RW, Kincaid CM, Varner JA, Cheresh DA (1995) Definition of two angiogenic pathways by distinct V integrins. *Science* 270: 1500–1502
58 Oppenheimer-Marks N, Lipsky PE (1997) Adhesion molecules and the regulation of the migration of lymphocytes. In: A Hamann (ed): *Adhesion Molecules and Chemokines in Lymphocyte Trafficking.* The Netherlands: Harwood Academic Publishers 55–88
59 van Dinther-Janssen AC, Horst E, Koopman G, Newmann W, Scheper RJ, Meijer CJ, Pals ST (1991) The VLA-4/VCAM-1 pathway is involved in lymphocyte adheison to endothelium n rheumatoid synovium. *J Immunol* 147: 4207–4210
60 Oppenheimer-Marks N, Davis LS, Lipsky PE (1990) Human T lymphocyte adhesion to endothelial cells and transendothelial migration. Alteration of receptor use relates to the activation status of both the T cell and the endothelial cell. *J Immunol* 145: 140–148
61 Springer TA (1990) Adhesion receptors of the immune system. *Nature* 346: 425–434
62 Tanaka Y, Albelda SM, Horgan KJ, van Seventer GA, Shimizu Y, Newman W, Hallam J, Newman PJ, Buck CA, Shaw S (1992) CD31 expressed on distinctive T cell subsets is a preferential amplifier of 1 integrin-mediated adhesion. *J Exp Med* 176: 245–253
63 Oppenheimer-Marks N, Brezinschek RI, Mohamadzadeh M, Vita R, Lipsky PE (1998) Interleukin-15 is produced by endothelial cells and increases the transendothelial migration of T cells in vitro and in the SCDI mouse-human rheumatoid arthritis model *in vivo*. *J Clin Invest* 101: 1261–1272
64 Altmann DM, Hogg N, Trowsdale J, Wilkinson D (1989) Cotransfection of ICAM-1 and HLA-DR reconstitutes human antigen-presenting cell function in mouse L cells. *Nature* 338: 512–514
65 Davis LS, Oppenheimer-Marks N, Bednarczyk JL, McIntyre BW, Lipsky PE (1990) Fibronectin promotes proliferation of naive and memory T cells by signaling through both the VLA-4 and VLA-5 integrin molecules. *J Immunol* 145: 785–793
66 Shimizu Y, van Seventer GA, Horgan KJ, Shaw S (1990) Costimulation of proliferative responses of resting $CD4^+$ T cells by the interaction of VLA-4 and VLA-5 with fibronectin or VLA-6 with laminin. J. Immunol 145: 59–67
67 van Seventer GA, Shimizu Y, Horgan KJ, Shaw S (1990) The LFA-1 ligand ICAM-1 provides an important costimulatory signal for T cell receptor-mediated activation of resting T cells. *J Immunol* 144: 4579–4586
68 van Seventer GA Newman W, Shimizu Y, Nutman TB, Tanaka Y, Horgan KJ, Gopal TV, Ennis E, O'Sullivan D, Grey H, Shaw S (1991) Analysis of T cell stimulation by superantigen plus major histocompatability complex class II molecules or by CD3 monoclonal antibody: Costimulation by purified adhesion ligands VCAM-1, ICAM-1, but not ELAM-1. *J Exp Med* 174: 901–913
69 Damle NK, Klussman K, Leytze G, Ochs HD, Aruffo A, Linsley PS, Ledbetter JA (1993)

Costimulation via vascular cell adhesion molecule-1 induces in T cells increased responsiveness to the CD28 counter-receptor B7. *Cell Immunol* 148: 144–156

70 Kavanaugh AF, Davis LS, Nichols LA, Norris SH, Rothlein R, Scharschmidt LA, Lipsky PE (1992) Treatment of refractory rheumatoid arthritis with a monoclonal antibody to intercellular adhesion molecule-1. *Arthritis Rheum* 37: 992–999.

71 Paleolog EM, Hunt M, Elliott MJ, Feldmann M, Maini RN, Woody JN (1996) Deactivation of vascular endothelium by monoclonal anti-tumor necrosis factor alpha antibody in rheumatoid arthritis. *Arthritis Rheum* 39: 1082–1091

72 Lawrence MB, Springer, TA (1991) Leukocytes roll on a selectin at physiologic flow rates: Distinction from and prerequisite for adhesion through integrins. *Cell* 65: 859–873

73 Butcher EC (1991) Leukocyte-endothelial cell recognition: Three (or more) steps for specificity and diversity. *Cell* 67: 1033–1036

74 Picker LJ, Warnock RA, Burns AR, Doerschuk CM, Berg EL, Butcher EC (1991) The neutrophil selectin LECAM-1 presents carbohydrate ligands to the vascular selectins ELAM-1 and GMP-140. *Cell* 66: 921–933

75 Kishimoto TK, Warnock RA, Jutila MA, Butcher EC, Lane C, Anderson DC, Smith CW (1991) Antibodies against human neutrophil LECAM-1 (LAM-1/Leu-8/Dreg 56 antigen) and endothelial cell ELAM-1 inhibit a common CD18-independent adhesion pathway *in vitro*. *Blood* 78: 805–811

76 Huber AR, Kunkel SL, Todd III RF, Weiss SJ (1991) Regulation of transendothelial neutrophil migration by endogenous interleukin-8. *Science* 254: 99–102

77 Smith CW, Rothlein R, Hughes BJ, Mariscalco MM, Rudloff HE, Schmalsteig FC, Anderson DC (1988) Recognition of an endothelial determinant for CD18-dependent human neutrophil adherence and transendothelial migration. *J Clin Invest* 82: 1746–1756

78 Smith WC, Marlin SD, Rothlein R, Toman C, Anderson DC (1989) Cooperative interactions of LFA-1 and Mac-1 with intercellular adhesion molecule-1 in facilitating adherence and transendothelial migration of human neutrophils *in vitro*. *J Clin Invest* 83: 2008–2017

79 Muller WA, Weigel SA, Deng X, Phillips DM (1993) PECAM-1 is required for transendothelial migration of leukocytes. *J Exp Med* 178: 449–460

80 Kansas GS, Spertini O, Stoolman LM, Tedder TF (1991) Molecular mapping of functional domains of the leukocyte receptor for endothelium, LAM-1. *J Cell Biol* 114: 351–358

81 Lasky LA, Singer MS, Yednock TA, Dowbenko D, Fennie C, Rodriguez H, Nguyen T, Stachel S, Rosen SD (1989) Cloning of a lymphocyte homing receptor reveals a lectin domain. *Cell* 56: 1045–1055

82 Masumoto A, Hemler ME (1993) Multiple activation states of VLA-4. Mechanistic differences between adhesion to CS1/fibronectin and to vascular cell adhesion molecule-1. *J Biol Chem* 268: 228–234

83 Alon R, Kassner PD, Carr MW, Finger EB, Hemler ME, Springer TA (1995) The inte-

grin VLA-4 supports tethering and rolling in flow on VCAM-1. *J Cell Biol* 128: 1243–1252.
84 Lalor PF, Clements JM, Pigott R, Humphries MJ, Spragg JH, Nash GB (1997) Association between receptor density, cellular activation, and transformation of adhesive behavior of flowing lymphocytes binding to VCAM-1. *Eur J Immunol* 27: 1442–1426
85 Berg EL, Robinson MK, Warnock RA, Butcher EC (1991) The human peripheral lymph node vascular addressin is a ligand for LECAM-1, the peripheral lymph node homing receptor. *J Cell Biol* 114: 343–349
86 Kotovouri P, Tontti E, Pigott R, Shepard M, Kiso M, Hasegawa A, Renkonen R, Nortamo P, Altieri DC, Gahmberg CG (1993) The vascular E-selectin binds to the leukocyte integrins CD11/CD18. *Glycobiology* 3: 131–136
87 Sako D, Chang XJ, Barone KM, Vachino G, White HM, Shaw G, Veldman GM, Bean KM, Ahern TJ, Furie B, et al (1993) Expression cloning of a functional glycoprotein ligand for P-selectin. *Cell* 75: 1179–1186.
88 Fuhlbrigge RC, Kieffer JD, Armerding D, Kupper TS (1997) Cutaneous lymphocyte antigen is a specialized form of PSGL-1 expressed on skin-homing T cells. *Nature* 389: 978–981
89 Galea P, Brezinschek R, Lipsky PE, Oppenheimer-Marks N (1994) Phenotypic characterizatin of CD4(-)/ TCR(+) and TCR(+) T cells with a transendothelial migratory capacity. *J Immunol* 153: 529–542
90 Baggiolini M, Dewald B, Moser B (1997) Human chemokines: An update. *Annu Rev Immunol* 15: 675–705
91 Kelner GS, Kennedy J, Bacon KB, Kleyensteuber S, Largaespada DA, Jenkins NA, Copeland NG, Bazan JF, Moore KW, Schall TJ et al (1994) Lymphotactin: A cytokine that represents a new class of chemokine. *Science* 266: 1395–1399
92 Timothy N, Wells C, Peitsch MC (1997) The chemokine information source: identification and characterization of novel chemokines using the World Wide Web and Expressed Sequence Tag Databases (1997) *J Leuk Biol* 61: 545–550
93 Baggiolini M, Dewald D, Moser B (1994) Interleukin-8 and related chemotactic cytokines: CXC and CC chemokines. *Adv Immunol* 55: 97–179
94 Benbaruch A, Michiel DF, Oppenheim JJ (1995) Signals and receptors involved in recruitment of inflammatory cells. *J Biol Chem* 270: 11703–11706
95 Brennan FM, Zachariae COC, Chantry D, Larsen CG, Turner M, Maini RN, Matsushima K, Feldmann M (1990) Detection of interleukin 8 biological activity in synovial fluids from patients with rheumatoid arthritis and production of interleukin 8 mRNA by isolated synovial cells. *Eur J Immunol* 20: 2141–2144
96 Schall TJ, Bacon K, Toy K.J, Goeddel DV (1990) Selective attraction of monocytes and T lymphocytes of the memory phenotype by cytokine RANTES. Nature 347: 669–671
97 Lipes MA, Napolitano M, Jeang K-T, Chang NT, Leonard WJ (1988) Identification, cloning, and characterization of an immune activation gene. *Proc Natl Acad Sci USA* 85: 9704–9708
98 Schall TJ, Bacon K, Camp RDR, Kaspari JW, Goeddel DV (1993) Human macrophage

inflammatory protein-1 (MIP-1) and MIP-1 chemokines attract distinct populations of lymphocytes. *J Exp Med* 177: 1821–1825

99 Rathanaswami P, Hachicha M, Sadick M, Schall TJ, McColl SR (1993) Expression of the cytokine RANTES in human rheumatoid synovial fibroblasts. *J Biol Chem* 268: 5834–5839

100 Streiter RM, Polverini PJ, Arenberg DA, Kunkel SL (1995) The role of CXC chemokines as regulators of angiogenesis. *Shock* 4: 155–160

101 Streiter RM, Polverini PJ, Kunkel SL (1995) The functional role of the ELR motif in CXC chemokine-mediated angiogenesis. *J Biol Chem* 270: 27348–27357

102 Ebnet K, Kaldijian EP, Anderson AO, Shaw S (1996) Orchestrated information transfer underlying leukocyte endothelial interactions. *Annu Rev Immunol* 14: 155–177

103 Wilkinson PC, Liew FY (1995) Chemoattraction of human blood T lymphocytes by interleukin-15. *J Exp Med* 181: 1255–1259

104 McInnis IB, Al-Mughales J, Field M, Leung BP, Huang F-P, Dixon R, Sturrock RD, Wilkinson PC, Liew FY (1996) The role of interleukin-15 in T-cell migration and activation in rheumatoid arthritis. *Nature Med* 2: 175–182

T cell reactivity to Epstein-Barr virus in rheumatoid arthritis

Marc Bonneville, Emmanuel Scotet, Marie-Alix Peyrat, Annick Lim[1], *Jacques David-Ameline and Elisabeth Houssaint*

INSERM U463, Institut de Biologie, 9 quai Moncousu, F-44035 Nantes, France
[1]INSERM U277, Institut Pasteur, 25 rue du Dr Roux, F-75724 Paris, France

Introduction

The notion that T cells could play a central role in rheumatoid arthritis (RA) emerged in the late 70's with the demonstration of massive T cell infiltration in inflamed joints from RA patients [1]. Support for this hypothesis later came from studies showing (i) an increased susceptibility to RA associated with expression of particular HLA-DR alleles [2], (ii) an increased expression of activation and memory markers by joint-infiltrating lymphocytes [3–6], (iii) T cell repertoire biases within joint-infiltrating lymphocytes when compared to peripheral blood T cells (reviewed in [7, 8]), and (iv) beneficial effects of T cell-depleting or suppressive treatments in RA patients [9–11]. However, in the absence of any direct evidence for a pathogenic role of T cells in RA and in light of the limited therapeutic effects of antibody-mediated T cell depletion in some clinical trials, the paradigm of RA as a T cell-mediated disease has more recently been put into question [12, 13]. Here we would like to present and discuss recent observations from our laboratory that may revive this paradigm and support an implication of common intracellular parasites, such as Epstein-Barr virus (EBV), in the perpetuation of T cell-dependent joint erosion during chronic RA. At the present stage our observations, which demonstrate the frequent occurrence of EBV-reactive T cells in inflamed joints from chronic RA patients [14, 15], raise many more questions than they provide answers. However, several testable hypotheses may account for these findings and these will be presented here.

Frequent recognition of EBV epitopes by synovial T lymphocytes from chronic RA patients

The controversy around the role, dispensable or mandatory, of T cells in RA pathogenesis has been based on the inability to demonstrate the existence of synovial T cell responses to identifiable antigens in most RA patients [12, 13]. Furthermore,

T Cells in Arthritis, edited by P. Miossec, W.B. van den Berg and G.S. Firestein

although an expansion of "private" (i.e. specific to a given individual) T cell clonotypes in inflamed joints are in evidence in most repertoire analyses of RA synovial lymphocytes (SL) [8], the existence of synovial T cell subsets with inter-individual recurrent T cell receptor (TCR) features, which would sign the existence of T cell responses directed against "public" (i.e. eliciting similar T cell responses in distinct individuals) antigens in RA, has been suggested in some but not all studies (reviewed in [7, 8]). In addition, since the recurrent SL TCR features (common V region or related TCR junctional sequences) noted by some groups generally differed from one study to another [7, 8], the general physiopathological significance of these repertoire biases has been put into question. Three major reasons could explain these controversial results. First, these differences may originate from the different ways T cell repertoire and specificity were analyzed (e.g. through either qualitative or quantitative assessment of TCR structural features and antigenic reactivity). The second reason may lie in the heterogeneity of the T cell populations analyzed in different studies (e.g. synovial fluid or synovial membrane-derived, CD4 or CD8, activated or resting, naive or memory, etc.). Finally, the third explanation might be linked to the heterogeneity of the clinical status of patients from which T cell samples were derived. Therefore, despite the wealth of data thus far obtained and because in most instances repertoire and specificity analyses have not been coupled, the generality of these synovial clonal expansions, their origin, and their pathological consequences have remained unclear.

Existence of expanded T cell clonotypes showing spatial and temporal recurrence in chronic RA patients

A few years ago, we initiated a study that aimed at determining whether T cell clonotypes with shared TCR motifs and definable specificity could be found in chronic RA patients, i.e. at stages where T cell independent inflammatory processes are thought to be the main mediators of disease perpetuation [12, 13, 16]. To this end, a group of patients with long-term aggressive disease (i.e. fulfilling at least five of the revised criteria proposed by the American Association of Rheumatology [17]) were selected, from which peripheral blood lymphocytes (PBL) and SL were isolated at different time points. To detect possible T cell clonotype expansions in the joints of these patients, four approaches were combined to allow both a qualitative and quantitative analysis of TCR features of complex mixtures of T cells (see a representative example in Fig. 1). TCR Vβ expression by $CD4^+$ and $CD8^+$ T cells was first evaluated by flow cytometry using a panel of mAb directed against 21 TCR Vβ regions covering about 70% of the peripheral T cell repertoire (Fig. 1A) [14]. TCR junctional features of PBL and SL were then studied in a global fashion through a recently developed methodology called "Immunoscope" [18, 19], which allows analysis of the distribution of junctional lengths of transcribed TCR β chain genes

(Fig. 1B–D). Using this technique, it was possible to estimate the frequency of T cells carrying TCR β chains with a given length and a given TCR Vβ and Jβ composition in a semi-quantitative fashion (Fig. 1C, D). The frequency of TCR transcripts with a given sequence was then estimated in some patients by analyzing TCR junctional transcripts, amplified from fresh T cells using Vβ and Cβ primers. Finally, both TCR α and β transcripts from T cell clones derived either from total synovial populations or from expanded TCR Vβ subsets were fully characterized (Tab. 1).

This analysis ([14, 15] and J. David-Ameline, M.A. Peyrat and M. Bonneville, unpublished observations) led to several conclusions that confirmed and extended previously published data [7, 8]. First, our results indicated that synovial over-representation of T cell subsets carrying TCR β chains with identical Vβ/Jβ composition and length were detected in most of the patients studied (see for instance BV2, 4, 14 and 22 subsets in patient R1, Fig. 1), although all of them were at a chronic stage of the disease [14]. Second, synovial repertoire biases involved cells belonging to either $CD4^+$ or $CD8^+$ subsets, and using TCR Vβ regions that differed from one patient to another. This strongly suggested that these T cell expansions were driven by polymorphic MHC/peptide complexes rather than by superantigens. Also in agreement with this hypothesis, expanded T cell subsets, which represented up to 1/6 of synovial T cells in some patients, were oligo- or monoclonal as indicated by Immunoscope and clonal analyses [14], (Fig. 1C and D). Importantly, T cell clones with identical TCR sequences were frequently found in different joints from the same patient at a given time point, and persisted in inflamed joints for more than 2 years [14]. This spatial and temporal stability of the above synovial T cell repertoire biases strongly suggested a non-random trapping and/or intra-articular expansion of T cells following recognition of a highly restricted set of antigens in a given patient. Since we failed, however, to observe any recurrent TCR motifs shared by clonotypes derived from distinct individuals, no information regarding the inter-individual relatedness of the antigens responsible for these synovial T cell expansions could be obtained.

Recognition of EBV epitopes by T cell clones over-represented within inflamed joints from two patients

In light of the above results, the antigen specificity of T cell clones derived from expanded synovial subsets in two patients was analyzed. One should mention that the *in vitro* culture conditions used to clone and to amplify these cells do not alter the relative representation of T cell clones since they were previously shown to allow expansion of basically all T cells, regardless of their antigenic specificity [20, 21]. Accordingly the TCR features of most T cell clones isolated corresponded to those of expanded T cell subsets detected in fresh samples (A. Lim, J. David-Ameline, M.A. Peyrat and M. Bonneville, unpublished observations).

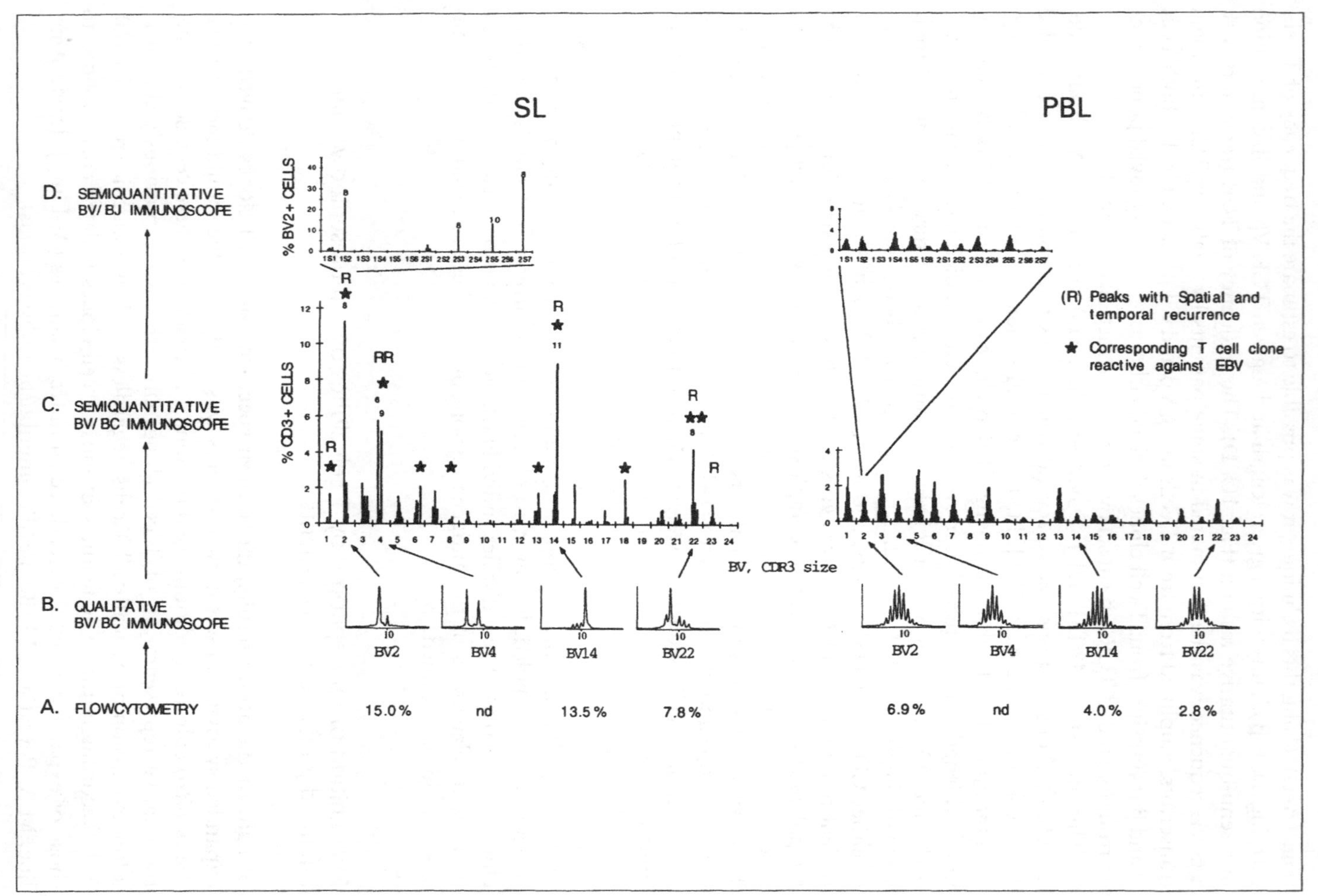
SL
PBL
D. SEMIQUANTITATIVE BV/BJ IMMUNOSCOFE
C. SEMIQUANTITATIVE BV/BC IMMUNOSCOFE
B. QUALITATIVE BV/BC IMMUNOSCOFE
A. FLOWCYTOMETRY
% BV2+ CELLS
% CD3+ CELLS
BV, CDR3 size
(R) Peaks with Spatial and temporal recurrence
★ Corresponding T cell clone reactive against EBV
BV2
BV4
BV14
BV22
15.0%
nd
13.5%
7.8%
BV2
BV4
BV14
BV22
6.9%
nd
4.0%
2.8%

Frequent recognition of autologous B lymphoblastoid cells by synovial T cell clones derived from patients R1 and R2

Since T cells potentially reactive against self articular components were being investigated, the rationale of the specificity analysis was to study the reactivity of SL-derived clones against autologous antigen presenting cells (APC) (either T cell blasts or EBV-transformed B lymphoblastoid cells (BLC)) loaded with extracts from joint tissues. In the course of several control experiments, most SL clones from a first patient (hereafter referred to as R1) unexpectedly recognized the autologous BLC, i.e. without any addition of tissue extracts. This peculiar behaviour (i) was observed with both $CD4^+$ and $CD8^+$ SL-derived clones but not with PBL clones derived from the patient, (ii) was major histocompatibility complex (MHC)-dependent since BLC recognition was blocked by mAb directed against framework regions of either human leukocyte antigen (HLA) class I or II isotypes and segregated with expression of particular HLA alleles and (iii) was BLC-specific since MHC-matched T cell blasts or myelomas were not recognized by BLC-reactive clones [14]. Furthermore, similar observations were made in a second RA patient (R2), thus suggesting frequent synovial enrichment of BLC-reactive T cells during RA [14].

Molecular identification of the antigens recognized by BLC-reactive SL clones

In order to identify the antigens recognized by SL-derived T cell clones, a molecular approach initially devised by Boon and colleagues, that had already led to successful cloning of several tumor antigens recognized by MHC class I-restricted melanoma-reactive T cell clones, was followed [22, 23]. In brief, this strategy con-

Figure 1
Example of T cell repertoire analyses performed on RA patients. Shown are representative data obtained on synovial lymphocyte (SL, left) and peripheral blood lymphocyte (PBL, right) from one patient (R1). From bottom to top are indicated results on 4 Vβ subsets (V2, V4, V14 and V22) obtained (i) by flowcytometry, (ii) by qualitative Immunoscope, (iii) by semiquantitative VβCβ Immunoscope and (iv) by semiquantitative VbJb Immunoscope. For more details about the technique and interpretation of the data, see text and [14, 15, 18, 19]. Note the gaussian distribution of the CDR3 size of TCR β chains expressed by PBL as compared to the presence of few dominant CDR3 β peaks in SL. In the example given for Vβ2, the dominant Vβ2Cβ peak, which represented close to 12% of SL, was composed of three major populations only, using either Jβ1.2, Jβ2.3 or Jβ2.7. By contrast a similar analysis performed on PBL-derived material amplified by Vβ2 and Jβ primers demonstrated a gaussian distribution of CDR3 sizes regardless of the Jβ studied. Importantly, all dominant peaks corresponded to clones reactive against EBV in this patient, and most clones were still detectable in joint samples drawn more than two years after the first analysis [14, 15].

Table 1 - Frequency and TCR diversity of synovial T cells reactive against a single MHC/viral peptide complex in a chronic RA patient

TCR Vβ analysis on total SL			**CDR3 β sequence of**
VJ combination	**size (aa)**	**% SL**	**corresponding T cell clones**
V1J2.5	10	1.8	SVGLTGQETQ
V2J2.3	8	1.5	SYLAGTTQ
V2J2.7	8	4.0	REDPSYEQ
V2J2.5	10	2.0	RAWRGPQETQ
V6.4J2.1	13	nd	SLEQGYRGSYNEQ
V8J1.2	11	nd	SLXNXATXLWQ
V14J2.3	11	8.8	SFNLGGLGDTQ
V18J2.7	9	nd	SPPLGTYEQ
V22J2.1	8	1.5	RTGERDEQ
V22J2.2	8	1.3	SGTYTGEL
V22J2.7	8	1.0	SHLGGGEQ
V22J1.2	12	<0.2	SPVPGQGENYGY
V22J2.3	12	<0.2	SGEVFTKITDTQ
total		≈22.0	

*The frequency of SL from a chronic RA patient (R1) carrying TCR β chains with a given VβJβ combination and CDR3 size was estimated by semi-quantitative Immunoscope on total SL (Fig. 1) and TCR β CDR3 sequences were determined on the corresponding T cell clones [14]. Shown are sequences derived from clones reactive against the same BZLF1-derived peptide (SENDRLRLL) presented by HLA-B*4002. Note the lack of obvious primary sequence homology between the TCR β chains expressed by these clones. Analysis of T cell clone-derived TCR α chains demonstrated a similar sequence heterogeneity (F. Davodeau, C. Courdel, M.A. Peyrat and M. Bonneville, unpublished data). Several T cell clones reacting against this antigen and expressing other Vβ regions (V5, V11 and V13) were also derived from the same patient but their CDR3 sequences were not determined.*

sists of testing the T cell response (as revealed by tumor necrosis factor (TNF) release) to COS cells cotransfected with DNA coding for the appropriate HLA allele and with cDNA derived from an expression library made from target cell RNA (Fig. 2). Since this technique does not allow characterization of MHC class II-restricted epitopes [22], BLC-reactive CD8$^+$ SL clones were exclusively evaluated, although several BLC-reactive CD4$^+$ synovial T cell clones from patient R1 were also available. Through this approach, pools of cDNA derived from an R1-BLC library were detected that were able to activate TNF release by an HLA-A*02-restricted synovial T cell clone derived from patient R1 [15]. This led to the identification of a first antigen derived from the BMLF1 protein, an EBV transactivator expressed during the early stage of the virus lytic cycle [24] (Tab. 1). Following a similar strategy, a second EBV epitope recognized by another synovial T cell clone from the same patient [15] was identified, which was again derived from a transactivator (BZLF1) expressed early during the virus lytic cycle [24] (Tab. 1). Subsequent analysis of the reactivity of the other BLC-reactive synovial T cell clones from patient R1 indicated that most of them recognized BZLF1 in the context of various HLA alleles (HLA-Cw*01 or -B *4002) [15] (Tab. 1). Furthermore, when screening BLC-reactive T cell clones derived from patient R2, several clones turned out to react against another BZLF1-derived epitope [15]. Taken together these results suggested that unlike PBL, a relatively high frequency of SL were EBV-reactive and directed against a restricted set of viral proteins.

Frequent synovial expansions of EBV-reactive T cells during chronic arthritis

Recognition of latent and lytic EBV proteins by synovial lymphocytes from chronic RA patients

In order to extend the above findings to a larger group of arthritis patients and to characterize the putative EBV antigens recognized by BLC-reactive clones with yet undefined specificity, we evaluated the reactivity of RA lymphocytes to COS cells cotransfected with cDNA encoding various HLA alleles and for most EBV proteins with known immunogenicity (i.e. six lytic proteins: BMLF1, BZLF1, BRLF1, BCRF1, BHRF1, BMRF1; and all latent proteins: EBNA-1, -2, -3A, -3B, -3C, -LP, LMP1 and LMP2) [24]. This analysis, which was performed either on T cell clones or directly on short term cultured PBL or SL lines, led to the following conclusions. Firstly, clonal analysis revealed recognition of both lytic and latent EBV proteins by several BLC-reactive clones from patient R2. Secondly, analysis of polyclonal cell lines demonstrated increased anti-EBV responses in synovial cell lines (as compared to PBL-derived lines) in 8/16 chronic RA patients. Thirdly, these responses were directed against diverse EBV lytic and latent proteins, whose epitopes were presented by various HLA class I alleles (Fig. 3). Hence it seemed that while EBV reactivity was a rather common feature of SL, there was no obvious immunodominance of a particular EBV protein or MHC/EBV epitope.

Synovial enrichment of EBV-reactive T cells: a general feature of chronic arthritis patients?

To test whether enrichment for EBV-reactive cells within inflamed joints was specific to RA patients, EBV reactivity of PBL and SL derived from two psoriatic arthritis (PA) and eight HLA-B*27-associated ankylosing spondylitis (AS) patients was then studied. Significant anti-EBV responses were detected in one synovial PA

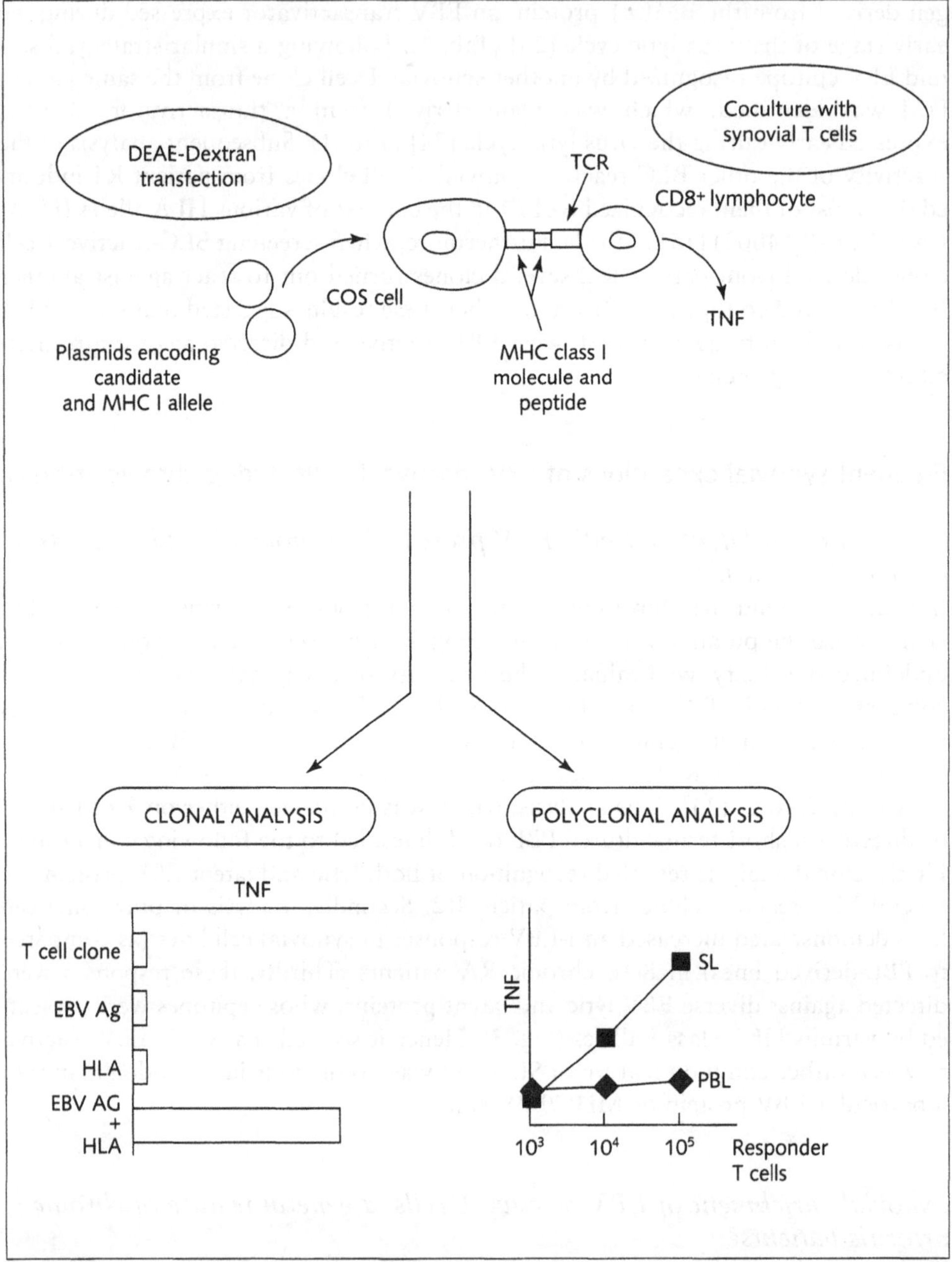

Figure 2
Rationale of the transient COS transfection assay used to detect anti-EBV T cell responses in chronic arthritis patients

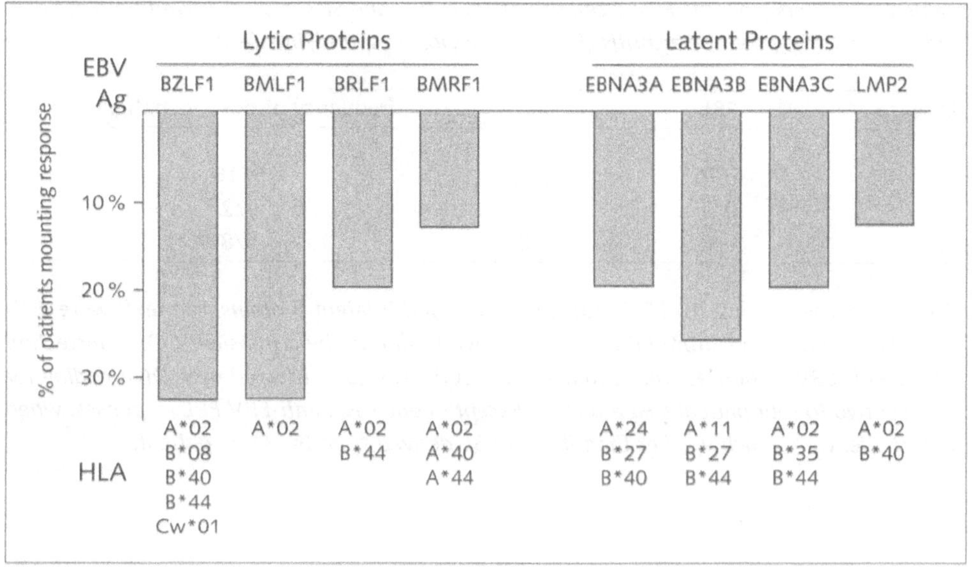

Figure 3
Features of anti-EBV T cell responses detected in RA synovial samples
Anti-EBV reactivity of SL was evaluated on short-term cultured T cells by transient COS transfection assay. In this figure are indicated (i) the fraction of EBV-responsive patients mounting a significant TNF response towards COS cells transfected with a given EBV protein and (ii) the HLA restriction of the responses.

sample and five synovial AS samples (Tab. 2) (E. Scotet et al., manuscript submitted). Noteworthy was that anti-EBV responses in AS patients were predominantly HLA-B27-restricted, although other HLA class I alleles were also involved. These preliminary observations would suggest that synovial trapping and expansion of EBV-reactive T cells is associated with chronic articular inflammation, regardless of its etiology. They may also reveal a peculiar antigen-processing behavior of HLA-B27 alleles that could account for their association with disease susceptibility.

Relationships between antigen specificity and TCR features of SL: implications for the interpretation of T cell repertoire studies

It is generally assumed that synovial over-representation of T cell subsets carrying a particular Vβ region and conserved junctional features reflects the occurrence of

Table 2 - Frequency of anti-EBV T cell responses in PBL and SL samples derived from patients with chronic RA, psoriatic arthritis (PA) and ankylosing spondylitis (AS)

Disease	PBL	SL	frequency of positive patients
RA	4/16	9/16	9/16
PA	0/2	1/2	1/2
AS	0/8	5/8	5/8

T cell responses against 16 EBV proteins (6 lytic and 9 latent proteins, see text) were estimated on short-term cultured PBL and SL-derived cell lines by a transient COS transfection assay. Anti-EBV responses were evaluated on COS cells cotransfected with DNA coding for at most two to four patient's HLA alleles. Except in one case, anti-EBV PBL responses, when detectable, were much weaker than those of SL derived from the same patient.

clonal expansions driven by nominal antigens [7, 8]. More generally, because of the structural constraints imposed by the antigen on TCR V regions, T cell clonotypes directed against a given MHC/peptide complex are expected to share recurrent motifs on their TCR antigen binding loops (e.g. common Vα or Vβ regions and/or common residues at particular positions on their junctional loops) [7, 8]. A corollary to this second assumption is that the diversity of the TCR expressed by a given T cell population should grossly correlate with the diversity of its recognized antigens. Putting together the extensive repertoire and specificity analyses performed on one RA patient (R1) allowed us to directly address the above issues (Fig. 1 and Tab. 1). Most synovial T cell clones derived from over-represented TCR Vβ subsets in patient R1 were reactive against EBV. Hence, synovial repertoire alterations seen in this patient appeared to be closely associated with an EBV-driven selection of synovial clonotypes. Strikingly, most over-represented synovial T cell clones from patient R1 were directed against the same MHC/peptide complex (i.e. the BZLF1 peptide SENDRLRLL associated with HLA-B*4002), although they generally expressed TCR with weakly homologous Vβ and Vα regions and unrelated TCR junctional sequences (Tab. 1). This kind of situation, where a given MHC/peptide complex is recognized by a set of TCR without any obvious primary sequence homology, is probably very common since similar observations were made with a variety of peptide antigens presented by either MHC class I or class II isotypes [25, 26]. Hence, in light of the lack of correlation between the homogeneity of the TCR repertoire of an antigen-selected T cell population and that of the selecting antigens, interpretations of SL repertoire studies without knowing SL specificity should be viewed with caution: while the presence of clones with shared

TCR features is certainly a good indication for an ongoing selection by a particular MHC/peptide complex, lack of such recurrent TCR motifs within synovial T cells should not be taken as evidence against the occurrence of a local antigen-driven T cell selection.

Importance of anti-EBV T cell responses in RA, as compared to previously described T cell specificities

How frequent are EBV-specific immune responses in arthritis patients?

These observations suggest that enrichment of EBV-reactive T cells within inflamed joints occurs in about half of chronic RA patients and in 2/3 of SA patients ([14, 15], manuscript submitted). This frequency is certainly underestimated because responses directed against EBV were evaluated for 16 EBV proteins only, in the context of at most half of the patient's HLA class I alleles. Nevertheless, this increased frequency of EBV-reactive T cells is clearly in line with the numerous previous observations linking EBV to RA, and in particular with the demonstration of elevated titers of anti-EBV antibodies, increased frequency of EBV-infected B cells, increased viral loads, and the frequent presence of EBV genome in synovial tissues in RA patients (reviewed in [27–29]. It is thus surprising that synovial T cell responses against EBV have not been previously reported.

Several reasons might account for these apparent failures. First, EBV-reactive synovial T cell lines or clones might have been erroneously referred to as "autoreactive", such as the $CD4^+$ synovial T cell clones obtained by Friedman et al. [30] directed against HLA-DRB1*04$^+$ BLC [30], or the $CD8^+$ synovial T cell clones derived from several AS patients by Hermann et al. [31] which recognized in an HLA-B*27-restricted fashion autologous BLC. Indeed, in both cases, recognition of EBV epitopes could not be ruled out since T cell clone reactivity towards EBV-negative targets was not evaluated. Secondly, it is also possible that EBV recognition is a feature more specific to $CD8^+$ than to $CD4^+$ synovial T cells. Since most studies have focused on the analysis of $CD4^+$ clones, they might have missed this kind of antiviral response. This hypothesis, however, seems rather unlikely because $CD4^+$ SL recognizing autologous BLCs were systematically found in patients developing synovial anti-EBV responses ([14] and E. Scotet, X. Saulquin, M.A. Peyrat, M. Bonneville, E. Houssaint, unpublished observations). A third explanation might be linked to the clinical status of the groups of patients studied. We selected patients with long-term aggressive disease but we do not have any data yet from patients at earlier stages of the disease. Thus, the possibility that anti-EBV synovial T cell responses are a specific feature of late, chronic RA patients cannot be excluded and, in fact, would be in agreement with studies suggesting that anti-EBV serological alterations are preferentially found within groups developing more aggressive RA [32].

Frequency of EBV-reactive synovial T cells as compared to that of SL when recognizing previously-described antigens

An obvious way to determine the relative importance of anti-EBV responses in RA pathogenesis, as compared to those directed against other endogenous or exogenous determinants, is to assess the respective frequencies of T cells reactive against the above antigens. However, such comparisons are rather difficult to make because the clinical status of the patients studied is seldom well defined. The choice of T cell samples (PBL or SL) and the way *in vitro* specificity assays have been performed (antigen preparation, T cell culture conditions, etc.) are also obvious critical parameters and here again it is sometimes difficult to determine whether or not the approach chosen allowed an optimal detection of T cells reactive against a given antigen. All these considerations may explain to a large extent the controversies regarding the relative importance of T cell responses to several candidate antigens such as type II collagen or mycobacterial heat shock proteins in RA patients (reviewed in [7]). Finally, the main reason that makes comparisons between T cell responses to viral antigens or other candidate antigens impossible or difficult is the current lack of T cell frequency data for most synovial samples studied so far. Results from our laboratory indicated that, in two patients, EBV-reactive SL represented at least 20 to 40% of $CD8^+$ T cells and close to 100% of clones derived from over-represented TCR Vβ subsets [14, 15]. Hence, this leaves little room for $CD8^+$ SL with other specificities in these two patients. However, comparable frequencies of type II collagen-reactive clones were previously described in one RA patient (33), thus indicating that the dominant antigens recognized by SL can be highly heterogeneous. As mentioned earlier, such a heterogeneity could be related to the stage of the disease but additional studies will definitely be required to address this issue.

Possible origin and physiopathological consequences of anti-EBV T cell responses during RA

Distinct scenarios can be proposed to account for the frequent presence of EBV-reactive T cells within SL and to explain how these could take part in RA pathogenesis, depending on whether EBV cross-activates self-reactive T cells or exclusively triggers virus-specific T cells.

EBV-mediated expansion of self-reactive T cells

Several major mechanisms of activation of self-reactive T cells following exposure to environmental antigens have been described which involve either cross-activation of autoreactive T cells by environmental antigens (e.g. following recognition of nominal epitopes (molecular mimics) or superantigens (SAg)) or upregulation of endogenous proteins recognized by self-reactive T cells. Observations suggesting that EBV could break T cell tolerance to "self" through either of these mechanisms are listed below.

Activation of autoreactive T cells by EBV-derived molecular mimics

In support of this hypothesis the motifs QKRAA or QRRAA, which are specifically shared by MHC class II alleles associated with RA susceptibility [34], have also been found on the gp110 EBV protein [35]. Furthermore, a recent study suggests the occurrence of elevated RA PBL responses to target cells pulsed with QKRAA-containing peptides derived from gp110 [36]. Taken together, these results support a model in which EBV cross-activates T cells reactive against RA susceptibility alleles [28]. Such a hypothesis would remain compatible with the observed diversity of the antigenic specificities of EBV-reactive $CD8^+$ SL [15]. However, a more restricted recognition pattern of EBV-reactive $CD4^+$ SL would be expected, and this remains to be demonstrated. In addition, several observations argue against the central importance of cross-activation of QKRAA-reactive T cells in RA pathogenesis. In particular, recent findings from Roudier and colleagues suggest that the presence of RA motifs, which are recognized by some heat shock proteins, may result in altered routage of the corresponding MHC class II alleles [37]. Hence, these results provide an explanation for the link between the presence of RA motifs and disease susceptibility which does not invoke a direct T cell recognition of such motifs.

Activation of autoreactive T cells by EBV-derived SAg

The implication of SAg in autoimmunity has recently been strengthened by an elegant study demonstrating the existence of human endogenous retroviruses specifically transcribed in type I diabetes patients and able to activate in a superantigenic fashion a Vβ T cell subset known to be enriched within β islet-infiltrating T cells from diabetes patients [38, 39]. In a similar fashion, SAg known to be expressed by EBV (40) may cross-activate self-reactive pathogenic T cells carrying the appropriate TCR Vβ region. Currently available data, however, do not really support an implication of SAg (either of viral or endogenous origin) in RA pathogenesis. In particular, none of the initial studies suggesting recurrent expansion of T cells with particular Vβ regions during RA have, as yet, been confirmed [7, 8]. Furthermore, none of the expanded TCR Vβ subsets described to date seem to correspond to those directed against known EBV SAg [7, 8, 40].

Activation of autoreactive T cells following virus-mediated transactivation of endogenous protein expression

This hypothesis is supported by recent observations showing that the p40 tax transactivator derived from HTLV-1, a retrovirus with arthritogenic properties [41], is able to upregulate expression of some autoantigens recognized by sera of systemic sclerosis patients [42]. It could be hypothesized that EBV transactivators may similarly upregulate expression of endogenous articular components, thus possibly resulting in breakage of T cell tolerance to the corresponding protein(s). Here again, although supported by preliminary observations, such a possibility remains to be directly and formally demonstrated.

In conclusion, although an EBV-mediated activation of T cells reactive against articular antigens or against RA susceptibility alleles cannot be formally ruled out, this hypothesis, whose corollary would be an implication of EBV in early stages of RA, is not supported by strong experimental evidence. Furthermore, several studies showing that anti-EBV serological alterations and increased virus loads are mainly found within patients developing aggressive chronic RA [32] would rather favour a late, indirect role for EBV in RA pathogenesis (see below).

Joint destruction mediated by virus-specific T cells

The role of environmental factors, like viruses and bacteria, in autoimmunity is well explained by models of reactive arthritis [43]. According to these models, modification of the homing and chemotactic properties of peripheral T cells upon recognition of common pathogens will result in their preferential migration to already inflamed synovia and lead to subsequent aggravation of articular-structure erosion [13, 43]. Such a model allows several predictions regarding the nature and diversity of the inducing pathogens (viruses or bacteria), the generality of the phenomenon, and the way pathogen-specific T cells could take part in the perpetuation of the autoimmune process.

Diversity of the pathogens possibly involved in chronic arthritis

Frequent enrichment of EBV-reactive T cells during chronic arthritis could merely be the consequence of peripheral reactivation of EBV-specific memory cells, which would then non-specifically migrate to chronically inflamed joints. In support of this, several *in vivo* models have shown (i) that activated T cell blasts, regardless of their antigen specificity, home preferentially to inflamed synovia [44] and (ii) that HTLV-I-infected T cells can migrate directly to affected joints in patients with polyarthritis [45]. If this homing process is simply linked to chronic inflammation of the synovium [44], one would expect that synovial enrichment of EBV-reactive cells would not be restricted to rheumatoid arthritis but would rather be observed in most arthritic processes, regardless of their etiology. Accordingly, increased frequency of EBV-reactive SL was found not only in RA patients, but also in psoriatic arthritis and AS patients. One would also expect that synovial T cells reactive against other common pathogens would also be enriched in some arthritic patients. Although this prediction remains to be tested in RA, several bacterial and viral candidates (*Yersinia*, *Shigella*, *Chlamidia*, HTLV-I, etc.) have already been implicated in AS and other arthritides [43]. Such heterogeneity of the cofactors possibly involved in chronicity of the inflammatory process could explain the apparent lack of EBV-reactive SL in some RA and AS patients. In these cases it might be worth testing the reactivity of SL towards common pathogens whose involvement in chronic arthritis has been previously suspected (e.g. HHV6, HHV8, parvo- and retroviruses) [41, 46, 47].

Possible pathogenic role of virus-specific SL

Once in inflamed joints, T cells specific for EBV or other pathogens could exert a direct pathogenic role without necessarily recognizing articular self-antigens. For instance, EBV-reactive SL may directly recognize virus-infected synovial cells, which would then result in T cell-mediated destruction of articular tissues and local release of inflammatory cytokines and chemokines. In this respect, a recent study suggests that major synovial T cell targets like type I synoviocytes can be productively infected by EBV and corresponding virus-infected synoviocyte lines can be isolated from RA patients [48]. Furthermore, although the presence of EBV genome in inflamed joints during RA has long been a controversial issue [49–51], a recent analysis performed by Posnett and colleagues [29] confirms that this virus is detectable in most synovial samples from RA patients. Alternatively, since both EBV-specific T cells and EBV-infected B cells are expected to be colocalized in synovial tissues [27, 28], T cell independent erosion processes could be triggered by T cell-derived factors released upon recognition of virus-infected B cells. In support of this second possibility, mice transgenic for a TCR reactive against a B cell-derived antigen were shown to develop an autoimmune disease very similar to rheumatoid arthritis, thus indicating that chronic T cell activation by systemic antigens can result in an organ-specific autoimmune disease [51].

Conclusion and perspectives

The demonstration of frequent recognition of EBV by synovial T cells from RA and AS patients has revived the connection between infection and autoimmunity and the paradigm of a central role played by T cells in autoimmune arthritides. Although available data would favour the hypothesis of an indirect pathogenicity of virus-specific T cells, it remains unclear whether these findings reflect a primary implication of EBV in RA etiology or a secondary function of this and other pathogens in disease perpetuation. In this respect, more extensive and systematic analyses of both $CD4^+$ and $CD8^+$ synovial subsets towards proteins derived from a larger set of candidate infectious agents will be required to directly address the above issues. Such studies may help in devising new therapeutic strategies in RA and other chronic inflammatory diseases should synovial T cell recognition of a restricted set of recurrent pathogens be confirmed.

Acknowledgements
We thank Dr François Lang for critical reading of the manuscript and helpful comments.

References

1 Van Boxel JA, Pagel SA (1975) Predominately T cell infiltrate in rheumatoid synovial membranes. *N Engl J Med* 293: 517–520
2 Stastny P (1978) Association of the B-cell alloantigen Drw4 with rheumatoid arthritis. *N Engl J Med* 298: 867–871
3 Burmester GR, Yu DTY, Irani AM, Kunkel HG, Winchester R (1981) Ia+ T cells in synovial fluid and tissues of patients with rheumatoid arthritis. *Arthritis Rheum* 24: 1370–1376
4 Hemler ME, Glass D, Coblyn JS, Jacobson JG (1986) Very late activation antigens on rheumatoid synovial fluid T lymphocytes: association with stages of T cell activation. *J Clin Invest* 78: 696–702
5 Thomas R, McIlraith M, Davis LS, Lipsky PE (1992) Rheumatoid synovium is enriched in CD45Bdim mature memory T cells that are potent helpers for B cell differentiation. *Arthritis Rheum* 35: 1455–1465
6 Kohem CL, Brezinschek RI, Wisbey H, Tortorella C, Lipsky PE, Oppenheimer-Marks N (1996) Enrichment of differentiated CD45 RBdim, CD27-memory T cells in the peripheral blood, synovial fluid, and synovial tissue of patients with rheumatoid arthritis. *Arthritis Rheum* 39: 844–854
7 Sakkas LI, Chen PF, Platsoucas CD (1994) T cell antigen receptors in rheumatoid arthritis. *Immunol Res* 13: 117–138
8 Struyk L, Hawes GE, Chatila MK, Breedveld FC, Kurnick JT, van der Elsen PJ (1995) T cell receptors in rheumatoid arthritis. *Arthritis Rheum* 38: 577–599
9 Kotzin BL, Strober S, Engleman EG, Calin A, Hoppe RT, Kansas GS, Terrel CP, Kaplan HS (1981) Treatment of intractable rheumatoid arthritis with total lymphoid irradiation. *N Engl J Med* 305: 969–976
10 Yocum DE, Klippel JH, Wilder RL, Gerber NL, Austin HA, Wahl SM, Lesko L, Minor

JR, Preuss HG, Yarboro C et al (1988) Cyclosporin A in treatment of severe refractory rheumatoid arthritis: a randomized study. *Ann Intern Med* 109: 863–869

11 Horneff G, Burmester GR, Emmrich F, Kalden JR (1991) Treatment of rheumatoid arthritis with an anti-CD4 monoclonal antibody. *Arthritis Rheum* 34: 129–140

12 Firestein GS, Zvaifler NJ (1990) How important are T cells in chronic rheumatoid arthritis? *Arthritis Rheum* 33: 768–773

13 Fox DA (1997) The role of T cells in the immunopathogenesis of rheumatoid arthritis: new perspectives. *Arthritis Rheum* 40: 598–609

14 David-Ameline J, Lim A, Davodeau F, Peyrat MA, Berthelot JM, Semana G, Pannetier C, Gaschet J, Vié H, Even J et al (1996) Selection of T cells reactive against autologous B lymphoblastoid cells during chronic RA. *J Immunol* 157: 4697–4707

15 Scotet E, David-Ameline J, Peyrat MA, Moreau-Aubry A, Pinczon D, Lim A, Even J, Semana G, Berthelot JM, Breathnach R et al (1996) T-cell response to Epstein-Barr virus transactivators in chronic rheumatoid arthritis. *J Exp Med* 184: 1791–1800

16 Koopman WJ (1994) The future of biologics in the treatment of rheumatoid arthritis. *Sem Arthritis Rheum* 23: 50–67

17 Arnett FC, Edworthy SM, Bloch DA, McShane DJ, Fries JF, Cooper NS, Healey LA, Kaplan SR, Liang MH, Luthra HS et al (1988) The American Rheumatism Association 1987 revised criteria for the classification of rheumatoid arthritis. *Arthritis Rheum* 31: 315–324

18 Even J, Lim A, Puisieux I, Ferradini L, Dietrich PY, Toubert A, Hercend T, Triebel F, Pannetier C, Kourislky P (1995) T cell repertoires in healthy and diseased human tissues analyzed by T cell receptor b chain CDR3 size determination: evidence for clonal expansions in tumors and inflammatory diseases. *Res Immunol* 146: 65–85

19 Pannetier C, Delassus S, Darche S, Saucier C, Kourislky P (1993) Quantitative titration of nucleic acids by enzymatic amplification reactions run to saturation. *Nucl Acids Res* 21: 577–586

20 Vié H, Chevalier S, Garand R, Moisan JP, Praloran V, Devilder MC, Moreau JF, Soulillou JP (1989) Clonal expansion of lymphocytes bearing the gamma/delta receptor in a patient with a large granular lymphocyte disorder. *Blood* 74: 285–296

21 Davodeau F, Peyrat MA, Gaschet J, Hallet MM, Triebel F, Vié H, Kabelitz D, Bonneville M (1994) Surface expression of functional T cell receptor chains formed by interlocus recombination on human T lymphocytes. *J Exp Med* 180: 1685–1694

22 Brichard V, van Pel A, Wölfel T, Wölfel C, DePlaen E, Lethé B, Coulie P, Boon T (1993) The tyrosinase gene codes for an antigen recognized by autologous cytolytic T lymphocytes on HLA-A2 melanomas. *J Exp Med* 178: 489–495

23 Seed B, Aruffo A (1987) Molecular cloning of the CD2 antigen, the T cell erythrocyte receptor, by a rapid immunoselection procedure. *Proc Natl Acad Sci USA* 84: 3365–3369

24 Kieff E (1996) Epstein-Barr virus and its replication. In: Fields BN, Knipe DM, Howley PM (eds) *Field Virology*. Philadelphia: Lippincott-Raven Publishers, 2343–2395

25 de Campos-Lima PO, Levitsky V, Imreh MP, Gavioli R, Masucci MG (1997) Epitope-

dependent selection of highly restricted or diverse T cell receptor repertoires in response to persistent infection by Epstein-Barr virus. *J Exp Med* 186: 83–89

26 Shanmugam A, Copie-Bergman C, Falissard B, Delrieu O, Jais JP, Rebibo D, Bach JF, Tournier-Lasserve E (1996) TCR αβ gene usage for myelin basic protein recognition in healthy monozygous twins. *J Immunol* 156: 3747–3754

27 Fox RI, Luppi M, Pisa P, Kang HI (1992) Potential role of Epstein-Barr virus in Sjögren's syndrome and rheumatoid arthritis. *J Rheumatol* 19: 18–24

28 Venables P (1988) Epstein-Barr virus infection and autoimmunity in rheumatoid arthritis. *Ann Rheum Dis* 47: 265–269

29 Posnett DN, Edinger J (1997) When do microbes stimulate rheumatoid factor? *J Exp Med* 185: 1721–1723

30 Li X, Sun GR, Tumang JR, Crow MK, Friedman SM (1994) CDR3 sequence motifs shared by oligoclonal rheumatoid arthritis synovial T cells: evidence for an antigen-driven response. *J Clin Invest* 94: 2525–2534

31 Hermann E, Yu DT, Meyer zum BŸschenfelde KH, Fleischer B (1993) HLA-B27-restricted CD8 T cells derived from synovial fluids of patients with reactive arthritis and ankylosing spondylitis. *Lancet* 342: 646–650

32 Jokinen EI, Mottonen TT, Hannonen PJ, Makela M, Arvilommi HS (1994) Prediction of severe rheumatoid arthritis using Epstein-Barr virus. *Br J Rheumatol* 33: 917–922

33 Londei M, Savill CM, Verhoef A, Brennan F, Leech ZA, Duance V, Maini RN, Feldmann M (1989) Persistence of collagen type II-specific T cell clones in the synovial membrane of a patient with rheumatoid arthritis. *Proc Natl Acad Sci USA* 86: 636–640

34 Nepom GT, Byers P, Seyfried C (1989) HLA genes associated with rheumatoid arthritis: identification of susceptibility alleles using specific oligonucleotide probes. *Arthritis Rheum* 32: 15–21

35 Lotz M, Roudier J (1989) Epstein-Barr virus and rheumatoid arthritis: cellular and molecular aspects. *Rheumatol Int* 9: 147–152

36 La Cava A, Carson DA, Albani S (1994) The QKRAA susceptibility sequence to RA, as expressed on the EDV protein gp110, is a target of immune responses in patients with RA. *Arthritis Rheum* 37: S312–314

37 Auger I, Escola JM, Gorvel JP, Roudier J (1996) HLA-DR4 and HLA-DR10 motifs that carry susceptibility to rheumatoid arthritis bind 70-kD heat shock proteins. *Nature Med* 2: 306–310

38 Conrad B, Weidmann E, Trucco G, Rudert WA, Behboo R, Ricordi C, Rodriquez-Rilo H, Finegold D, Trucco M (1994) Evidence for superantigen involvement in insulin-dependent diabetes mellitus aetiology. *Nature* 371: 351–355

39 Conrad B, Weissmahr RN, Böni J, Arcari R, SchŸpbach J, Mach B (1997) A human endogenous retroviral superantigen as candidate autoimmune gene in type I diabetes. *Cell* 90: 303–313

40 Sutkowski N, Palkana T, Ciurli C, Sekaly RP, Thorley-Lawson DA, Huber BT (1996) An Epstein-Barr virus-associated superantigen. *J Exp Med* 184: 971–980

41 Iwakura Y, Tosu M, Yoshida E, Takiguchi M, Sato K, Kitajima I, Nishioka K, Yamamo-

to K, Takeda T, Hatanaka M et al (1991) Induction of inflammatory arthropathy resembling rheumatoid arthritis in mice transgenic for HTLV-I. *Science* 253: 1026–1028

42 Iwakura Y, Saijo S, Kioka Y, Nakayama-Yamada J, Itagaki K, Tosu M, Asano M, Kanai Y, Kakimoto K (1995) Autoimmunity induction by human T cell leukemia virus type I in transgenic mice that develop chronic inflammatory arthropathy resembling rheumatoid arthritis in humans. *J Immunol* 155: 1588–1598

43 Sieper J, Kingsley G (1996) Recent advances in the pathogenesis of reactive arthritis. *Immunol Today* 17: 160–163

44 Liao HX, Haynes BF (1995) Role of adhesion molecules in the pathogenesis of rheumatoid arthritis. *Rheum Dis Clin North Am* 21: 715–740

45 Yoshida M (1993) HTLV-I Tax: regulation of gene expression and disease. *Trends in Microbiology* 1: 131–134

46 Newkirk MM, Watanabe-Duffy KN, Leclerc J, Lambert N, Shiroky JB (1994) Detection of cytomegalovirus, Epstein-Barr virus and Herpes virus-6 in patients with rheumatoid arthritis with or without Sjögren's syndrome. *Br J Rheumatol* 33: 317–322

47 Simpson RW, McGinty L, Simon L, Smith CA, Godzeski CW, Boyd RJ (1984) Association of parvoviruses with rheumatoid arthritis in humans. *Science* 223: 1425–1428

48 Koide J, Takada K, Sugiura M, Sekine H, Ito T, Saito K, Mori S, Takeuchi T, Uchida S, Abe T (1997) Spontaneous establishment of an Epstein-Barr virus-infected fibroblast line from the synovial tissue of a rheumatoid arthritis patient. *J Virol* 71: 2478–2481

49 Zhang L, Nikkari S, Skurnik M (1993) Detection of herpes viruses by polymerase chain reaction in lymphocytes from patients with rheumatoid arthritis. *Arthritis Rheum* 36: 1080–1086

50 Newkirk MM, Watanabe-Duffy KN, Paleckova A, Ivaskova E, Galianova A, Seeman J, Vojtechovsky K, Dostal T (1995) *J Rheumatol* 22: 2055–2061

51 Kouskoff V, Korganow AS, Duchatelle V, Degott C, Benoist C, Mathis D (1996) Organ-specific disease provoked by systemic autoimmunity. *Cell* 87: 811–822

T cell responses in reactive and Lyme arthritis

Joachim Sieper and Jürgen Braun

Department of Medicine, Division of Nephrology and Rheumatology, Klinikum Benjamin Franklin, Free University, Hindenburgdamm 30, D-12200 Berlin, Germany

Introduction

In reactive arthritis (ReA) and Lyme arthritis the triggering antigen is known, which is in contrast to that for rheumatoid arthritis. Thus, in these two arthritides the antigen-specific T cell response can be investigated in detail and lessons learned for other rheumatic diseases: not only for rheumatoid arthritis but also for ankylosing spondylitis where T cells are also believed to play an important role in the pathogenesis.

T cell response in reactive arthritis

Reactive arthritis can occur after bacterial or viral infection with a variety of different pathogens. In this overview we will concentrate on the form of reactive arthritis that has an association with the major histocompatibility complex (MHC) class I antigen human leukocyte antigen (HLA)-B27 of between 50 and 80%. The main bacteria in this context are *Chlamydia trachomatis,* infecting the urogenital tract, and Yersinia, Salmonella, Shigella, and Campylobacter in the gut [1]. Other bacteria, such as *Chlamydia pneumoniae* [2], are also uncommon triggers of HLA-B27-associated ReA [3].

Bacterium-specific T cell response in synovial fluid

Dennis Ford was the first to describe a proliferative response of synovial mononuclear cells (MNC) to the triggering bacteria in ReA [4]. The presence of this specific T cell response was subsequently confirmed by others [5, 6, 7]. The detection of bacterial antigen in the joint by various methods in the last 10 years [8, 9, 10, 11] suggests that locally persisting antigen drives this immune response in the joint. Comparable T cell proliferation can also be observed in peripheral blood (PB) cells,

T Cells in Arthritis, edited by P. Miossec, W.B. van den Berg and G.S. Firestein

albeit in only about 20% of those patients who show the response in synovial fluid (SF) [12]). Such a response in PB seems to be time dependent, because it was detectable at the high value of up to 50% of patients between weeks two and four after the start of arthritis [12]. Both T cells and macrophages are highly activated in SF compared to PB and, furthermore, there is a wide variation in the T cell/macrophage ratio in SF of ReA patients [13]. It has therefore been speculated that part of the observed T cell response in ReA might be non-specific, resulting from recruitment of circulating T cells from the peripheral blood [14, 15].

Limiting dilution to determine the antigen-specific T cell frequency in synovial fluid yielded a value between 1/600 and 1/5000, clearly higher than in peripheral blood (mean 1/7350) [16]. The higher response in SF compared to PB was independent of whether the antigen presenting cells were taken from SF or PB, suggesting that the antigen specific T cell frequency is indeed higher in the joint, contrary to the proposal that the source of the antigen presenting cells is the critical variable [17, 18]. In serial investigations of synovial T cell responses in ReA and Lyme arthritis, antigen specificity remained constant over time, further supporting the concept of a local antigen-specific T cell response [19]. The higher T cell proliferation in SF is not simply due to a higher proportion of $CD45RO^+$ T cells compared to PB because the same difference was found in the $CD45RD^+$ T cell subsets in SF and PB [20]. The presence of an antigen-specific oligoclonal T cell expansion in the joint is also suggested by the finding of limited T cell receptor (TCR) usage in HLA-B27 restricted $CD8^+$ cytotoxic T cell clones [21] or in fresh T cells [22] derived from the synovial fluid of ReA patients. Although it is doubtful whether synovial lymphocyte proliferative responses provide a useful diagnostic test [23, 24] because of unclear sensitivity and specificity [3, 19], it is important as a tool for investigating the T cell response in ReA.

About twice as many CD4 T cells as CD8 T cells are present in the synovial fluid of ReA patients [25]. The relative role of these two T cell subsets for the immune response in ReA is not clear. Furthermore, MHC-unrestricted gamma delta-T cells specific for Yersinia have also been reported in ReA [26].

Thus, based on the presence of an antigen-specific T cell response in synovial fluid it was logical to investigate the specificity of the bacterial epitopes recognized by synovial T cells and the cytokine pattern.

Bacterial epitopes in the CD4 T cell response

The synovial T cell proliferative response to bacteria is predominantly one of CD4 cells [5]. Although this response is mainly specific for the triggering bacterium, it is less clear which are immunodominant among the approximately 2000 proteins present in a bacterium. Previous attempts to identify the target antigens in ReA have concentrated on Yersinia [27, 28, 29] and *Chlamydia trachomatis* [30, 31, 32]. We and others had started to test biochemically purified proteins for immunodominance; the 19 kDa urease β-subunit and 13 kDa ribosomal protein have been identified as stimulatory for synovial CD4 T cells in Yersinia-induced ReA patients [27, 28, 29]. Subsequently this apporach was extended by including a range of Yersinia-recombinant proteins [33]. We could confirm that the 19kd urease β-subunit is a T cell antigen in Yersinia-induced ReA, and we found three other Yersinia-antigens to be highly reactive: the 18 kDa OMP H, the 32 kDa ribosomal L2 protein, and heat shock protein (hsp)60. All these proteins are highly conserved and therefore good targets for a cross-reactive immune reponse among bacteria and between bacteria and autologous antigens.

Among the Yersinia-proteins, the 19 kDa protein was not recognized by synovial T cells from patients with arthritis of different etiology and might therefore be suitable for future diagnosis of Yersinia-induced ReA. The strongest immunodominant antigen was clearly the Yersinia hsp60, although previous reports regarding the role of hsp60 in Yersinia-induced ReA are contradictory [34, 35]. Using the recombinant homologues from Yersinia, Chlamydia, Borrelia, and the human counterpart we could demonstrate a broad recognition of the different bacterial and human hsp60's by SF T cells from all patients with Yersinia ReA tested. This demonstrates cross-recognition of hsp through conserved epitopes. Recognition of conserved epitopes within the hsp60-family members seems to be confined to patients with Yersina-ReA, since two patients with Chlamydia-ReA recognized only the Chlamydia-hsp but no other hsp60's in the same study.

Gaston et al have described synovial $CD4^+$ T cell clones specific for an 18 kDa histone-like protein and for the 57 kDa hsp of *Chlamydia trachomatis*, in patients with Chlamydia-induced ReA [30, 31, 32]. The hsp60-specific T cell clone recognized only hsp60 from *Chlamydia trachomatis* and *Chlamydia pneumoniae* but not hsp60 derived from enterobacteria. The epitope for the $CD4^+$ T cell response was indeed found only on chlamydial hsp60 but not on others [36].

The antigen-specific $CD8^+$ T cell response in reactive arthritis

Although there is a clear CD4 response to different antigens derived from ReA-associated bacteria, the CD8 response is of special interest in ReA and related diseases such as ankylosing spondylitis because of the high association of the MHC class I antigen HLA-B27 with reactive arthritis (50–80% positivity) and ankylosing spondylitis (95% positivity). The prinicipal function of MHC molecules is the presentation of antigenic peptides to T cells. While MHC class II molecules present peptides to $CD4^+$ T cells, CD8 T cells respond to the MHC class I/peptide complex. One attractive explanation for the HLA-B27 association is that presentation of a bacterial peptide and/or cross-reacting peptide by HLA-B27to $CD8^+$ T cells might be a crucial step in the pathogenesis of the disease [1, 37].

The relative importance of CD4+ and CD8+ T cells in resisting infections with ReA-associated bacteria is unclear. Proteins from pathogens such as Yersinia, Chlamydia, and Salmonella are normally presented via the MHC class II antigen presentation pathway to CD4+ T cells, while pathogens with access to the cytoplasm (viruses, Listeria, or Shigella) by pathway I [38]. However, it has been shown in humans or mice that the ReA-triggering bacteria Yersinia [39, 40], Salmonella [41], and Chlamydia [42, 43, 44] can also induce a CD8+ T cell response. Although the exact mechanism by which bacterial antigens gain access to pathway I is not known, several possibilities have been discussed [45].

The first major study indicating that bacteria-specific CD8+ T cells are indeed present in the joint of ReA patients was that of Hermann et al [39]. They raised Yersinia-specific CD8+ T cell clones from synovial fluid, which recognized Yersinia-infected target cells in an HLA-B27 restricted manner. Subsequently, we too raised Yersinia-specific CD8+ T cell lines from SF in ReA patients [40]. Investigation of pools of peptides derived from proteins known to be relevant to the CD4 response, and fulfilling the HLA-B27 binding motif, revealed that mainly the pool of peptides from the Yersinia hsp60 was recognized in an HLA-B27-restricted fashion. Furthermore, we could identify a single peptide (amino acid sequence 321–329) derived from this protein which was recognised by cytotoxic CD8+ T cells from three patients. Futhermore, synovial T cell lines, from patients with Yersinia-induced ReA, raised by repeated stimulation with the pool of peptides from the hsp60 and specific for the very same peptide could indeed lyse target cells infected with Yersinia, suggesting that this peptide is naturally processed [40].

For *Chlamydia trachomatis* the role of CD8+ T cells in ReA is less clear. An earlier study [46] failed to show any cytotoxic T cell response against target cells infected with *Chlamydia trachomatis*. Using an HLA-B27 transgenic mouse model we raised a CD8+ T cell response against Chlamydia, which was HLA-B27 restricted [44]. In this model it was also possible to induce a CD8+ T cell response to the chlamydial 57 kDa hsp by immunisation with it. However, the protein was not a major target of the Chlamydia-specific CD8 response. This model makes it possibile to identify single peptides from Chlamydia presented by HLA-B27; their relevance could then be tested in patients with Chlamydia-induced ReA.

Cytokine pattern in reactive arthritis

Cytokines play an important role in the regulation and outcome of an immune response. T helper type (Th) 1 and Th2 subsets have been implicated in the regulation of many immune responses (overview in [47]). The Th1-type cytokines interferon (IFN)-γ and tumor necrosis factor (TNF)-α are required for an effective cellular immune response against intracellular bacteria, while Th2 cells (secreting IL-4 and IL-5) are responsible for the induction of a humoral response. Two other important cytokines which regulate the Th1 and Th2 responses are interleukin (IL)-12 and IL-10. IL-12 selectively induces a Th1 cytokine pattern against which IL-10 is an important negative regulator.

In infections with intracellular microbes such as Leishmania and *Mycobacterium leprae*, a Th1 response is essential for elimination of bacteria while a Th2 response is associated with susceptibility and dissemination. For the ReA-associated bacteria, animal models and *in vitro* experiments indicate that Th1-type cytokines such as IFN-γ, IL-12, and TNF-α are also crucial for effective elimination of these bacteria [48, 49, 50]. Since persistent bacteria/bacterial antigen can be detected in the joint of ReA patients it is an obvious question as to whether T cells fail to eliminate bacteria. In context with the Th1/Th2 dichotomy this asks whether a Th2 pattern in ReA patients, locally and/or systemically, contributes to bacterial persistence. Earlier studies using Yersinia- [51] and Chlamydia-specific [52] T cell clones derived from synovial fluid of ReA patients suggested the presence of a Th1 pattern in the joint. However, this might have been due to the *in vitro* culture conditions during the cloning procedure.

Subsequently we reported that the key cytokine for a Th2 response, IL-4, was found in synovial membrane of ReA patients more frequently than in rheumatoid arthritis patients using the technique of PCR and *in situ*-hybridisation [53]. In another study the Th1/Th2 cytokine secretion pattern upon stimulation of synovial fluid mononuclear cells with the triggering bacterium was investigated in ReA patients [54]. These cells secreted low amounts of IFN-γ and TNF-α but high amounts of IL-10 also hinting towards a Th2 pattern in ReA. Interestingly, IL-10 was responsible for suppression of IFN-γ and TNF-α, as judged by the effect of adding either anti-IL-10 or exogenous IL-10 to these cultures. Adding neutralizing anti-IL-12 completely abolished the effects of anti-IL-10 suggesting that inhibition of the Th1-like cytokines by IL-10 was mediated through suppression of IL-12. Exogenous IL-12 clearly enhanced IFN-γ and TNF-α secretion. The cytokine pattern became even clearer by comparison with Lyme-arthritis [55]. Here a clearly higher TNFα/IL-10 ratio could be found than in ReA. A significantly higher IL-10/TNFα ratio was also detected in peripheral blood mononuclear cells (MNC) in 53 patients with early reactive arthritis (disease duration less than 8 weeks) compared to patients with early Lyme arthritis or patients with untreated, early rheumatoid arthritis after mitogenic stimulation [56].

Investigating synovial membrane by immunohistology the ratio of cells positive for the Th2-cytokine, IL-4, to cells positive for IFNγ was higher in ReA than in rheumatoid arthritis or in Lyme-arthritis [55, 57, 58]. Other researchers also reported recently a smaller number of IFNγ$^+$ cells in ReA synovial membrane compared to rheumatoid arthritis [58]. In contrast, using a nested PCR for the detection of cytokine mRNA in synovial membrane from patients with different forms of arthritis, less IFNγ was detected in RA compared to ReA [59]. IL-4 was rarely detected.

In our experience, it is methodologically difficult to demonstrate small differences in T cell cytokines using PCR for synovial membrane biopsies [54]. By analysing T cells from synovial fluid at the single cell level we showed that the ratio of IL-4 to IFNγ^+ T cells was indeed higher in ReA than in RA [58] using the method of intracellular cytokine staining after mitogenic *in vitro* stimulation with subsequent analysis by flow cytometry [60].

Interestingly, using bulk cultures from synovial fluid or peripheral blood a Th2-like pattern could only be detected by analysing IL-10/TNFα ratios but not for the typical Th1/Th2-cytokines Il-4/IFNγ while at the single cell level a more Th2-like pattern was found analysing the latter two cytokines. In bulk cultures the differences in T cell cytokine secretions might be too small to be detectable by enzyme linked immuno sorbent assay (ELISA) but might be sufficient to drive the monocyte secretion pattern due to close cell contacts towards Th1 (TNFα) or Th2 (IL-10). It has been reported that Th1-like cells induce high TNFα secretion in monocytes while, after being stimulated in the presence of Th2-like cells, monocytes secrete lower levels of TNFα [61].

Taken together, these data seem to indicate that a Th2-type cytokine pattern predominates in the joint of ReA. As Th1-type cytokines are necessary for elimination of ReA-associated bacteria, Th2-cytokines might contribute to bacterial persistence in the joint. Furthermore, the IL-10/IL-12 balance appears to be crucial for regulation of the cytokine pattern in the joint of ReA patients.

Pathogenesis of reactive arthritis

How can this data be used to explain the pathogenesis of reactive arthritis? The described Th-2 pattern might contribute to the persistence of bacterial antigen in ReA. It has been described by several authors that the cellular immune response of reactive arthrits patients measured in the peripheral blood is lower when compared to healthy controls or to patients with an infection of the urogenital tract or the gut who do not develop arthritis [62, 63, 64]. These findings could be explained, at least partly, by the high IL-10 secretion found in ReA [54, 56] which might suppress antigen-specific T cell proliferation [65]. By comparing synovial Chlamydia-specific T cell proliferation with the detection of *Chlamydia trachomatis* in synovial fluid by the PCR technique, an inverse relationship for the dection of antigen and the cellular response to the same antigen was found [3]. Thus, a strong T cell response might lead to an effective elimination of Chlamydia while a weak cellular response might result in persistence. Whether such a Th2 response is determined by genetical factors or is due to environmental influences has to be investigated in the future.

Interestingly, we have recently also found a Th2-like pattern in the peripheral blood of patients with the ReA-related disease ankylosing spondylitis (AS) (J. Braun and J. Sieper, unpublished observations). Only a minority of patients with AS show evidence of exposure to bacteria such as a former episode of ReA or the presence of inflammatory bowel disease which might result in a constant stimulation of the immune system by gut bacteria through the damaged gut mucosa. However, it has been speculated that the majority of patients with so called idiopathic AS might have had a preceding asymptomatic infection or an asymptomatic gut lesion [1]. Therefore, difficulties in handling bacteria due to the presence of a Th2-like pattern could play a pathogenetic role not only in ReA but also in other spondylarthropathies such as AS.

Whether a Th1- or Th2-response results after encounter of the immune system with a pathogen seems also to be antigen-dependant. In our study already mentioned above we could show at the clonal level that cross-reacting T cell clones recognizing both the Yersinia hsp60 and the human hsp60 produced relatively high amounts of IL-10 and IL-4 (Th2-like response) after antigen-specific stimulation while a clone reacting specifically with the Yersinia hsp60 showed more of a Th1-like cytokine secretion [33]. In mice immunized with both autologous and chlamydial hsp60 the antigen-specific T cell response to murine hsp60 was Th1-like while in mice immunized only with the murine one T cells stimulated with the same protein showed no proliferation but secreted IL-10 [66]. Thus, epitopes on autologous hsp60 seem to favour a Th2 response while epitopes specific for bacterial hsp60 a Th1 response. If such an antigen-dependant balance or imbalance in the Th1/Th2 response exists it might offer the opportunity to drive the immune response in the wanted direction. Such an antigen-specific manipulation of the Th1/Th2 balance is an exciting possibility and would avoid the disadvantage of altering the whole immune system would have [61, 67].

The first successes in identifying antigen-specific T cell epitopes derived from bacteria in ReA will make it possible to investigate the antigen-specific cytokine release in more detail [33]. The response to the bacterial hsp60 seems to be relevant both for the CD4 and the CD8 T cell response and need to be further investigated. The relative contribution of the $CD4^+$ and the $CD8^+$ T cell subsets in the pathogenesis of ReA is not yet known. It seems to be likely that CD4 T cells are important in acute ReA and that the cytokine pattern produced by these cells might contribute to elimination or persistence of pathogens [1, 68]. The Th1/Th2 dichotomy has also been described for $CD8^+$ T cells [47]. Whether this is relevant for the immunopathology or not is not clear. An HLA-B27 restricted CD8-response might be mainly relevant for chronic courses because chronicity and some features such as sacroiliitis, enthesitis, and uveitis are strongly linked to HLA-B27. Whether the arthritogenic peptide hypothesis or other hypotheses [reviewed in [1] and [69, 70] can explain the HLA-B27-association has to be determined. Once a bacterium persists this might finally lead to the manifestation of AS if HLA-B27 is present. In any case the identification of T cell epitopes for CD4 and CD8 T cells is a major step forward and allows further investigations looking for cross-reactivity among bacteria and between bacteria and self antigens.

At the moment there are few animal models available (apart from the one mentioned above) that are of some interest in the context of this discussion, two are transgenic for HLA-B27 [71, 72]. In the HLA-B27 transgenic rat [71] and in the HLA-B27 transgenic mice lacking β2-microglobulin [72], arthritis/spondylitis occurs only if animals are raised in an environment which is not germ-free suggesting that interaction of the immune system with pathogens is essential for the manifestation of rheumatic symptoms. However, until now it has neither been possible to identify the crucial bacterium/bacteria or single bacterial antigens in these models nor is the relative contribution of the CD4 and CD8 T cell subsets to the immunopathology clear. When Lewis rats (non-transgenic) are injected intravenously with *Yersinia enterocolitica*, about 70% of the animals develop arthritis resembling human ReA. This model has been used to investigate the effect of antibiotic treatment on the course of arthritis [73]. However, the role of the T cell response is less clear in this model.

T cell response in Lyme arthritis

Lyme borreliosis is a multisystem disease caused by the tickborne spirochetes *Borrelia burgdorferi* (Bb) *sensu strictu*, *Borrelia garinii*, and *Borrelia afzelli* [74, 75]. In Europe all three species are present, while Bb *sensu strictu* has so far only been isolated in North America. Arthritis is a major manifestation which occurs in about 55% of infected, untreated American patients [76]. Similar to ReA Bb persists in the joint making it likely that it drives the local immune response, at least initially. Bb can be detected, by polymerase chain reaction, in the joint of up to 96% of untreated patients, rarely also by culture [77]. While most patients respond to antibiotic therapy, about 10% develop treatment-resistant chronic arthritis. It is not clear why these patients do not respond to antibiotics. Persistent infection and Bb-induced autoimmunity have both been discussed as possible explanations [78, 79].

Infection with Bb does not induce reliable immunity. The earliest detectable serological response is to Bb flagellin while antibodies against outer surface protein A (OspA) can be detected only in some patients with late disease. However, the presence of anti-OspA antibodies is associated with a chronic course of the disease [75]. The humoral immune response seems to play a dominant role in effectively fighting infections with Bb. Most interestingly, antibodies against OspA or OspB protect mice from Lyme borreliosis [75].

$CD4^+$ Borrelia-specific T cells in Lyme arthritis

The role of T cells in Bb infection has been less well investigated compared to that of the humoral immune response. Similar to ReA, synovial fluid MNC proliferate specificly to whole Bb antigen and this response is stronger compared to peripheral blood [24, 80]. Furthermore, the synovial fluid T cell response to Bb remained specific over time in patients with chronic Lyme arthritis [19]. A Bb-specific T cell proliferation has also been reported in peripheral blood of patients with Lyme arthritis [81, 82, 83] but also in healthy controls [84].

CD4$^+$ T cell responses to a variety of Bb-derived antigens such as flagellin, OspA, OspB, OspC, p39, p93, hsp 60 and hsp 70 have been described [78, 81, 85, 86]. However, due to the protective role of OspA-specific antibodies interest has focussed on the T cell response to OspA although the role of OspA-specific T cells is less clear. Despite the fact that a CD4$^+$ T cell clone specific for Bb could induce resistance to Bb infection [87], T cells seem not to be sufficient for the elimination of Bb but rather for an optimal induction of protective antobodies since T cells were unable to confer protection in severe combined immuno deficiency (SCID) mice [88]. After vaccination of mice with OspA a possible protective T cell epitope was identified on the OspA molecule (residues 186–203) [89]. A very similar epitope derived from the OspA molecule was also found to be immunodominant for a CD4$^+$ T cell response both after infection with Bb and after immunization with OspA [90]. Interestingly, this epitope induced IL-4 release by stimulated T cells [90] why this was not the case in the former study [89].

Epitopes on OspA have also been identified in patients with Lyme arthritis. T cell clones from three patients with Lyme arthritis recognized several epitopes on the C-terminal and on the N-terminal part of the molecule [91]. Investigating peripheral blood MNC from patients with Lyme arhritis the strongest response was directed against OspB in patients with both limited and chronic disease [78]. However, OspA was the most frequently recognized antigen by T cell lines from patients with treatment-resistant arthritis, while it was less frequently recognized by treatment-responders. Thus, it was speculated that a T cell response to OspA could be a bad prognostic sign. Whether T cells specific for OspA-epitopes are themselves relevant for the chronicity of the immune response, or whether the detection of such T cells is simply due to longer exposure to Bb, is not clear at the moment. Subsequently, the same authors described that the OspA epitope recognized by these T cells is located at the N-terminal end within amino acid sequence 84–113 [92]. Based on these results the authors have speculated that this epitope might be arthritogenic. In contrast, the OspA epitope described above, at the C-terminal end, might be protective [89].

CD8$^+$ Borrelia-specific T cells in Lyme arthritis

The role of CD8$^+$ T cells in Lyme arthritis is even less clear than that of CD4$^+$ T cells. Provided that Bb is located mainly extracellularly and that the humoral response for which T cell help is necessary is protective [75] there might be no role at all. However, it could be shown in animal experiments that depletion of CD8$^+$ T cells led to a reduced incidence of arthritis, suggesting that $CD8^+$ T cells might be relevant for the generation of protective immunity or alternatively, that $CD8^+$ T cells do play a role as effector cells in the chronic immune response against Bb [93]. Recently it could be demonstrated in humans that a cytotoxic $CD8^+$ T cell against different Bb-derived antigens such as OspA, OspB, and flagellin, is present in PB and SF from patients with Lyme arthritis [94]. However, these experiments were also unable to answer the question as to whether the $CD8^+$ T cells are simply innocent bystanders or part of the immune response which causes immunopathology.

Cytokine pattern in Lyme arthritis

Similar to ReA, the concept of Th1/Th2 balance has attracted much interest recently in attempts to understand the pathogenesis of Lyme disease. Useful data was gained in animal experiments. Depending on the genetic background, infection of inbred mice with Bb resulted in strain-specific disease manifestatins that were associated with polarized lymphokine patterns. The Th2 pattern (in BALB/c mice) was correlated with disease resistance whereas the Th1 cytokine patteren (in C3H mice) was correlated with disease susceptibility [95]. Furthermore, treatment with anti-IL-4 worsened disease in both strains [96], while administration of IL-4 favoured a positive effect [97]. Based on these results it seems to be likely that a Th2 cytokine response protects against Bb infection in mice.

Accumulating evidence in humans suggest that a Th1 pattern can be found in patients with Lyme arthritis and that Lyme arthritis therefore resembles the susceptible strain in animal models. The first study reported in humans found that 16 out of 18 clones prepared from the PB and two clones derived from the SF of four Lyme arthritis patients produced Th1-type cytokines upon stimulation by Bb antigen [85]. In another study spontaneous and Bb-stimulated IFNγ secretion of PB MNC was higher, and IL-4 secretion lower, in patients with Lyme borreliosis compared with healthy controls [98]. We investigated the cytokine pattern in the joints of patients with Lyme arthritis using different methods. Synovial fluid MNC produced high amounts of IFNγ and TNFα, but little IL-10 and little or no IL-4, after stimulation with Bb [55]. The presence of a Th1 pattern became even clearer after comparison with ReA: the TNFα/IL-10 and the IFNγ/IL-10 ratio after antigen-specific stimulation were significantly higher than in ReA using the corresponding triggering bacterial antigens [54]. Using the methods of semi-quantitative PCR and immunohistology, more IFNγ than IL-4 could also be detected in synovial membrane [55]. The Th1 response, especially the production of TNFα, could be down-regulated *in vitro* by IL-10, but not by IL-4 or anti-IL-12, suggesting insufficient IL-10 production *in vivo*.

In general, it is not clear what directs the immune system towards a Th1 response or a Th2 response after encountering microbes. Several factors possibly relevant for this "decision" have been discussed [47]. Using αβ T cell receptor (specific for ovalbumin) transgenic mice it could be shown that Bb itself induced a Th1 response why ReA-associated bacteria such as Yersinia and Salmonella induced a Th2 response [99]. Thus, bacteria try to induce a response which permits their own survival but is harmful to the host.

HLA class II association in Lyme arthritis

The reported association of HLA-DR4 and HLA-DR2 with chronic courses of Lyme arthritis would also support a role for T cells in the pathogenesis of Lyme arthritis [100]. However, DR4Dw4-transgenic mice were not predisposed to the development of chronic Lyme arthrits compared to non-transgenic litter mates [101]. Thus, the role of HLA-DR4 in Lyme arthritis requires further investigation.

Summary and conclusions

A bacterium-specific T cell response to the triggering bacterium is present both in reactive arthritis and Lyme arthritis. A cellular immune response from the host is essential in fighting the ReA-associated bacteria effectively. Therefore, the T cell response found in ReA might not be strong enough to eliminate bacteria but still enough to cause synovitis. This seems to be mediated, at least partly, by a "wrong" Th2-like cytokine pattern found in patients with reactive arthritis. The relative role of the $CD4^+$ and the $CD8^+$ T cell response in ReA is not clear. Both subtypes are present in the joint of ReA patients and both subtypes can recognize the triggering bacterium. Interestingly, $CD8^+$ T cells which are Yersinia-specific and HLA-B27 restricted are present in the joint of patients with Yersinia-induced ReA. T cell responses to bacteria-derived antigens have been identified for Yersinia and *Chlamydia trachomatis* in ReA patients. Among various proteins the 60 kDa hsp seems to be of importance. Different epitopes located on this protein seem to be associated with different cytokine secretion patterns.

In contrast, in Lyme arthritis the humoral immune response is essential for the elimination of *Borrelia burgdorferi*. Thus, the "wrong" Th1-like T cells found in patients with Lyme arthritis might permit persistence of Bb in the joint and might also, by acting as effector cells, cause immunopathology. Since antibodies against the Bb-derived protein OspA are protective the T cell response against this protein is of great interest. Different OspA-specific T cell epitopes have been identified which have been linked either to protection or to chronic courses of the disease.

Further analysis of epitope-specific T cell responses might allow to change the immune response towards a wanted action. Although antibiotics are normally effective in the treatment of Lyme arthritis this is less clear for ReA. Thus, based on new insights into the pathogenesis of Lyme and ReA immunotherapies might also become a therapeutical option for chronic cases of ReA and Lyme arthritis. With regard to the cytokine secretion pattern ReA seems to be similar to ankylosing spondylitis while Lyme arthritis resembles rheumatoid arthritis.

References

1 Sieper J, Braun J (1995) Pathogenesis of spondylarthropathies. Persistent bacterial antigen, autoimmunity, or both? *Arthritis Rheum* 38: 1547–1554

2 Braun J, Laitko S, Treharne J, Eggens U, Wu P, Distler A, Sieper J (1994) Chlamydia pneumoniae—a new causative agent of reactive arthritis and undifferentiated oligoarthritis. *Ann Rheum Dis* 53: 100–105

3 Wilkinson NZ, Kingsley GH, Sieper J, Braun J, Wared ME (1998) The detection of Chlamydia trachomatis but not Chlamydia pneumoniae in the synovium of patients with a range of rheumatic diseases. *Arthritis Rheum, in press*

4 Ford DK, da Roza DM, Shah P (1981) Cell-mediated immune responses of synovial mononuclear cells to sexually transmitted, enteric and mumps antigens in patients with Reiter's syndrome, rheumatoid arthritis and ankylosing spondylitis. *J Rheumatol* 8: 220–232

5 Gaston JS, Life PF, Granfors K, Merilahti Palo R, Bailey L, Consalvey S, Toivanen A, Bacon PA (1989) Synovial T lymphocyte recognition of organisms that trigger reactive arthritis. *Clin Exp Immunol* 76: 348–353

6 Sieper J, Kingsley G, Palacios Boix A, Pitzalis C, Treharne J, Hughes R, Keat A, Panayi GS (1991) Synovial T lymphocyte-specific immune response to Chlamydia trachomatis in Reiter's disease. *Arthritis Rheum* 34: 588–598

7 Sieper J, Braun J, Wu P, Hauer R, Laitko S (1993) The possible role of Shigella in sporadic enteric reactive arthritis. *Br J Rheumatol* 32: 582–585

8 Schumacher HR, Jr., Magge S, Cherian PV, Sleckman J, Rothfuss S, Clayburne G, Sieck M (1988) Light and electron microscopic studies on the synovial membrane in Reiter's syndrome. Immunocytochemical identification of chlamydial antigen in patients with early disease. *Arthritis Rheum* 31: 937–946

9 Granfors K, Jalkanen S, von Essen R, Lahesmaa Rantala R, Isomaki O, Pekkola Heino K, Merilahti Palo R, Saario R, Isomaki H, Toivanen A (1989): Yersinia antigens in synovial-fluid cells from patients with reactive arthritis. *N Engl J Med* 320: 216–221

10 Granfors K, Jalkanen S, Lindberg AA, Maki Ikola O, von Essen R, Lahesmaa Rantala R, Isomaki H, Saario R, Arnold WJ, Toivanen A (1990): Salmonella lipopolysaccharide in synovial cells from patients with reactive arthritis. *Lancet* 335: 685–688

11 Bas S, Griffais R, Kvien TK, Glennas A, Melby K, Vischer TL (1995) Amplification of plasmid and chromosome Chlamydia DNA in synovial fluid of patients with reactive arthritis and undifferentiated seronegative oligoarthropathies. *Arthritis Rheum* 38: 1005–113

12 Fendler C, Braun J, Eggens U, Laitjo S, S^rensen H, Distler A, Sieper J (1997) Bacteria-specific lymphocyte proliferation in peripheral blood in reactive arthritis and related disease. *Brit J Rheumatol. in press*

13 Sieper J, Braun J, Wu P, Kingsley G (1992) Alteration in T cell/macrophage ratio may reveal lymphocyte proliferation specific for the triggering antigen in reactive arthritis. *Scand J Immunol* 36: 427–434

14 Keat AC, Knight SC (1990): Do synovial fluid cells indicate the cause of reactive arthritis? *J Rheumatol* 17: 1257–1259

15 Hermann E, Mayet WJ, Lohse AW, Grevenstein J, Meyer zum Buschenfelde KH, Fleischer B (1990): Proliferative response of synovial fluid and peripheral blood mononuclear cells to arthritogenic and non-arthritogenic microbial antigens and to the 65-kDa mycobacterial heat-shock protein. *Med Microbiol Immunol Berl* 179: 215–224

16 Sieper J, Braun J, Wu P, Kingsley G (1993) T cells are responsible for the enhanced synovial cellular immune response to triggering antigen in reactive arthritis. *Clin Exp Immunol* 91: 96–102

17 Life PF, Viner NJ, Bacon PA, Gaston JS (1990) Synovial fluid antigen-presenting cells unmask peripheral blood T cell responses to bacterial antigens in inflammatory arthritis. *Clin Exp Immunol* 79: 189–194

18 Stagg AJ, Hughes RA, Keat AC, Elsley WA, Knight SC (1996) Antigen-presenting cells but not lymphocytes in the joint may indicate the cause of reactive arthritis. *Br J Rheumatol* 35: 1082–1090

19 Fendler C, Wu P, Eggens U, S^rensen H, Distler A, Braun J, Sieper J (1997) Longitudinal investigation of bacterium-specific synovial lymphocyte proliferation in reactive arthritis and Lyme arthritis. *Brit J Rheumatol, in press*

20 Braun J, Grolms M, Distler A, Sieper J (1994) The specific antibacterial proliferation of reactive arthritis synovial T cells is not due to their higher proportion of $CD45RO^+$ cells compared to peripheral blood. *J Rheumatol* 21: 1702–1707

21 Duchmann R, May E, Ackermann B, Goergen B, Meyer zum Buschenfelde KH, Marker Hermann E (1996) HLA-B27-restricted cytotoxic T lymphocyte responses to arthritogenic enterobacteria or self-antigens are dominated by closely related TCRBV gene segments. A study in patients with reactive arthritis. *Scand J Immunol* 43: 101–108

22 Allen RL, Gillespie JMA, Hall F, Edmonds S, Hall MA, Wordsworth BP, McMichael AJ, Bowness P (1997) Multiple T cell expansion are found in the blood and synovial fluid of patients with reactive arthritis. *J Rheumatol* 24: 1750–1757

23 Sieper J, Braun J, Doring E, Wu P, Heesemann J, Treharne J, Kingsley G (1992) Aetiological role of bacteria associated with reactive arthritis in pauciarticular juvenile chronic arthritis. *Ann Rheum Dis* 51: 1208–1214

24 Sieper J, Braun J, Brandt J, Miksits K, Heesemann J, Laitko S, Sorensen H, Distler A, Kingsley G (1992) Pathogenetic role of Chlamydia, Yersinia and Borrelia in undifferentiated oligoarthritis. *J Rheumatol* 19: 1236–1242

25 Braun J, Grolms M, Sieper J (1994) Three-colour flowcytometric examination of

CD4/CD45 subsets reveals no differences in peripheral blood and synovial fluid between patients with reactive arthritis and rheumatoid arthritis. *Clin Exp Rheumatol* 12: 17–22

26 Hermann E, Ackermann B, Duchmann R, Meyer zum Buschenfelde KH (1995) Synovial fluid MHC-unrestricted gamma delta-T lymphocytes contribute to antibacterial and anti-self cytotoxicity in the spondylarthropathies. *Clin Exp Rheumatol* 13: 187–191

27 Viner NJ, Bailey LC, Life PF, Bacon PA, Gaston JS (1991): Isolation of Yersinia-specific T cell clones from the synovial membrane and synovial fluid of a patient with reactive arthritis. *Arthritis Rheum* 34: 1151–1157

28 Mertz AK, Daser A, Skurnik M, Wiesmuller KH, Braun J, Appel H, Batsford S, Wu P, Distler A, Sieper J (1994) The evolutionarily conserved ribosomal protein L23 and the cationic urease beta-subunit of Yersinia enterocolitica O: 3 belong to the immunodominant antigens in Yersinia-triggered reactive arthritis: implications for autoimmunity. *Mol Med* 1: 44–55

29 Probst P, Hermann E, Meyer zum Buschenfelde KH, Fleischer B (1993) Identification of the Yersinia enterocolitica urease beta subunit as a target antigen for human synovial T lymphocytes in reactive arthritis. *Infect Immun* 61: 4507–4509

30 Hassell AB, Reynolds DJ, Deacon M, Gaston JS, Pearce JH (1993) Identification of T-cell stimulatory antigens of Chlamydia trachomatis using synovial fluid-derived T-cell clones. *Immunology* 79: 513–519

31 Deane KH, Jecock RM, Pearce JH, Gaston JS (1997) Identification and characterization of a DR4-restricted T cell epitope within chlamydia heat shock protein 60. *Clin Exp Immunol* 109: 439–445

32 Gaston JS, Deane KH, Jecock RM, Pearce JH (1996) Identification of 2 Chlamydia trachomatis antigens recognized by synovial fluid T cells from patients with Chlamydia induced reactive arthritis. *J Rheumatol* 23: 130–136

33 Mertz AKH, Ugrinovic S, Lauster R, Wu P, Grolms M, B^ttcher U, Appel H, Yin Z, Schiltz E, Batsford S, et al (1998) Charcterization of the synovial T cell response to various recombinant Yersinia antigens in Yersinia-triggered reactive arthritis: the hsp60 drives a major immune response. *Arthritis Rheum* 41: 315–326

34 Hermann E, Lohse AW, Van der Zee R, Van Eden W, Mayet WJ, Probst P, Poralla T, Meyer zum Buschenfelde KH, Fleischer B (1991) Synovial fluid-derived Yersinia-reactive T cells responding to human 65-kDa heat-shock protein and heat-stressed antigen-presenting cells. *Eur J Immunol* 21: 2139–2143

35 Probst P, Hermann E, Meyer zum Buschenfelde KH, Fleischer B (1993) Multiclonal synovial T cell response to Yersinia enterocolitica in reactive arthritis: the Yersinia 61-kDa heat-shock protein is not the major target antigen. *J Infect Dis* 167: 385–391

36 Deane KHO, Jecock RM, Pearce JH (1996) Mapping a DR4-restricted T cell epitope in Chlamyida HSP60-implications for reactive arthritis pathogenesis. *Arthritis Rheum* 39: S115

37 Benjamin RJ, Parham P (1997) Guilt by association: HLA-B27 and ankylosing spondylitis. *Immunol Today* 11: 137–142

38 Germain RN (1994) MHC-dependent antigen processing and peptide presentation: providing ligands for T lymphocyte activation. *Cell* 76: 287–299
39 Hermann E, Yu DT, Meyer zum Buschenfelde KH, Fleischer B (1993) HLA-B27-restricted CD8 T cells derived from synovial fluids of patients with reactive arthritis and ankylosing spondylitis. *Lancet* 342: 646–650
40 Ugrinovic S, Mertz A, Wu P, Braun J, Sieper J (1997) A single nonamer from the Yersinia 60kd heat shock protein is the target of HLA-B27 restricted CTL response in Yersinia-induced reactive arthritis. *J Immunol* 159: 5715–5723
41 Pfeifer JD, Wick MJ, Roberts RL, Findlay K, Normark SJ, Harding CV (1993) Phagocytic processing of bacterial antigens for class I MHC presentation to T cells. *Nature* 361: 359–362
42 Beatty PR, Stephens RS (1994) $CD8^+$ T lymphocyte-mediated lysis of Chlamydia-infected L cells using an endogenous antigen pathway. *J Immunol* 153: 4588–4595
43 Starnbach MN, Bevan MJ, Lampe MF (1994) Protective cytotoxic T lymphocytes are induced during murine infection with Chlamydia trachomatis. *J Immunol* 153: 5183-5189
44 Kuon W, Lauster R, Bottcher U, Koroknay A, Ulbrecht M, Hartmann M, Grolms M, Ugrinovic S, Braun J, Weiss EH, Sieper J (1997) Recognition of chlamydial antigen by HLA-B27-restricted cytotoxic T cells in HLA-B*2705 transgenic CBA (H-2k) mice. *Arthritis Rheum* 40: 945–954
45 Rock KL, Clark K (1996) Analysis of the role of MHC class II presentation in the stimulation of cytotoxic T lymphocytes by antigens targeted into the exogenous antigen-MHC class I presentation pathway. *J Immunol* 156: 3721–372647.
46 Hassell AB, Pilling D, Reynolds D, Life PF, Bacon PA, Gaston JS (1992) MHC restriction of synovial fluid lymphocyte responses to the triggering organism in reactive arthritis. Absence of a class I-restricted response. *Clin Exp Immunol* 88: 442–447
47 Abbas AK, Murphy KM, Sher A (1996) Functional diversity of helper T lymphocytes. *Nature* 383: 787–793
48 Autenrieth IB, Beer M, Bohn E, Kaufmann SH, Heesemann J (1994) Immune responses to Yersinia enterocolitica in susceptible BALB/c and resistant C57BL/6 mice: an essential role for gamma interferon. *Infect Immun* 62: 2590–2599
49 Yang X, HayGlass T, Brunham RC (1996) Genetically determined differences in IL-10 and IFNγ-responses correlate with clearance of Chlamydia trachomatis mouse pneumonitis infection. *J Immunol* 156: 4338–4344
50 Summersgill JT, Sahney NN, Gaydos CA, Quinn TC, Ramirez JA (1995) Inhibition of Chlamydia pneumoniae growth in HEp-2 cells pretreated with gamma interferon and tumor necrosis factor alpha. *Infect Immun* 63: 2801–2803
51 Schlaak J, Hermann E, Ringhoffer M, Probst P, Gallati H, Meyer zum Buschenfelde KH, Fleischer B (1992) Predominance of Th1-type T cells in synovial fluid of patients with Yersinia-induced reactive arthritis. *Eur J Immunol* 22: 2771–2776
52 Simon AK, Seipelt E, Wu P, Wenzel B, Braun J, Sieper J (1993) Analysis of cytokine profiles in synovial T cell clones from chlamydial reactive arthritis patients: predominance of the Th1 subset. *Clin Exp Immunol* 94: 122–126

53 Simon AK, Seipelt E, Sieper J (1994) Divergent T-cell cytokine patterns in inflammatory arthritis. *Proc Natl Acad Sci USA* 91: 8562–8566

54 Yin Z, Braun J, Neure L, Wu P, Liu L, Eggens U, Sieper J (1997) Crucial role of interleukin-10/interleukin-12 balance in the regulation of the type 2 T helper cytokine response in reactive arthritis. *Arthritis Rheum* 40: 1788–1797

55 Yin Z, Braun J, Neure L, Wu P, Eggens U, Krause A, Kamradt T, Sieper J (1997) T cell cytokine pattern in the joints of patients with Lyme arthritis and its regulation by cytokines and anticytokines. *Arthritis Rheum* 40: 69–79

56 Braun J, Yin Z, Krause A, Liu L, Spiller I, Sieper J (1997) Peripheral blood cells of reactive arthritis patients secrete more IL-10 and less TNF-alpha than patients with Lyme- or rheumatoid arthritis. *Arthritis Rheum* 40: S79

57 Yin Z, Neure L, Grolms M, Eggens U, Radbruch A, Braun J, Sieper J (1997) Th1/Th2 cytokine patteren in the joint of rheumatoid arthrits and reactive arthritis patients: analysis at the single cell level. *Arthritis Rheum* 40: S37

58 Tak PP, Smeets TJM, Dolhain RJEM, Thurkow EW, Breedveld FC (1997) Analysis of the synovial infiltrate and expression of cytokines in rheumatoid arthritis compared with Yersinia-induced arthritis patients in relation to disease duration. *Arthritis Rheum* 40: S252

59 Shigeru K, Schumacher HR, Yarboro CH, Arayssi TK, Pando JA, Kanik KS, Gourley MF, Klippel JH, Wilder RL(1997) In vivo gene expression of type 1 and type 2 cytokines in synovial tissues from patients in early stages of rheumatoid, reactive, and undifferentiated arthritis. *Proc Ass Am Phys* 109: 286–302

60 Sornasse T, Larenas PV, Davis KA, de Vries JE, Yssel H (1996) Differentiation and stability of T helper 1 and 2 cells derived from naive human neonatal $CD4^+$ T cells, analyzed at the single cell level. *J Exp Med* 184: 473–483

61 van Roon JA, Van Eden W, van Roy JL, Lafeber FJ, Bijlsma JW (1997) Stimulation of suppressive T cell responses by human but not bacterial 60-kD heat-shock protein in synovial fluid of patients with rheumatoid arthritis. *J Clin Invest* 100: 459–463

62 Leino R, Vuento R, Koskimies S, Viander M, Toivanen A (1983) Depressed lymphocyte transformation by yersinia and Escherichia coli in yersinia arthritis. *Ann Rheum Dis* 42: 176–181

63 Inman RD, Chiu B, Johnston ME, Vas S, Falk J (1989) HLA class I-related impairment in IL-2 production and lymphocyte response to microbial antigens in reactive arthritis. *J Immunol* 142: 4256–4260

64 Chieco Bianchi F, Hedley K, Weissensteiner T, Panayi GS, Kingsley GH (1995) Reactive arthritis-associated bacteria can stimulate lymphocyte proliferation in non-exposed individuals and newborns. *Clin Exp Immunol* 102: 551–559

65 Groux H, O'Garra A, Bigler M, Rouleau M, Antonenko S, De Vries JE, Roncarolo MG (1997) $CD4^+$ T cell subset inhibits antigen-specific T cell responses and prevents colitis. *Nature* 389: 737–742

66 Yi Y, Yang X, Brunham RC (1997) Autoimmunity to heat shock protein 60 and antigen-specific production of interleukin-10. *Infect Immun* 65: 1669–1674

67 Prakken AB, van Hoeij MJ, Kuis W, Kavelaars A, Heynen CJ, Scholtens E, de Kleer IM, Rijkers GT, Van Eden W (1997) T-cell reactivity to human HSP60 in oligo-articular juvenile chronic arthritis is associated with a favorable prognosis and the generation of regulatory cytokines in the inflamed joint. *Immunol Lett* 57: 139–142

68 Sieper J, Kingsley G (1996) Recent advances in the pathogenesis of reactive arthritis. *Immunol Today* 17: 160–163

69 Lopez de Castro JA (1997) The pathogenetic role of HLA-B27 in chronic arthritis. *Curr Op Immunol, in press*

70 Märker-Hermann E, Meyer zum B¸schenfelde K-H, Wildner G (1997) HLA-B27-derived peptides as autoantigens for T lymphocytes in ankylosing spondylitis. *Arthritis Rheum* 40: 2047–2054, 1997

71 Taurog JD, Richardson JA, Croft JT, Simmons WA, Zhou M, Fernandez Sueiro JL, Balish E, Hammer RE (1994) The germfree state prevents development of gut and joint inflammatory disease in HLA-B27 transgenic rats. *J Exp Med* 180: 2359–2364

72 Khare SD, Luthra HS, David CS (1995) Spontaneous inflammatory arthritis in HLA-B27 transgenic mice lacking beta 2-microglobulin: a model of human spondyloarthropathies. *J Exp Med* 182: 1153–1158

73 Zhang Y, Gripenberg-Lerche C, Soderstrom KO, Toivanen A, Toivanen P (1996) Antibiotic prophylaxis and treatment of reactive arthritis. Lessons from an animal model. *Arthritis Rheum* 39: 1238–1243

74 Burmester GR, Daser A, Kamradt T, Krause A, Mitchison NA, Sieper J, Wolf N (1995) Immunology of reactive arthritides. *Annu Rev Immunol* 13: 229–250

75 Sigal LH (1997) Lyme disease: a review of aspects of its immunology and immunopathogenesis. *Annu Rev Immunol* 15: 63–92

76 Steere AC (1989) Lyme disease. *N Engl J Med* 321: 586–596

77 Nocton JJ, Dressler F, Rutledge BJ, Rys PN, Persing DH, Steere AC (1994) Detection of Borrelia burgdorferi DNA by polymerase chain reaction in synovial fluid from patients with Lyme arthritis. *N Engl J Med* 330: 229–234

78 Lengl Janssen B, Strauss AF, Steere AC, Kamradt T (1994) The T helper cell response in Lyme arthritis: differential recognition of *Borrelia burgdorferi* outer surface protein A in patients with treatment-resistant or treatment-responsive Lyme arthritis. *J Exp Med* 180: 2069–2078

79 Kamradt T, Krause A, Burmester GR (1995) A role for T cells in the pathogenesis of treatment-resistant Lyme arthritis. *Mol Med* 1: 486–490

80 Sigal LH, Steere AC, Freeman DH, Dwyer JM (1986) Proliferative responses of mononuclear cells in Lyme disease. Reactivity to Borrelia burgdorferi antigens is greater in joint fluid than in blood. *Arthritis Rheum* 29: 761–769

81 Krause A, Brade V, Schoerner C, Solbach W, Kalden JR, Burmester GR (1991) T cell proliferation induced by Borrelia burgdorferi in patients with Lyme borreliosis. Autologous serum required for optimum stimulation. *Arthritis Rheum* 34: 393–402

82 Krause A, Burmester GR, Rensing A, Schoerner C, Schaible UE, Simon MM, Herzer P, Kramer MD, Wallich R (1992) Cellular immune reactivity to recombinant OspA and

flagellin from Borrelia burgdorferi in patients with Lyme borreliosis. Complexity of humoral and cellular immune responses. *J Clin Invest* 90: 1077–1084

83 Dattwyler RJ, Volkman DJ, Luft BJ, Halperin JJ, Thomas J, Golightly MG (1988) Seronegative Lyme disease. Dissociation of specific T- and B-lymphocyte responses to *Borrelia burgdorferi. N Engl J Med* 319: 1441–1446

84 Roessner K, Fikrig E, Russell JQ, Cooper SM, Flavell RA, Budd RC (1994) Prominent T lymphocyte response to *Borrelia burgdorferi* from peripheral blood of unexposed donors. *Eur J Immunol* 24: 320–324

85 Yssel H, Shanafelt MC, Soderberg C, Schneider PV, Anzola J, Peltz G (1991) *Borrelia burgdorferi* activates a T helper type 1-like T cell subset in Lyme arthritis. *J Exp Med* 174: 593–601

86 Lahesmaa R, Shanafelt MC, Allsup A, Soderberg C, Anzola J, Freitas V, Turck C, Steinman L, Peltz G (1993) Preferential usage of T cell antigen receptor V region gene segment V beta 5.1 by *Borrelia burgdorferi* antigen-reactive T cell clones isolated from a patient with Lyme disease. *J Immunol* 150: 4125–4135

87 Rao TD, Frey AB (1995) Protective resistance to experimental *Borrelia burgdorferi* infection of mice by adoptive transfer of a $CD4^{+}$ T cell clone. *Cell Immunol* 162: 225–234

88 Schaible UE, Wallich R, Kramer MD, Nerz G, Stehle T, Museteanu C, Simon MM (1994) Protection against *Borrelia burgdorferi* infection in SCID mice is conferred by presensitized spleen cells and partially by B but not T cells alone. *Int Immunol* 6: 671–681

89 Zhong W, Wiesmuller KH, Kramer MD, Wallich R, Simon MM (1996) Plasmid DNA and protein vaccination of mice to the outer surface protein A of *Borrelia burgdorferi* leads to induction of T helper cells with specificity for a major epitope and augmentation of protective IgG antibodies *in vivo. Eur J Immunol* 26: 2749–2757

90 Bockenstedt LK, Fikrig E, Barthold SW, Flavell RA, Kantor FS (1996) Identification of a *Borrelia burgdorferi* OspA T cell epitope that promotes anti-OspA IgG in mice. *J Immunol* 157: 5496–5502

91 Shanafelt MC, Anzola J, Soderberg C, Yssel H, Turck CW, Peltz G (1992) Epitopes on the outer surface protein A of *Borrelia burgdorferi* recognized by antibodies and T cells of patients with Lyme disease. *J Immunol* 148: 218–224

92 Kamradt T, Lengl Janssen B, Strauss AF, Bansal G, Steere AC (1996) Dominant recognition of a Borrelia burgdorferi outer surface protein A peptide by T helper cells in patients with treatment-resistant Lyme arthritis. Infect Immun 64: 1284–1289

93 Lim LC, England DM, DuChateau BK, Glowacki NJ, Schell RF (1995) Borrelia burgdorferi-specific T lymphocytes induce severe destructive Lyme arthritis. Infect Immun 63: 1400–1408

94 Busch DH, Jassoy C, Brinckmann U, Girschick H, Huppertz HI (1996) Detection of *Borrelia burgdorferi*-specific $CD8^{+}$ cytotoxic T cells in patients with Lyme arthritis. *J Immunol* 157: 3534-3541

95 Matyniak JE, Reiner SL (1995) T helper phenotype and genetic suscept ibility in experimental Lyme disease. *J Exp Med* 181: 1251–1254

96 Keane Myers A, Nickell SP (1995) Role of IL-4 and IFN-gamma in modulation of immunity to *Borrelia burgdorferi* in mice. *J Immunol* 155: 2020–2028

97 Keane Myers A, Maliszewski CR, Finkelman FD, Nickell SP (1996) Recombinant IL-4 treatment augments resistance to *Borrelia burgdorferi* infections in both normal susceptible and antibody-deficient susceptible mice. *J Immunol* 156: 2488–2494

98 Oksi J, Savolainen J, Pene J, Bousquet J, Laippala P, Viljanen MK (1996) Decreased interleukin-4 and increased gamma interferon production by peripheral blood mononuclear cells of patients with Lyme borreliosis. *Infect Immun* 64: 3620–3523

99 Infante-Duarte C, Kamradt T (1997) Lipopeptides of *Borrelia burgdorferi* outer surface proteins induce TH1 phenotype development in ab T-cell receptor transgenic mice. *Infect Immun* 65: 4094–4099

100 Steere AC, Dwyer E, Winchester R (1990) Association of chronic Lyme arthritis with HLA-DR4 alleles. *N Engl J Med* 323: 219–223

101 Feng S, Barthold SW, Bockenstedt LK, Zaller DM, Fikrig E (1995) Lyme disease in human DR4Dw4-transgenic mice. *186* 172: 286–289

T cell directed therapies and biologics

Ferdinand C. Breedveld

Leiden University Medical Center, Department of Rheumatology, C4-R, P.O.B. 9600, NL-2300 RC Leiden, The Netherlands

Introduction

One result of the growing evidence that T cells are responsible for the initiation and perpetuation of chronic arthritis is that therapies aimed at downregulating the effects of lymphocytes may prove to be beneficial for arthritis patients. Thoracic duct drainage, lymphapheresis, total lymphoid irradiation and cyclosporin treatment, whose principal action is assumed to be confined to lymphocytes, have been reported to be effective in patients with rheumatoid arthritis (RA) [1–5]. The association of some of these therapies with serious side-effects and their failure to induce permanent remission warranted the development of new therapies that would more specifically downregulate disease-relevant T cells. Based on promising results in experimental autoimmune disease models [6], and pilot studies in human subjects [7], clinical trials using biological agents targeted at T cell surface antigens were initiated. These included both monoclonal antibodies (mAb) and recombinant fusion proteins. Another approach involved targeting the trimolecular complex of antigen, human leucocyte antigen (HLA) molecule, and T cell receptor (TCR) to selectively influence the response to a specific autoantigen without compromising normal immune function. Cohen et al. demonstrated in experimental autoimmune disease models that disease-inducing T cell clones could be employed to induce immunity following attenuation of the T cells before inoculation. This procedure, designated T cell vaccination (TCV), was assumed to be based on the interference of a network of T cells that recognize cell surface structures expressed by certain other T cells [8, 9]. Analogous to the animal experiments, "vaccines" have been prepared of T cells, or of T cell receptor peptides, and used in clinical trials. Others used oral administration of antigens to induce a state of specific unresponsiveness to the antigen, termed oral tolerance. As such it is a form of antigen-driven peripheral immune tolerance. Recent work by Hafler and Weiner two pathways could be delineated by which oral tolerization results in a systemic hyporesponsiveness. Low doses of oral antigen favour the generation of active suppression whereas higher dosages favour anergy driven tolerance [10]. This review will

T Cells in Arthritis, edited by P. Miossec, W.B. van den Berg and G.S. Firestein

describe available information on clinical trials that have used biological agents directed against T cell surface antigens and biological agents aimed at the induction of a specific immune response that attenuates autoreactive T cells.

Intervention targeted at T cell surface antigens

Most information has been obtained with mAb against the CD4 surface antigen which plays a critical role in T cell activation and the induction of specific responses.

Immunopharmacological aspects of CD4-mAb

The half-life of unbound CD4 monoclonal antibodies was found to vary considerably depending on the dose and the individual antibody used. After infusion of 20 mg of the murine CD4 mAb MAX.16H5 [11] the half-life was found to be three hours, and twelve hours after the infusion mAb were no longer detectable. The half-life of chimerized antibodies was found to be 15 hours [12]. The apparent half-life of humanized CD4-mAb is longer and increases with the dose to a mean value of 80 hours at 10 mg/kg [13]. The half-life of CD4 mAb seems to be considerably shorter than that of mAb that bind to antigens in the extravascular space. This suggests that CD4-mAb meets continuously with unoccupied antigens in the circulation. Saturation of CD4 binding sites in the circulation occurs with dosages above 10 mg. With higher dosages there is an incremental increase in the duration of CD4 saturation. Specific enrichment of CD4-mAb was demonstrated in organs with a high number of $CD4^+$ cells and in arthritic joints [14]. Higher dosages also lead to more intense coating of lymphocytes in the arthritic joint [15]. Several studies reported that the percentage of peripheral blood- and synovial fluid lymphocytes coated with CD4-mAb correlated with the clinical response seen in patients [12, 15]. This suggests that a careful study of pharmacodynamics is necessary to determine the appropriate dose of mAb for an optimal clinical effect.

The most impressive immediate effect seen during the first trials of CD4-mAb administration was the clearance of $CD4^+$ lymphocytes from the circulation. After application of several murine CD4-mAb, the number of CD4+ lymphocytes reached pretreatment levels within 24 hours but others such as the MAX 16H5, and in particular the chimeric cM-T412, induced a prolonged depletion of $CD4^+$ lymphocytes lasting for several years. To date, the mechanisms responsible for the prolonged depletion of circulating $CD4^+$ T cells have not been elucidated. The most obvious explanation is that the depletion is due to trapping of antibody-coated cells in the mononuclear phagocyte system. Evidence for direct complement-mediated lysis was not found [12]. Recent studies with primatized and humanized CD4-mAb of the

IgG1 and IgG4 class induced no lymphocytopenia, or only transient lymphocytopenia, in a limited number of patients.

Evidence was provided that CD4-mAb selectively eliminates the resting naive $CD4^+$ population. Cells expressing HLA molecules, Interleukin (IL)-2 receptors, CD27, and the $CD45RO^+$ subset are relatively spared from depletion following CD4-mAb therapy [16]. Observations in RA patients [17] did not confirm those in mice that CD4-mAb increases IL4 and decreases interferon (IFN)γ production by mononuclear cells [18].

Therapeutic efficacy of CD4-mAb

CD4-mAb treatment was mainly studied in RA patients refractory to conventional therapeutic regimens. The initial trials were of an open, uncontrolled design, with the primary aim of assessing safety and objective biological effects. These studies used murine and chimeric mAb. More recent studies had a placebo-controlled design. To decrease the immunogeneicity and lymphocytopenia, non-depleting primatized as well as humanized antibodies were applied.

Interestingly, the doses of CD4-mAb used in RA were generally lower and the treatment durations shorter than those used in animal models. The differences in the design of the interventions in the clinical and experimental situation may explain some of the apparent discrepancies in efficacy.

CD4-mAb administration in dosages between 10 and 700 mg/week was not associated with serious toxicity. Allergic reactions as a result of repeated treatment were reported in only two murine CD4-mAb treated patients and in none of the chimeric, primatized or humanized CD4-mAb treated patients [11, 19]. Leukocytoclastic vasculitis of the skin was observed in RA patients treated with 2x 140 mg/week of a primatized CD4-mAb [20]. One patient died six months after infusion of 100 mg CD4-mAb as a result of *Pneumocystis Carinii* and *Staphylococcus aureus* pneumonia in association with cardiovascular failure while being treated concomitantly with methotrexate and high doses of prednisolone [21]. Despite the induction of significant lymphocytopenia in some studies no increase in the number of infective episodes or lymphomas has been recorded [22].

Placebo-controlled double-blind studies were initially performed with cM-T412, a chimerized IgG1 mAb. In the first study, single dose infusions with placebo, 5, 10 or 50 mg CD4-mAb were given in three consecutive months in 64 Methotrexate-treated RA patients [13]. In another study two patients were randomized to placebo and seven to single dose infusions with 50 mg cM-T412 [23]. In the third study, 60 RA patients with less than one year disease duration received five daily infusions of placebo, 10, 25 or 50 mg cM-T412. Thirty patients entered a nine month continuation phase in which single, monthly doses of 50 mg of cM-T412 were given [24]. Clinical responses showed no difference between active and placebo-treated groups in these three studies. A correlation between the clinical response and the changes in circulating CD4+ cells was not found.

In two more recent studies of which the results were presented in abstract form, RA patients were treated with multiple dosages of non-depleting CD4-mAb. Patients with active RA (n=136) received, over four weeks, twice weekly placebo, 40, 80 or 140 mg of IDEC-CE9.1. 77% of the patients in the 140 mg cohort met the predefined response criteria, 47 and 42% in the 80 mg and 40 mg dose cohort respectively, and 20% in the placebo group [20]. In an open label extension study those patients that experienced a flare received 280 mg of the mAb intravenously [25]. Overall, 73% of the patients showed 20% responses according to the criteria of the American College of Rheumatology (ACR) while 32% of the patients showed a 50% response. In the second study, with an open design, 24 RA patients received on five consecutive days 10, 30, 100 or 300 mg/day of the CD4-mAb 4162W94. In contrast to the patients receiving the lower dosages, 3/6 and 5/5 in the 100 mg and 300 mg cohorts fulfilled the response criteria, respectively, beginning as early as day seven and lasting in some patients for more than three months [26]. Of interest is the observation that clinical improvement was accompanied by a significant reduction in the synovial fluid concentrations of IL-6 and tumor necrosis factor (TNF)α [27]. This observation is in line with previous observations in synovial biopsies taken before and after CD4-mAb treatment [28]. Decreasing scores for T cells, B cells, and macrophages as well as decreased expression of adhesion molecules was found following CD4-mAb treatment. These observations suggest that CD4-mAb therapy suppress synovial inflammation by decreasing the cytokine-induced upregulation of adhesion molecules and thereby the further influx of inflammatory cells. The therapeutic efficacy of the most recent studies with antibodies that deplete the T cells relatively weakly, applied in high dosages, suggests that previous studies did not use the appropriate dosage or duration of treatment.

mAb and fusion proteins binding other T cell surface antigens

An immunoconjugate of murine IgG1 mAb against CD5 antigen coupled to ricine (a ribosomal inhibitory protein) was investigated in RA. CD5 is present on the majority of T cells and a subset of B cells. Following two positive open label trials, a placebo-controlled, randomized trial on 104 patients failed to show efficacy [29]. The responses in the placebo cohort exceeded the active treatment group. This agent is no longer under development. Monoclonal antibodies against the CD7 and CDw52 (Campath-1H) proteins, both present on the majority of T cells, have been investigated for antirheumatic properties in open studies [30, 31]. Despite the induction of T lymphocytopenia by both antibodies there was only modest and short-lived improvement in the clinical state and no significant change in the acute phase response. Campath-1H fixes complement effectively and hence it is very lytic for

CDw52-positive cells. Following infusions, severe lymphokine release syndromes have been reported. In addition, after Campath-1H treatment, several patients were found to develop life-threatening infections and malignant lymphoma's indicating that clinical experiments with mAb against components of the immune system should be performed with great caution [32].

Another strategy employed DAB interleukin-2 (IL-2) which is a fusion protein of the enzymatically active fragment of diphtheria toxin, the membrane-translocating portion, and sequences for human IL-2, produced by recombinant expression in *E. coli*. DAB IL-2 binds specifically to the high affinity IL-2-receptor (R) and is rapidly internalized via receptor-mediated endocytosis. Once internalized into an acidic vesicle the enzymatically active fragment is released into the cytosol and inhibits protein synthesis, resulting in cell death. Only activated T cells express IL-2 receptors and will therefore be specifically killed.

DAB IL-2 has been evaluated in short-term, placebo-controlled trials in patients with long-standing refractory RA [33, 34]. In an initial blinded study, a five day course of DAB IL-2 was compared to placebo. No responders were observed in the placebo group (n=23) compared to 4/22 in the treatment group (p=0.05) as defined by ≥25% improvement in both swollen and tender joint count. In another placebo-controlled study of DAB IL-2 no difference was observed between the active (n=33) and placebo (n=32) treatment after one month.

Future prospects

Following the disappointing results of the initial controlled studies on the effect of depleting CD4-mAb in RA, encouraging results are now being presented by investigators that use non-depleting CD4-mAb. It is not yet clear as to what extent antibody characteristics determine the clinical observation. More information on the optimal characteristics for a therapeutic CD4-mAb would certainly allow a more appropriate usage of this therapeutic tool. Such information would also provide surrogate measures of outcome for patients undergoing therapy. Experience with CD4-mAb in animal models shows that the clinical response strongly depends on the timing and dose of administration.

In this respect the observation of a synergistic effect of CD4-mAb and a TNFα-blocking agent in an animal model is of interest. Based on the assumption that re-induction of self tolerance would be more difficult to achieve in an inflammatory setting, Isaacs and colleagues treated RA patients with soluble P55 TNF receptors and a humanized IgG1 CD4-mAb. The combination appeared to be safe and induced a prolonged period of reduced disease activity [35]. Further studies on this strategy are in progress. Clinical activity of CD4-mAb can only be judged in relatively large and costly clinical trials. In order to allow the best choice between these potentially effective immunotherapeutic reagents, future studies should focus not only on clinical efficacy but also on the relationship between antiarthritic, pharmacological and immunological parameters. Such observations will not only support the development of this therapeutic strategy but will also provide important information about the pathogenesis of the disease.

Specific immunotherapy

T cell and T cell receptor peptide vaccination

Animal experiments on T cell vaccination opened up new pathways for the treatment of human autoimmune disease. RA was a logical choice, since the T cell population present in the joint was supposed to contain disease-relevant T cell clones and these cells were easily accessible for removal. In addition, analysis of the central portions of the antigen binding site of TCR (CDR3 region) revealed an altered composition of amino acids in the CDR3 regions of TCRs derived from the site of inflammation compared to those of the periphery, suggesting that these T cells selectively accumulated in the synovium [36].

In an open study, 13 RA patients have been treated by means of a subcutaneous inoculation with attenuated, autologous T cells [37]. None of the patients developed a clear cellular or humoral immune response to the vaccine. Responses of peripheral blood mononuclear cells (PBMC) cells against irradiated, activated T cells from the inoculum could be detected but, with the possible exception of one patient, did not differ from pre-treatment levels. Nevertheless, several findings suggested immunomodulatory effects of the procedure. Interestingly, this was most pronounced in the patient with a recent onset of disease who was inoculated with the *M. tuberculosis* reactive T cell clone.

Although the study was not designed to evaluate the clinical effectiveness of the treatment, a preliminary impression of the influence on disease activity could be obtained. Taken as a group, mean values of all parameters indicated an improvement in disease activity during the first two months after treatment. However, variability of the responses among the individual patients was high and a remission of disease was not observed in any of the patients.

Another approach to eliminating putative pathogenic T cells is vaccination with peptides derived from portions of T cell receptors. Since several studies have reported overrepresentation of Vβ14 and Vβ17 T cell receptor utilization in synovial T cell populations, the first open label studies have been conducted in RA patients using immunization with a 17 amino acid sequence peptide derived from the CDR2 region of human Vβ17 T cell receptor with incomplete Freund's adjuvant. After six weeks a cellular immune response against the peptide was detected in ±50% of the patients [38]. In several patients a significant decrease from baseline values of activated $V\beta17^+$ T cells occurred clinical assessments showed trends towards improvement on safety. Recently the same investigators reported the results of a placebo-controlled phase II trial in RA using a combination of the T cell receptor peptides assumed to be important in RA, namely Vβ3, Vβ14 and Vβ17. Three groups of 33 patients received either incomplete Freuds adjuvant alone, 90 mg, or 300 mg injections at week 0, 4, 8 and 20. The results showed *in vitro* proliferative immune responses against the vaccine in the majority of the patients. The treatment was well tolerated and safe. Furthermore, a statistically significant higher percentage of patients fulfilled the 20% ACR response criteria compared to the control group [39].

Oral tolerance

Although the role of immune responses to collagen in the pathogenesis of RA has not been elucidated, anti-collagen antibodies and anti-collagen T cell reactivity are present in patients with RA. Collagen has been suggested to be one of the inciting antigens in the initiation and/or perpetuation of synovitis. Oral administration of an antigen has been demonstrated to induce a state of specific immune unresponsiveness to the antigen, a procedure termed oral tolerance. Feeding of collagen type II was shown to be effective in the prevention and treatment of the adjuvant and collagen models of arthritis. A placebo-controlled, randomized-controlled trial utilized oral doses of chicken collagen type II in 60 patients with active RA [40]. Results revealed a greater reduction in the mean number of tender and swollen joints in collagen-treated patients compared to controls, although at three months only 14% of the active group and 13% of the placebo group were considered responders. No toxicity was reported and no biological effect was apparent. This study has been criticized for its short duration and the absence of a wash-out period from dosing with second-line agents prior to initiating oral treatment. Recently the results of a second study on oral administration of collagen have been presented [41]. In this study there was no significant difference in the response rate between the groups. Further work will be necessary to better elucidate the potential clinical role of this well-tolerated therapy.

Conclusion

The initial clinical interventions with T cell-targeted biological agents or immune-specific interventions have been met with great enthusiasm which has not been confirmed in subsequent controlled clinical trials. With the possible exception of CDw52 mAb therapy, major toxic side-effects have not been observed. Despite the prolonged peripheral blood lymphocytopenia observed after treatment with chimeric CD4 mAb no clear evidence of an immune compromized state has been obtained. For the further development of T cell-targeted therapies several fundamental questions still need to be answered. These include: how does one define and select disease-inducing T cells or the immune reaction that drives the chronic inflammation in RA ? What is an efficient way to block T cell functions or to induce an immune response against those T cells that are relevant for the disease ? How can one reliably measure the effect of a particular intervention on the pivotal immune mechanisms of the rheumatoid inflammation ? Some of these questions may be addressed in animal models but it has become quite clear during the studies discussed above that it is a long way from an experimental rodent model to the treatment of a patient.

References

1 Paulus HE, Machleder HI, Levine S, Yu DTY, MacDonald NS (1977) Lymphocyte involvement in rheumatoid arthritis: studies during thoracic duct drainage. *Arthritis Rheum* 20: 1249

2 Karsh J, Klippel SH, Plotz PH, Decker JL, Wright DR, Flye MW (1981) Lymphapheresis in rheumatoid arthritis: a randomized trial. *Arthritis Rheum* 24: 867

3 Kotzin BL, Strober S, Engelman EG, Calin A, Hoppe RT, Kansas GS, Terrell CP, Kaplan HS (1981) Treatment of intractable rheumatoid arthritis with total lymphoid irradiation. *N Engl J Med* 305: 969

4 Trentham DE, Belli JA, Andersson RJ, Buckley JA, Goetzl EJ, David JR, Austen KF (1981) Clinical and immunological effect of fractionated total lymphoid irradiation in refractory rheumatoid arthritis. *N Engl J Med* 305: 976

5 Tugwell P, Bombardieri C, Gent M, Bennett KJ, Bensen WG, Carette S, Chalmers A, Esdaile JM, Klinkhoff AV, Kraag GR, Ludwin D, Roberts DS (1990) Low-dose cyclosporin versus placebo in patients with rheumatoid arthritis. *Lancet* 335: 1051

6 Cobbold SP, Qin S, Leong LYW, Martin G, Waldmann H (1992) Reprogramming the immune system for peripheral tolerance with CD4 and CD8 monoclonal antibodies. *Immunol Rev* 129: 165

7 Hertzog C, Walker C, Müller W, Rieber P, Riethmüller G, Wassmer P, Stockinger H, Madic O, Pichler WJ (1989) Anti-CD4 antibody treatment of patients with rheumatoid arthritis: I. effect on clinical course and circulating T cells. *J Autoimmun* 2: 627

8 Ben-Nun A, Wekerle H, Cohen IR (1981) Vaccination against autoimmune encephalomyelitis with T lymphocyte line cells reactive against myelin basic protein. *Nature* 292: 60

9 Cohen IR (1989) Physiological basis of T cell vaccination against autoimmune disease. *Cold Spring Harbor Symp Quant Biol* 154: 879

10 Hafler DA, Weiner HL (1995) Immunological mechanisms and therapy in multiple sclerosis. *Immunol Rev* 144: 75–107

11 Horneff G, Burmester GR, Emmrich F, Kalden JR (1991) Treatment of rheumatoid arthritis with an anti CD4 monoclonal antibody. *Arthritis Rheum* 34: 129–140

12 Van der Lubbe PA, Reiter C, Miltenburg AMM, Krüger K, de Ruyter AN, Rieber EP, Bijl JA, Riethmüller G, Breedveld FC (1994) Treatment of rheumatoid arthritis with a chimeric CD4 monoclonal antibody (cM-T412): immunopharmacological aspects and mechanisms of action. *Scand J Immunol* 39: 286–294

13 Moreland LW, Pratt PW, Mayes MD, Postlethwaite A, Weisman MH, Schnitzer T, Lightfoot R, Calabrese L, Zelinger DJ, Woody JN, Koopman WJ (1995) Double-blind, placebo-controlled multicenter trial using chimeric monoclonal antibody, cM-T412, in rheumatoid arthritis patients receiving concomitant methotrexate. *Arthritis Rheum* 38: 1581–1588

14 Kinne RW, Becker W, Simon G, Paganelli G, Palombo-Kinne E, Wolski A, Block S, Schwarz A, Wolf F, Emmrich F (1993) Joint uptake and body distribution of a Technetium-99m-labeled anti-rat CD4 monoclonal antibody in rat adjuvant arthritis. *J Nucl Med* 34: 92–98

15 Choy EHS, Pitzalis C, Cauli A, Bijl JA, Schantz A, Woody J, Kingsley GH, Panayi GS (1996) Percentage of anti-CD4 monoclonal antibody-coated lymphocytes in the rheumatoid joint is associated with clinical improvement: Implications for the development of immunotherapeutic dosing regimens. *Arthritis Rheum* 39: 52–56

16 Jamali I, Field EH, Fleming A, Cowdery JS (1992) Kinetics of anti-CD4-induced T helper cell depletion and inhibition of function: activation by the CD3 pathway inhibits and-CD4-mediated T cell elimination and down-regulation of cell surface CD4. *J Immunol* 148: 1613–1619

17 Van der Lubbe PA, Breedveld FC, Tak PP, Schantz A, Woody J, Miltenburg AMM (1997) Treatment with a chimeric CD4 monoclonal antibody is associated with a relative loss of $CD4^+/CD45RA^+$ cells in patients with rheumatoid arthritis. *J Autoimmun* 10: 87–97

18 Field EH, Rouse TM, Fleming AL, Jamali I, Cowdery J (1992) Altered IFN-γ and IL-4 pattern lymphokine secretion in mice partially depleted of CD4 T cells by anti-CD4 monoclonal antibody. *J Immunol* 149: 1131–1137

19 Reiter C, Kakavand B, Rieber EP, Schattenkrichner M, Riethmüller G, Krüger K (1991) Treatment of rheumatoid arthritis with monoclonal CD4 antibody M-T151. *Arthritis Rheum* 34: 525

20 Levy R, Weisman M, Wiesenhutter C, Yocum D, Schnitzer T, Goldman A, Schiff M, Breedveld F, Solinger A, MacDonald B et al (1996) Results of a placebo-controlled multicenter trial using a primatized® non-depleting, anti-CD4 monoclonal antibody in the treatment of rheumatoid arthritis. *Arthritis Rheum* 39 (suppl): S122

21 Moreland LW, Bucy RP, Tilden A, Pratt PW, LoBuglio AF, Khazaeli M, Everson MP, Daddona P, Ghrayeb J, Kilgarriff C et al (1993) Use of a chimeric monoclonal anti-CD4 antibody in patients with refractory rheumatoid arthritis. *Arthritis Rheum* 36; 307

22 Moreland LW, Bucy PR, Jackson B, James T, Koopman WJ (1996) Long-term (5 years) follow-up of rheumatoid arthritis patients treated with a depleting anti-CD4 monoclonal antibody, cM-T412. *Arthritis Rheum* 39 (suppl): S244

23 Choy EHS, Chikanza IC, Kingsley GH, Corrigall V, Panayi GS (1992) Treatment of

rheumatoid arthritis with single dose or weekly pulses of chimaeric anti-CD4 monoclonal antibody. *Scand J Immunol* 36: 291
24 Van der Lubbe PA, Dijkmans BAC, Markusse HM, Nässander U, Breedveld FC (1995) A randomized double-blind placebo-controlled study of CD4 monoclonal antibody therapy in early rheumatoid arthritis. *Arthritis Rheum* 38: 1097
25 Tesser JRP, Wiesenhutter C, Levy R, Schiff M, Lipani J, Solinger A, MacDonald B, Elliot M, Singh K (1997) Treatment of rheumatoid arthritis with a primatized anti-CD4 monoclonal antibody, SB-210396 (IDEC-CE9.1) – results of an open label extension study in patients responding to induction therapy. *Arthritis Rheum* 40 (suppl): S224
26 Panayi GS, Choy EHS, Connolly DJA, Regan T, Manna VK, Rapson N, Kingsley GH, Johnston JM (1996) T cell hypothesis in rheumatoid arthritis (RA) tested by humanized non-depleting anti-CD4 monoclonal antibody (mAb) treatment I: suppression of disease activity and acute phase response. *Arthritis Rheum* 39 (suppl): S244
27 Choy EHS, Connolly DJA, Rapson N, Kingsley GH, Johnston JM, Panayi GS (1997) Effect of a humanised non-depleting anti-CD4 monoclonal antibody (mAb) on synovial fluid (SF) in rheumatoid arthritis (RA). *Arthritis Rheum* 40 (suppl): S52
28 Tak PP, van der Lubbe PA, Cauli A, Daha MR, Smeets TJM, Kluin PhM, Meinders AE, Yanni G, Panayi GS, Breedveld FC (1995) Reduction of synovial inflammation after anti-CD4 monoclonal antibody treatment in early rheumatoid arthritis. *Arthritis Rheum* 38: 1457
29 Olsen NJ, Cush JJ, Lipsky PE, St. Clair EW, Matteson E, Cannon G, McCune WJ, Strand V, Lorenz T (1994) Multicentre trial of an anti CD5 immunoconjugate in rheumatoid arthritis. *Arthritis Rheum* 37: S295
30 Kirkham BW, Thien F, Pelton BK, Pitzalis C, Amlot P, Denman AM, Panayi GS (1992) Chimeric CD7 monoclonal antibody therapy in rheumatoid arthritis. *J Rheumatol* 19: 1348–1352
31 Isaacs JB, Watts RA, Hazleman BL, Hale G, Keogan MT, Cobbold SP, Waldman H (1992) Humanized monoclonal antibody therapy for rheumatoid arthritis. *Lancet* 340: 748–752
32 Isaacs JB, Manna VK, Hazleman BL, Schnitzer TJ, St. Clair EW, Matteson EL, Bulpitt KJ, Johnston JM (1993) Campath 1H in rheumatoid arthritis. *Arthritis Rheum* 36: S40
33 Sewell KL, Parker KP, Woodworth TG, Reuben J, Swartz W, Trentham D (1993) DAB_{486}IL-2 fusion toxin in refractory rheumatoid arthritis. *Arthritis Rheum* 26: 1223–1233
34 Moreland LW, Sewell KL, Sullivan WF, Shmerling H, Parker KC, Swartz WG, Woodworth TG, Trentham DE, Koopman WJ (1993) Double-blind placebo-controlled phase II trial of diphtheria-interleukin-2 fusion toxin (DAB486IL2) in patients with refractory rheumatoid arthritis (RA). *Arthritis Rheum* 36: S39
35 Morgan AW, Hale G, Rebello P, Richards S, Waldmann H, Emery P, Isaacs JD (1997) Combination therapy with a TNF antagonist and a CD4 monoclonal antibody in rheumatoid arthritis. A pilot study. *Arthritis Rheum* 40 (suppl): S81
36 Struyk L, Hawes GE, Dolhain RJEM, van Scherpenzeel A, Godthelp B, Breedveld FC,

van den Elsen PJ (1994) Evidence for selective *in vivo* expansion of synovial tissue infiltrating $CD4^+CD45RO^+$ T-lymphocytes on the basis of CDR3 diversity. *Int Immunol* 6: 897–907

37 Laar van JM, Miltenburg AMM, Verdonk MJA, Leow A, Elferink BG, Daha MR, Cohen IR, de Vries RRP, Breedveld FC (1993) Effects of inoculation with attenuated autologous T cells in patients with rheumatoid arthritis. *J Autoimmun* 6: 159–167

38 Moreland LW, Heck Jr LW, Koopman WJ, Saway PA, Adamson TC, Fronek Z, O'Connor RD, Morgan EE, Brostoff SW (1994) Vβ17 T-cell receptor peptide vaccine: results of a phase I dose finding study in patients with rheumatoid arthritis. *Arthritis Rheum* 37: S337

39 Moreland L, Adamson T, Calabrese L, Markenson J, Matsumoto A, Matteson E, Weyand C, Carlo D, Morgan E et al (1997) Results of a phase II rheumatoid arthritis clinical trial using T cell receptor peptides. *Arthritis Rheum* 40 (suppl): S223

40 Lohse AW, Bakker NPM, Hermann E, Poralla T, Jonker M, Meyer zum Buschenfelde KH (1993) Induction of an anti-vaccine response by T cell vaccination in non-human primates and humans. *J Autoimmun* 1: 121–130

41 Sieper J, Kay S, Eggens U, Zink A, Michison NA (1995) Treatment of rheumatoid arthritis with oral collagen type II: results of a double-blind placebo-controlled randomized trial. *Arthritis Rheum* 38 (suppl): S957

T Cells as primary players in rheumatoid arthritis

Michael T. Falta and Brian L. Kotzin

Departments of Medicine and Pediatrics, National Jewish Medical and Research Center, 1400 Jackson Street, Denver, CO 80206, USA; and Departments of Medicine and Immunology, University of Colorado Health Sciences Center, 4200 East Ninth Ave, Denver, CO 80262, USA

Introduction

The sequence of events required for the development of rheumatoid arthritis (RA) remains poorly defined. Evidence strongly supports a genetic predisposition for disease development, and an association between certain class II major histocompatibility complex (MHC) alleles and the development and severity of RA has been established. Clearly, environmental factors are also likely to contribute to the disease process, although these etiological agents in RA have not been identified. Early histopathological alterations in the RA joint include morphological and phenotypic changes in the vascular endothelium, and hypertrophy of the synovial lining cells. However, also present at this stage is a modest perivascular accumulation of lymphocytes, including T lymphocytes. As disease progresses, this T cell infiltration becomes more pronounced and frequently more organized, and is accompanied by an influx of B lymphocytes, macrophages, dendritic cells and fibroblasts. Cytokines, primarily of macrophage and fibroblast origin, are secreted in abundance within the synovia and contribute in multiple ways to the progression of chronic inflammation, synovial cell proliferation and expansion, and cartilage destruction.

In this context, attempts to model the pathogenesis of RA based on the available data have been plagued with difficulty. Numerous studies have investigated various aspects of this disease. However, clarifying cause and effect relationships remains a key challenge. Adding to this complexity is that mechanisms involved in the perpetuation of disease may be different and may even obscure mechanisms related to disease onset. Nevertheless, two competing hypotheses have emerged as contenders for explaining the pathogenesis of RA. The T cell paradigm maintains that T cell activation and subsequent interactions play the primary role in the initiation and perpetuation of synovitis. In the most favored model, antigen presenting cells present arthritogenic antigens via disease-associated human histocompatibility leukocyte antigen (HLA) -DR molecules to $CD4^+$ T cells, thereby activating them and setting into motion the inflammatory process. An alternate hypothesis, mostly premised on the observation that macrophage/fibroblast-derived cytokines are the most abun-

T Cells in Arthritis, edited by P. Miossec, W.B. van den Berg and G.S. Firestein

dant in the synovial lining, argues that these non-T cells and their products are the most important in the disease process [1]. In this model, T cells accumulate non-specifically in the joint, and T cell independent production of cytokines and synovial proliferation account for nearly all pathology. As will become evident, alternative interpretations of the same data are frequently used to support the T cell paradigm or to criticize it.

Table 1 presents the most frequently cited evidence to support the role of T cells as primary players in RA. The association of disease susceptibility with particular MHC class II alleles is particularly noteworthy. As will be discussed below, a number of different models have been proposed to explain this association. However, all invoke a primary role for $CD4^+$ T cells. Furthermore, the genes that predispose to autoimmunity must, *ipso facto*, be related to primary events in pathogenesis, further emphasizing the importance of $CD4^+$ T cells in the pathogenesis of RA. The same line of argument can be used if disease is confirmed to be associated with particular genes within the T cell receptor (TCR) gene complexes. Importantly, RA-associated HLA-DR alleles also appear to predict progression and severity of disease, implying a central role for $CD4^+$ T cells in the progression of joint involvement and extra-articular manifestations.

Table 1 also cites histopathological studies of inflammatory synovium in RA, which frequently show a marked infiltration with T cells, especially $CD4^+$ T cells (reviewed in [2]). This infiltration frequently predominates in perivascular areas of the tissue under the synovial lining, but it can also be diffuse and/or organized into aggregates. When the infiltration and aggregation is extensive, the sub-synovial lining area can resemble peripheral lymphoid tissue. A large fraction of synovial $CD4^+$ T cells express markers of activation, such as HLA-DR, lymphocyte function associated antigen-1 (LFA-1, CD11a/CD18), very late activation antigen 1 (VLA-1), CD69, and CD40 ligand ([3–7]; reviewed in [2]). However, only a small minority of synovial T cells express interleukin (IL)-2 receptor [3, 4]. In addition, very few of

Table 1 - Evidence for a primary role for T cells in the pathogenesis of RA

- Association of disease susceptibility and/or disease severity with particular class II MHC alleles (i.e. HLA-DRB1 shared epitope)
- Infiltration of synovial tissue with T cells, including activated $CD4^+$ T cells
- Studies of T cell receptor (TCR) repertoire showing TCR $V\beta^+$ subset expansions, oligoclonal expansions, and accumulation of related T cell clonotypes
- Association of disease with TCR gene complex alleles
- Role of T cells in the production of cytokines by non-T cells
- Improvement of disease with therapies directed against T cells or T cell products
- Improvement of RA in some individuals with HIV infection and development of AIDS
- Role of T cells in experimental models of inflammatory arthritis

these cells can be demonstrated to be actively dividing, and several studies have shown that synovial T cells have diminished proliferation and IL-2 release in response to recall antigens and mitogens [8, 9]. Although synovial $CD4^+$ T cells appear to have undergone activation at some time in the past, it is not clear if this stimulation has occurred in the synovium.

Some of the evidence listed in Table 1 is discussed in great detail in other chapters of this book and will not be covered in detail herein. For example, the role of T cells in the continued production of cytokines secreted by synovial macrophages and fibroblasts has been extensively investigated (see chapter by D. Burger and J.-M. Dayer, this volume). T cell cytokines are sparse in the synovium, especially compared to the large amount of non-T cell derived factors such as tumor necrosis factor-α (TNF-α), IL-1, IL-1 receptor antagonist (IL-1ra), granulocyte/ macrophage colony stimulating factor (GM-CSF), IL-6, fibroblast growth factors (FGF), and transforming growth factor-β (TGF-β) [1]. Still, T cells may be critically involved in their production. It is important to emphasize that a small and histologically imperceptible number of activated T cells with Th1-type cytokine production might be adequate to drive the synovial inflammatory response. There are other pathological conditions in which the disease process is mediated by non-T cell inflammatory cytokines, but $CD4^+$ T cells are critical for the pathological response. For instance, exposure to the bacterial toxin, toxic shock syndrome toxin-1, results in massive release of TNF-α and other cytokines from non-T cells, which are primarily responsible for the clinical manifestations of toxic shock syndrome. Studies have shown that these bacterial toxins are superantigens which cause marked TCR Vβ-specific T cell stimulation, and that this T cell stimulation is required for the release of non-T cell cytokines [10].

Other chapters in this book review therapies directed against T cells (see chapter by F.C. Breedveld, this volume) as well as animal models of inflammatory arthritis (see chapter by W.B. van den Berg, this volume). From the perspective of T cells, animal studies demonstrate the requirement for $CD4^+$ T cells in the induction of arthritis after immunization with type II collagen, cartilage gp39, or components of cartilage proteoglycans [11–14]. However, the relevance of these models to RA is currently unclear because the target antigens for T cells in RA are unknown. In the case of multiple sclerosis, evidence supports the disease-relevance of antigens such as myelin basic protein used in the induction of experimental autoimmune encephalomyelitis (EAE). Perhaps the most relevant animal model of RA is the MRL-*lpr/lpr* mouse [15, 16]. A number of these animals spontaneously develop a hind limb destructive arthropathy associated with elevated serum levels of rheumatoid factor [17]. Interestingly, pathological changes are characterized by early synovial cell proliferation with progressive destruction of articular cartilage, followed by synovial infiltration with lymphocytes and other inflammatory cells [18]. The early synovial proliferation and destruction without inflammation is different to that observed in RA, and perhaps is related to deficient Fas expression and defects in synovial cell apoptosis in MRL-*lpr/lpr* mice. Relevant to the theme of this review, however, depletion of CD4+ T cells still prevents the development and progression of arthritis in these mice [19].

As noted above, some of the same pieces of evidence used to support the T cell paradigm have been used to argue against it (Tab. 2). For example, studies of TCR expression have not consistently demonstrated one type of expansion in the joint among different patients. In addition, although therapies directed against T cells and T cell products have shown some efficacy, the effects have been weak, especially when compared to therapies directed against TNF-α. The most frequently cited arguments in opposition to the T cell paradigm relate to studies showing that T cell-derived cytokines are much less abundant compared to other pro-inflammatory cytokines in chronically inflamed joints [1] (see chapter by K.H.Y. Nguyen and G.S. Firestein, this volume). Perhaps most problematic is the failure to identify one or a few common stimulating antigen(s) in patients' joints, which would be predicted if the HLA-DR shared epitope is presenting a common arthritogenic peptide.

Table 2 - Evidence against a primary role for T cells in the pathogenesis of RA

• Failure to identify the antigen(s) that stimulate the majority of synovial CD4+ T cells
• T cell receptor (TCR) repertoire studies of synovial T cells showing marked heterogeneity of TCR expression, different TCR V regions expanded in different patients, lack of clonal expansions in some patients, and lack of related TCRs in the same individual and among different patients
• Paucity of T cell-derived cytokines in synovium, especially in relation to the abundance of non-T cell-derived cytokines
• Relative lack of efficacy for therapies directed against T cells and T cell products
• Progression of disease in some patients with HIV infection and AIDS

Critical to the function of CD4+ T cells as primary players in RA is the trimolecular complex, which is created by the interaction of the TCR with class II MHC bound to peptide. The remainder of this review will focus on these components of T cell recognition in RA.

Interaction of MHC class II molecules with T cells in RA

The major genetic contribution to RA involves particular HLA-DRB1 alleles predominated by HLA-DRB1*0401 and *0404 in Caucasian populations, but also includes other DR4 subtypes (*0405, *0408), as well as DRB1*0101, *1402 and

*1001 (reviewed in [20]). These alleles all share a sequence motif at positions 67–74 (L-L-E-Q-R/K-R-A-A) of the third hypervariable region of the DRB1 gene termed the "shared epitope" [21]. The increased risk for disease development has been estimated to be five- to six-fold for DRB1*0404 and *0401, with absolute risks of 1 in 20 and 1 in 35, respectively. For individuals carrying both of these alleles (i.e. *0401/*0404), the increased risk has been estimated to be ~100-fold, with an absolute risk of 1 in 7 [20]. This HLA class II association with disease is commonly cited as the most compelling evidence for the important role of CD4$^+$ T cells in the inflammatory process since the major function of class II molecules is to present peptides in the thymus during selection of the CD4$^+$ T cell repertoire and to present antigens to mature CD4$^+$ T cells in the peripheral lymphoid tissues.

The crystal structure of the DRB1*0101 [22, 23] and DRB1*0401 molecules [24] confirmed structural models which had predicted that the shared epitope encodes a segment of the DR β-chain alpha helix bordering the antigen binding site [25]. From this structure, it was anticipated that variation in this region might profoundly influence peptide binding and T cell recognition of the MHC/peptide complex. This was especially true when the shared epitope sequences of disease-associated DRB1 molecules were compared to those not associated with disease, such as DRB1*0402. Therefore, a model of disease pathogenesis entailing the selective binding and presentation of arthritogenic peptides to CD4$^+$ T cells has provided a conceptual framework for understanding the shared epitope association with RA. However, over the last several years, provocative data have suggested other models for explaining the mechanism of the shared epitope. These are summarized in Table 3.

Table 3 - Potential mechanisms of the HLA-DRB1 shared epitope association with RA

- DRB1 molecule with shared epitope is critically involved in the presentation of arthritogenic peptides to autoreactive T cells in the periphery
- DRB1 molecule with shared epitope, via presentation of peptides in the thymus, is critically involved in shaping the TCR repertoire by increasing positive selection of autoreactive specificities or decreased negative selection of regulatory populations
- Shared epitope of DRB1 molecule itself (i.e. without presentation of a special peptide) affects thymic selection as described above and/or alters T cell recognition of arthritogenic peptides
- Molecular mimicry of shared epitope sequence with antigens expressed by particular pathogens allows recognition of the shared epitope as autoantigen or affects immunological response to the pathogen
- DR β-chain peptide encompassing the shared epitope is selectively bound and presented by HLA/DQ molecules, which affects thymic selection of the TCR repertoire as described above and/or alters T cell recognition of arthritogenic peptides

To investigate the association of the shared epitope with RA, one approach is to examine the structural nature of how peptides bind to the MHC, and determine if specific binding patterns segregate with RA-associated class II molecules. MHC molecules contain a deep cleft where peptides are bound, and side chains of the peptide interact with discrete pockets deep in the groove. The pockets within the MHC molecule are encoded by polymorphic segments of the class II genes, including the region of the shared epitope. The establishment of primary and secondary anchor residues which permit peptide binding to DR molecules has been a active area of research, and many studies have examined naturally processed or synthetic peptides which bind to DR4 molecules [26–33]. These peptides contain a particular motif of amino acid side chains, at relative peptide positions p1, p4, p6, and p9, which correspond to four separate pockets within the class II peptide-binding groove.

Recently, peptide binding motifs which discriminate between RA-associated and non-associated alleles, especially the different DRB1*04 alleles, have been described [34, 35]. These studies showed that peptides with negatively charged residues at the p4 position bound to the DRB1*0401 and *0404 molecules, but were not accepted by DRB1*0402, a DR4 subtype not associated with RA [34]. Conversely, a peptide containing a positive charge at position p4 did bind to DRB1*0402, but binding to the RA-associated DR molecules was minimal. This difference appeared to be mediated by the electrostatic charge of residue 71 in the DRβ chain. Thus, a site-directed mutant molecule of DRB1*0401 that exchanged a lysine for a glutamic acid at DRβ71 established a binding pattern similar to that of DRB1*0402, which has a glutamic acid at this position. The crystal structure of DRB1*0401 complexed with a peptide of human type II collagen (CII) has confirmed the close contact of DRβ71 with p4 (aspartic acid in the CII peptide), and the requirement for charge complementarity at these positions [24]. Based on these criteria, peptides having differential binding properties were identified from candidate autoantigens, suggesting the potential applicability of this kind of approach to the identification of autoantigenic peptides in RA [34]. It is emphasized, however, that the preference for negatively charged amino acids at position p4 may be favored for high-avidity interactions, but it is not obligatory for peptides to be bound by RA-associated class II molecules. Furthermore, the preference for particular peptide residues at other positions involved in binding is not so easily predicted for the different RA-associated versus RA-non-associated molecules.

Since the antigens (peptides) recognized by $CD4^+$ T cells in RA are not known, the relevance of the above discussion regarding peptide-binding motifs to disease pathogenesis remains theoretical. Recent studies have examined susceptibility to collagen-induced arthritis in transgenic mice expressing HLA-DR1 (DRB1*0101) or DR4 (DRB1*0401) molecules [36, 37]. Transgenic mice demonstrated enhanced development of arthritis compared to mice that expressed only murine class II MHC molecules. Furthermore, the dominant epitopes of type II collagen recognized by the murine T cells corresponded to the predicted shared epitope binding motifs as discussed above [36–38].

In addition to interactions with CD4+ T cells in the periphery, class II MHC/peptide contacts with T cells in the thymus are crucial for the development of a TCR repertoire restricted to antigens presented by the same class II MHC molecule and deleted of high-affinity autoreactive T cells. It has been proposed that DR shared epitope/self-peptide complexes presented in the thymus contribute to the pathogenesis of RA through the selection of the TCR repertoire [39]. Interactions between components of the trimolecular complex can vary in affinity and result in different selection pressures leading to the increased presence of potentially autoreactive T cells or the absence of regulatory specificities. The genetic control of TCR repertoire formation by the expression of distinct MHC haplotypes has been suggested by studies showing that TCR V gene usage is more similar among monozygotic twins and siblings sharing a MHC haplotype than among non-related individuals [40–42]. Individuals separated on the basis of DR shared epitope expression showed differences in their peripheral CD4+/CD45RO− (naive T cell) TCR repertoire [43, 44]. These differences could only be detected at the level of TCRBJ gene expression within a TCRBV subpopulation, and certain patterns clustered individuals in groups that correlated with their DR haplotypes. Interestingly, RA patients varied from HLA-matched normal controls perhaps hinting that other genetic components also contribute to the formation of the TCR repertoire [43].

Nepom and colleagues have proposed that particular residues within the shared epitope may play a role in susceptibility to RA by contacting the TCR of CD4+ T cells directly, independent of the specific peptide bound in the class II groove [45; G.T. Nepom, personal communication]. This model is based on several interesting observations. For example, these investigators have shown that amino acid substitutions at positions 67, 70, and 74 in the DRB1*0404 molecule can prevent recognition by alloreactive T cell clones, an effect that appeared to be independent of peptide presentation [46, 47]. In separate studies, recognition of a rubella peptide/DR4 complex by an antigen-specific clone was shown to be ablated by specific substitutions in the peptide's TCR contact residues. Interestingly, recognition could be recovered by a substitution at position 74 of the DRβ-chain, and the effect appeared to be independent of peptide binding [48]. Finally, molecular modeling of the interaction between DRB1*0404 and TCR predicted direct contacts between specific residues in all three complementarity determining regions (CDRs) of the TCR and shared epitope residues 70 and 71 of the DRβ-chain [45]. These modeling studies therefore suggested that particular TCR Vβs could preferentially interact with the disease-associated HLA-DR shared epitope region. It was hypothesized that this enhanced interaction could boost affinity interactions between the TCR and class II MHC in the thymus such that a new set of CD4+ T cells would be positively selected or a set of regulatory T cells would be deleted. The increased interaction of peripheral T cells with the shared epitope could also overcome the threshold for activation of autoreactive $CD4^+$ T cells. Interestingly, this model predicts the development of oligoclonal expansions that are not specific for a particular autoantigen or peptide, and predicts selective usage of particular TCR Vβs by activated synovial T cells. As discussed below, certain analyses of $CD4^+$ T cells and their TCR repertoire in RA patients are consistent with these predictions.

Separate models to explain the association of the shared epitope with RA involve molecular mimicry of the shared epitope sequence with antigens expressed by infectious agents. This mimicry is hypothesized to cause self class II expressing cells to be targeted by the immune response and/or to alter the immune response to a particular pathogen, similar to models of pathogenesis in HLA-B27-related diseases. Interestingly, the QKRAA sequence motif is over-represented in protein databases [49], and is contained in proteins from a number of pathogens including the Epstein-Barr virus (EBV) glycoprotein gp110 [50], and the dnaj heat shock protein of the microorganisms *E. coli*, *L. lactis* and *B. ovis* [51]. It has been proposed that T cells positively selected in the thymus based on low avidity interactions with shared epitope-derived peptides, might then respond as mature T cells to exogenous antigens mimicking the original selecting peptide [52]. Studies addressing this hypothesis showed that while DRB1*0401 expressing normal subjects and RA patients did not respond to DRβ peptides containing the shared epitope [53], only RA patients showed DQ-restricted peripheral T cell proliferation to QKRAA-containing peptides derived from EBV gp110 and the dnaj protein [51, 54]. Responses to *E. coli* dnaj peptide were also seen in synovial fluid T cells from RA patients [54]. In separate studies related to molecular mimcry, the QKRAA motif has been shown to bind heat shock proteins (HSPs) of both endogenous and bacterial origin [55, 56]. Although the significance of these findings is unclear, it is conceivable that the interaction of DRB1 molecules with HSPs may increase the expression and presentation of these HSPs and allow them to be targeted by the immune response. The interaction with HSPs, especially human HSP70s, could also alter DR protein expression or antigen processing. Overall, molecular mimicry models have been somewhat circuitous and complex as explanations for the shared epitope association in RA and at this time, there is no direct evidence for how mimicry leads to the disease process.

Another model for how the shared epitope is associated with RA is based on the fact that DRβ peptides encompassing the shared epitope can bind and be presented by HLA-DQ molecules [57]. In this model, the primary role of DRB1-encoded molecules would not be as a presenting element in the trimolecular complex; rather, a peptide from the third hypervariable region (HV3) of DR would itself be presented by susceptibility HLA-DQ molecules and potentially skew the immune response towards autoimmunity. It has been hypothesized that these DQ molecule/DR-peptide complexes would be involved in shaping the $CD4^+$ T cell repertoire and/or modifying peripheral $CD4^+$ T cell recognition. Protection from disease might be related to the capacity of peptides from RA-non-associated versus RA-associated DRB1 molecules to bind and be presented by a particular DQ molecule. Closely related to this model, studies suggest that susceptibility to RA may be associated with HLA-DRB1 alleles (with the shared epitope) in combination with closely linked HLA-DQ alleles [57]. The RA-associated DR4 alleles are in linkage disequilibrium with the DQ7 and DQ8 alleles [58], and in Japan, the DRB1*0405 allele is linked with DQ4 and DQ8. In contrast, the data suggest that DQ6, for example, is not associated with RA.

Studies of collagen-induced arthritis (CIA) in mice have been used to provide support for this DQ presentation model. For example, in DBA/1 or B10.Q mice, which do not express I-E class II molecules, development of CIA is dependent on the presentation of type II collagen (CII) peptides by the I-A^q molecule (murine equivalent of HLA-DQ). Introduction of a functional I-E (murine equivalent of HLA-DR) molecule resulted in a marked decrease in the incidence and severity of CIA [59]. Detailed studies showed that different I-E molecules provided varying degrees of protection from disease which correlated with sequence variations in the HV3 of the I-Eβ-chain [57]. Follow-up studies were conducted using a DQ8 (DQB1*0302/DQA1*0301) double-transgenic strain also carrying a knockout for the murine class II molecule. DQ8 transgenic mice developed severe arthritis following immunization with CII whereas transgenic mice expressing DQ6 were resistant to CIA induction [60, 61]. When DQ8 transgenic mice were immunized with various DRβ peptides, T cell proliferative responses to peptide p65-79 of the HV3 region from different HLA-DRB1 alleles varied markedly. Interestingly, peptides derived from RA-non-associated DRB1 molecules were highly immunogenic, whereas those from RA-associated alleles failed to induce a response [62]. Responses were DQ-restricted [62], and peptide immunogenicity depended on the presence of a DQ-binding motif (DERAA) at position p70-74 of RA-non-associated DRB1 alleles (such as *0402) [63]. These results imply that HV3 peptides with high affinity for presenting DQ molecules (i.e. derived from RA-non-associated DRB1 alleles) would be presented in the thymus and could efficiently delete potentially autoreactive T cells. In contrast, poor binders, such as those derived from RA-associated DRB1 alleles, could result in the positive selection of these cells, which may later become stimulated in the periphery in response to molecular mimics of the shared epitope (see above) or particular self antigens.

The correlation between the HLA genotype of RA patients with disease severity and other clinical manifestations has provided additional clues regarding the role of the shared epitope in disease susceptibility. It has become increasingly evident that there is a gene dosage effect, and a hierarchy of DRB1 allele combinations correlates with increased susceptibility, disease severity, and various extra-articular manifestations. With regards to susceptibility, two copies of the DRB1 shared epitope resulted in the highest degree of disease concordance in identical twins [64]. Patients expressing two copies of RA-associated DRB1 molecules also experienced an increased frequency of nodular destructive disease [65–68], whereas those carrying only one RA-associated allele showed no trend for destructive disease or extra-articular involvement [65]. Progression to the most severe forms of disease, including major organ involvement and Felty's syndrome, was associated with homozygosity for DRB1*0401. This allele combination has also been associated with an increased frequency of rheumatoid factor seropositivity and it appears to be the most potent of the RA shared epitope combinations [69]. Evidence has also been presented for synergism between DRB1*0401 and DRB1*0404 for disease severity. As DRB1*0401 is the only RA-associated allele having a lysine at position 71 of the DRβ chain (all other alleles have a conserved arginine substitution at this position), the clinical data supports a significant contribution from this position in disease expression. The weakest allele with the shared epitope appears to be DRB1*0101, which as a single or double copy rarely results in seropositive or erosive disease. Overall, these clinical associations suggest that the shared epitope association with RA more likely operates at the level of T cell repertoire formation in the thymus rather than solely peptide presentation in the periphery. Thus, a double dose of MHC/peptide might overcome a stimulation threshold for low affinity autoreactive T cells in the periphery, but MHC dosage has been consistently observed to be important in thymic T cell selection events [70]; this notion is in accordance with current models for negative and positive selection [71, 72].

It is clear from the above discussion that a more complete understanding is required for how particular class II HLA alleles are associated with RA. At this time, we favour a model in which autoreactive T cell responses in the joint are tied to genetic influences placed on the formation of the TCR repertoire. However, it is important to re-emphasize that all of the models invoke a primary role for $CD4^+$ T cells.

Genetic contributions from the T cell receptor (TCR) gene complexes

The association of RA with HLA class II alleles accounts for less than half of the genetic contribution to this disease. Since the TCR interacts with HLA molecules in the trimolecular complex, the TCR gene complexes are obvious candidates to search for other susceptibility loci. The TCR αβ heterodimer is encoded by genes within the α-chain (TCRA) locus on chromosome 14 and the β-chain (TCRB) locus on chromosome 7. Both TCR gene complexes contain numerous variable region (V) gene segments which are closely linked to joining (J), diversity (D) in the TCRB complex only, and constant (C) region gene segments. To be expressed as a functional gene in the T cell, a somatic rearrangement of V region gene segments to downstream TCRAJ or TCRBDJ genes must occur. Considerable polymorphism exists in the TCRA and TCRB gene complexes among different individuals, especially in the different V regions. In addition to affecting recognition of MHC/peptide complexes, various V region polymorphisms have been shown to markedly alter expression levels of their respective V region expressing T cell subsets. For example, low expressing or null alleles for TCRBV3.1, TCRBV6.1, and TCRBV20 have been shown to markedly decrease the percentage of peripheral blood cells expressing these Vβ regions (reviewed in [73]).

The influence of germline TCR genes on the development of RA has been investigated by both linkage and association studies. One linkage study of the TCRB locus in RA-affected sibling pairs from North American families suggested linkage to the tri-allelic TCRBV12S2 marker ($p = 0.005$) [74]. Association studies analyzing the TCRB locus have been suggestive but small [75]. Another group of investigators described a weak but significant association with a TCRAV8S1 allele (odds ratio 1.3, $p < 0.008$) in a large case control study involving nearly 800 RA patients and a similar number of controls from northwest Europe [76]. A follow-up linkage study in 184 RA families from the United Kingdom, however, found no significant linkage at the TCRA or TCRB locus [77]. As emphasized by these investigators, false-negative linkage analyses are expected to be frequent with relatively low numbers of families, especially when the contribution to risk is expected to be low (i.e. a locus specific lambda less than 1.5).

Related to these studies in adult RA are studies in pauciarticular-onset juvenile rheumatoid arthritis (JRA), in which a TCRBV6.1 gene polymorphism has been associated with disease in a subset of patients [78, 79]. Follow-up studies demonstrated reduced expression of the disease-associated TCRBV allele related to a loss of function cysteine to arginine mutation at position 92 of the β-chain [80]. These association studies in JRA await replication in separate data sets.

Studies of T cell receptor (TCR) repertoire in RA

A major effort over the past several years has been to describe the repertoire of the TCRs utilized by T cells infiltrating the synovium in RA patients. If synovial T cell responses to particular antigens are important in the pathogenesis of disease, these cells should demonstrate a pattern of TCR expression characteristic of antigen-stimulated populations (Tab. 4). It has been reasoned that the identification of synovial T cells selectively expanded by antigen and expressing a characteristic TCR pattern, could be exploited to identify disease-relevant antigens and define the immune response in RA. Validation of this approach comes from studies of murine experimental allergic encephalomyelitis (EAE). In this model, disease-causing, myelin basic protein specific T cell clones demonstrate restricted usage of selected TCRB and TCRA genes [81, 82]. These clonotypes can be isolated from the central nervous system and distinguished from bystander cells brought in non-specifically by the inflammatory response [83].

Early reports of the TCR repertoire in RA examined TCR gene rearrangements by Southern blot analysis and showed that the synovial T cell population is not dominated by a single or limited number of clones (Tab. 5) [84–90]. While several

Table 4 - Predicted TCR characteristics of disease-relevant T cells in RA

- Increased expression of particular TCR Vα and Vβ regions (or particular TCRAV and TCRBV gene segments) in the synovium compared to blood
- Presence of oligoclonal expansions in synovium
- Presence in synovium of multiple clonotypes expressing homologous TCRs, especially homologous CDR3 sequences, which is indicative of selection by a common antigen
- Oligoclonal expansions or sets of related T cells that are:
  - Enriched in a subpopulation of activated cells
  - Present in multiple joints from the same patient
  - Persistent in the same joint over an extended time of disease activity
  - Present among different RA patients

Table 5 - Features of the synovial TCR repertoire in RA

- Markedly heterogeneous TCR expression but different compared to peripheral blood
- Increased expression of particular TCRAV and BV gene segments in synovium relative to peripheral blood
  - Increased TCRV expression does not necessarily predict oligoclonal expansions
  - Results have not been consistent from patient to patient or study to study
  - Consensus of studies, however, implicate TCRBV2, 3, 6's, 8, 14, and 17
- Multiple oligoclonal expansions in synovium in both $CD4^+$ and $CD8^+$ T cell subsets
- Presence of some clonotypes in different joints of the same patient
- Persistence of oligoclonal expansions in active joints
- Sets of related T cells based on homologous TCRs, including homologous CDR3s

studies described "dominant" clones [85, 87, 88, 90], these were only observed following cell culture with IL-2 or IL-2 plus mitogens. Therefore, although in vivo activated IL-2 responsive clones may have been identified, this methodology does not quantitate the frequency of such clones in the synovia, nor does it account for the possibility of an in vitro bias in the results. In retrospect, these data are consistent with current information. Thus, clonal expansions within the joint are typically not large enough to consistently detect at the T cell population level. TCR subfamily analysis (e.g., BV-specific polymerase chain reaction (PCR)) or even more sensitive analytic techniques (e.g., BV-BJ specific PCR, CDR3 length analysis, or single-stranded conformational polymorphism analysis) are usually required to detect the majority of T cell expansions present in synovial tissue or fluid.

In contrast to the suggestion that the synovial TCR repertoire may be highly limited in diversity, the cumulative evidence describes a repertoire in established disease that is markedly heterogeneous, although skewed compared to peripheral blood.

The majority of recent studies have used PCR-based methodologies to analyze TCRAV, or more frequently TCRBV, expression in the synovium compared to peripheral blood. These studies have indicated that in most patients, a large number of TCRs are present, with nearly all AV and BV gene segments expressed at detectable levels. There is some indication that the repertoire may be more restricted in early disease [91, 92]. This observation is consistent with the idea that the early cellular infiltrate may be more dominated by local antigen-driven T cells, and that cells subsequently arriving will include non-specific T cell populations being recruited to the area of inflammation.

Within the heterogeneity of synovial T cells, biases in the TCRA and TCRB repertoire have been reported (see chapter by D.A. Fox and N.J. Singer, this volume). For TCRA, clusters of patients have shown increased expression of TCRAV1 [93], AV2 [94], AV10 [95], AV11 [96], AV14 [96], AV15 [95, 97], AV17 [93] and AV18 [95]. Other studies have shown no skewing [98–100]. Multiple studies have analyzed TCRBV expression, and some consensus among different studies has suggested preferential usage of BV2 [91, 98, 101–104], BV3.1 [91, 98, 101, 103, 105], BV6s [96, 102–104], BV14.1 [93, 101, 102, 105–107] and BV17.1 [93, 105, 108, 109]. One study noted increased expression of BV14 in RA synovial fluid compared to abnormally low levels in the blood of the same patients [106]. These investigators hypothesized that a Vβ14-specific superantigen could account for such findings. However, more detailed experiments showed prominent oligoclonal expansions within the TCRBV14 subset ([106]; see below), which would not be predicted to occur after stimulation by a superantigen. Furthermore, follow-up studies using a monoclonal antibody specific for Vβ14$^+$ T cells did not document low CD4$^+$ Vβ14$^+$ T cells in the peripheral blood of RA patients compared to controls [73]. Other investigators have also hypothesized a role for superantigens since BV3, BV14 and BV17 share the ability to be stimulated by particular superantigens, such as staphylococcal enterotoxin B (SEB) [105]. However, recent studies have not provided additional support for such a model, and as described below, the pattern of TCR expression in the joint suggests T cell stimulation by conventional peptide/MHC and not superantigen (see below). Although subsets of RA patients do show similar patterns of increased TCR V gene expression, many patients do not exhibit these patterns, leaving the prospect of a uniform TCR V gene bias in RA, whether secondary to stimulation by a superantigen or by a common peptide presented by DR4, as increasingly unlikely.

Perhaps the hallmark of the synovial TCR repertoire is the presence of multiple clonal expansions, and the presence of CD4$^+$ clonal expansions provides strong evidence for a previous or ongoing response to conventional antigen(s), i.e. peptides presented by class II MHC. Some of the preferential TCR V gene usages mentioned above are accounted for by the accumulation of expanded clonotypes. Furthermore, increasingly sensitive methods, such as CDR3 length and single-stranded conformational polymorphism (SSCP) analysis, have allowed for the detection of expansions previously missed by monoclonal antibody staining or BV-specific PCR [110–113]. Numerous recent studies applying these methods or performing extensive sequencing have demonstrated that the frequency of clonal expansions in the synovium is markedly increased relative to peripheral blood lymphocytes [112–115] (C.C. Striebich, M.T. Falta, B.L. Kotzin, unpublished observations). Expanded clonotypes have also been found in different areas of the same tissue, in more than one joint in the same patient, and have been shown to persist in the same joint over extended periods of continued disease activity [90, 103, 104, 104, 109, 112–116] (C.C. Striebich, M.T. Falta, B.L. Kotzin, unpublished observations). It is emphasized that many of these expansions are small when considering the entire population of synovial T cells. Thus, if a TCRBV subfamily constitutes 5% of the total TCRs present, and a clonotype represents 10% of this subfamily, the overall frequency of the clone will only be 0.5%. However, this clonal frequency is much greater than that found in the peripheral blood of normals, where the expected frequency of any clonotype is expected to be less than 1 in 10, 000. Recent studies from our laboratory have further documented that the synovial TCR repertoire is not a passive reflection of that in the circulating pool. Occasionally, identical expanded clonotypes have been found in both the blood and synovial compartments of individual RA patients [106, 112, 113, 117–119]. It is unclear whether these cells have been stimulated by systemic antigens and subsequently migrated to the joint, or whether they proliferated in the joint and subsequently spread systemically.

The best evidence for demonstrating that cells have TCRs characteristic of antigen-stimulation is to show that they express related CDR3s in the context of similar TCRV and J regions. The CDR3 is considered to be the key TCR element in antigen (peptide) recognition, making direct contact with the peptide presented by an appropriate MHC molecule. If independent T cell clones express highly related TCRs, it is inferred that they have been selectively stimulated by a common antigen. In RA, evidence for the presence of related clonotypes within individual patients has been limited, and evidence for homologous TCRs (i.e. homologous CDR3 motifs) among different RA patients has not been published. Several studies have presented evidence for homologous TCRs among different synovial clones ([96, 109, 113, 114, 120]; reviewed in [121]). However, many of the so-called related clones had significant non-conserved amino acid substitutions within the CDR3 sequence, and often differed in CDR3 length as well as BV and BJ usage. These differences can have profound effects on T cell specificity [122, 123]. Most importantly, the vast majority of these comparisons were made without knowledge of the co-expressed TCRA gene. Therefore, any conclusions regarding the similarity of these compared clones and the implication for recognition of the same antigen must be limited.

With the advent of rapid sequencing techniques, the search for related TCR structures has been greatly facilitated. In our laboratory, greater than 1600 cDNA clones were sequenced through the CDR3 in a multi-joint study of $CD4^+$ T cells in patients with established RA (C.C. Striebich, M.T. Falta, B.L. Kotzin, unpublished observations). While focusing on TCRBV gene segments implicated in RA by previous studies (BV2, 3, 8, 14, 17; see above), we frequently found examples of clones utilizing highly homologous TCRB genes, and these clones were usually present in different joints of the same patient. Furthermore, clones with identical TCR β-chain amino acid sequences, but encoded by different nucleotide sequences (i.e. derived from independent precursors) were observed in all patients. In instances where T cell clones cultured by limiting dilution could be obtained, the co-expressed TCRA chains also shared a number of conserved features, providing a firmer basis for concluding that these cells were selected by a common conventional antigen.

While the above holds promise that clonal expansions and related sets of T cells selected by a common antigen can be identified in RA synovium, investigators are also concerned regarding the lack of evidence that related TCRs are present in different patients [1, 39, 124]. If RA-associated HLA-DR4 molecules present a limited number of arthritogenic peptides to T cells in the synovium, a significant fraction of the synovial T cell response and their TCRs should be similar among different patients. Thus far, this does not appear to be the case. Several proposals have been made to explain the heterogeneous synovial repertoire in RA. One is that the T cell infiltrate is not related to the disease process of RA *per se*, but rather, is comprised of cells which have non-specifically migrated and been retained in the inflamed synovial tissue. These cells would represent a subpopulation of peripheral cells which had been activated at sites distant from the joint and acquired surface expression of adhesion molecules and memory markers allowing antigen-independent access to the synovium [1, 124]. These cells may be participating in the inflammatory response, but they provide no clue to synovial antigens being targeted in RA. The data thus far do suggest that a disease-specific synovial T cell population will constitute a small proportion of the total synovial T cell repertoire. This phenomenon has been observed in other T cell-mediated disorders. Studies of T cell responses to etiological antigens in tuberculoid leprosy, leishmaniasis, multiple sclerosis (and EAE), and allografts show that the frequency of antigen-specific T cells at the site of inflammation is extremely low, presumably diluted by the recruitment of non-specific T cells to the area of inflammation.

Other possible sources of confusion, both technical and biologic, may also be involved in the variability of TCR studies reported to date. For example, the levels of TCR expression determined by semi-quantitative PCR techniques and the size of clonal expansions are subject to PCR amplification artifacts. In contrast, related clones (rather than identical) selected by a common antigen cannot be accounted for by PCR artifact. In addition, studies have varied by analyzing synovial tissue versus synovial fluid and by studying cultured versus freshly isolated synovial T cells. We have found that the repertoire of synovial fluid $CD4^+$ T cells is greatly altered by short- and long-term culture. Another important source of confusion in some studies is the failure to separately analyze $CD4^+$ and $CD8^+$ populations. Repertoire biases confined to one subset will be obscured by the other. In addition, $CD4^+$ and $CD8^+$

cells are unequally distributed in different areas of the inflamed synovial membrane, and possible differences in CD4:CD8 ratios may invalidate comparisons of V region expression between the synovial fluid and blood. It has also been established that $CD8^+$ T cell clonal expansions commonly occur in the peripheral blood of normal individuals [125–127] and are even more frequent in RA patients [111, 127–129]. Since these peripheral $CD8^+$ expansions can be present in RA synovium [111], and clonal expansions within the synovia are dominated by $CD8^+$ cells [116], repertoire studies which do not separate $CD4^+$ cells may be primarily sampling $CD8^+$ clonal expansions. Finally, the heterogeneity of RA patients is also frequently underappreciated as a variable in TCR analyses. Characteristics that vary frequently include HLA type, disease duration and severity, and prescribed medications. Biological factors perhaps related to the duration of disease include intramolecular epitope spreading and the evolution of responses to newly released synovial antigens [130–132].

Other studies have suggested that the repertoire of peripheral blood $CD4^+$ cells in RA is also abnormal. In a study of patients with early disease, Goronzy et al. [117] found clonal expansions of peripheral $CD4^+$ T cells, with a preference for expression of BV3, BV14 and BV17. These expansions could not be demonstrated in HLA-DRB1*04 matched normals or psoriatic arthritis controls, however, they were present in unaffected siblings of RA patients. Furthermore, they did not express CD7 or CD28, proliferated in response to mitogens despite not expressing CD28, and demonstrated autoreactivity in autologous mixed lymphocyte reactions [118]. The frequency of CD7-/CD28- cells was shown to be increased in RA peripheral blood, and it was suggested that this phenotype is under genetic control [133]. The authors concluded that oligoclonality is a risk factor in RA rather than directly resulting from synovial inflammation, and that defects in clonal downsizing might be the operative mechanism.

The future challenge for studies of T cells in RA is to demonstrate the disease relevance of synovial or peripheral blood T cell expansions and other TCR repertoire alterations. The key experiments will be directed toward defining the specificity for antigen.

Target antigens in RA

Description of the antigens which stimulate T cell proliferation in the early stages of RA remains elusive. As the etiology of disease continues to be an unanswered question, debate has centered on whether the inciting antigens originate from endogenous proteins or if they are derived from microbial organisms following infection. As such, candidate antigens fall into two major categories. The first are self-proteins such as type II collagen (CII), cartilage glycoprotein gp39, and components of cartilage proteoglycan (aggrecan), which are expressed at the site of chronic inflammation in the joint. Antigenic determinants on these molecules might become available to functionally ignorant T cells if they are released from sequestered sites following tissue trauma or infection/inflammation [134, 135]. Alternatively, tissue damage may unveil cryptic epitopes to which tolerance has not been achieved during intrathymic development of T cells [130–132]. Cryptic epitope presentation may also be mediated by proinflammatory cytokines which induce quantitative and qualitative differences in the antigen-processing capabilities of professional and non-professional antigen presenting cells.

Generally, attempts to define synovial T cell specificity to various antigens have measured T cell proliferation by stimulating bulk cultures or, less frequently, at the clonal level by limiting dilution. Occasionally, clones have been established by selection with a candidate antigen. CII has attracted the most attention as a candidate autoantigen because it is a major cartilage constituent and can induce experimental arthritis in genetically susceptible rodents [11, 12], or mice transgenic for human HLA-DR1 [36] and DR4 [37] or DQ molecules [60]. Disease induction in these models always correlated with strong humoral and cellular responses to CII. In RA patients, CII-reactive T cell clones can be isolated [141, 142] and shown to persist over time [141], and peripheral blood responses to CII is a common finding in many, but not all, RA patients [143–146]. In controls demonstrating proliferation to CII, the kinetics were that of a primary response in contrast to RA patients whose kinetics suggested a recall response [146]. Responses to CII are DR-restricted [146], and an immunodominant p261-273 epitope has been identified [36-38]. Interestingly in one study, the TCRBV gene segment usage of RA synovial fluid T cells cultured with CII was biased toward usage of BV14, 17 and 8, gene segments previously shown to be overrepresented in the synovia of some RA patients (reviewed in [121]).

Other self-antigens which have been implicated in RA because of peripheral or synovial T cell proliferative responses or the capability of inducing inflammatory arthritis in animals include immunoglobulin [147], cartilage proteoglycan (aggrecan) components [14, 142, 145, 148–150], cartilage link protein [151], a 68 kDa antigenic target of antibodies occurring specifically in RA [152], and cartilage glycoprotein gp39 [13]. Human cartilage gp39 is of interest because it is a major secretory protein of synovial fibroblasts and articular chondrocytes [153, 154]. mRNA of gp39 was detectable in synovial specimens and cartilage of RA patients but not in healthy adult cartilage [154], and the serum levels of this protein correlated with joint disease [155], suggesting that this molecule may be a target in the RA joint. Using a DR4 peptide binding motif, Verheijden and coworkers identified gp39-derived peptides selectively recognized by peripheral blood T cells from RA patients [13]. Furthermore, immunization of BALB/c mice with whole protein resulted in the development of a chronic arthritis which could be modulated by intranasal administration of gp39 [13].

In another recent study, a set of CD4^{+} T cell clones isolated from the synovial membrane and fluid of two RA patients responded in a DR4- or DR9-restricted manner to autologous synovial cells [156]. These clones responded to solubilized HPLC-fractionated proteins derived from RA synovial cells, but they did not recognize autologous peripheral blood antigen presenting cells, nor solubilized antigens prepared from synovial cells from three non-RA controls.

The second category of disease-inciting candidate antigens is derived from infectious organisms. Multiple viruses have been implicated in autoimmune diseases and arthritis [136], and bacterial infections have been associated with chronic inflammatory arthritis such as in reactive arthritis and Lyme disease. Molecular mimicry may provide one link between immune responses to infectious agents and subsequent autoimmunity [136]. In this model of disease induction, T cells with degenerate specificity first properly respond to viral or bacterial antigens to clear the infection. However, they also inappropriately cross-react with endogenous antigens bearing conformational similarity to the original inciting antigen. These self-antigens are likely to be cryptic as well since the responding T cells are not deleted in the thymus [137]. The crystal structure of a human TCR-MHC/peptide complex provides a structural basis for the degeneracy of TCR binding as there are only a few contact points made between the peptide and TCR [138]. Other recent studies have directly demonstrated the existence of autoreactive T cells capable of being activated by peptides from different viruses and bacteria [139, 140].

Immune responses to foreign epitopes also have the potential to contribute to the synovial inflammation. As discussed above, bacterial heat shock proteins (HSPs) and the EBV glycoprotein gp110 contain the QKRAA amino acid motif in common with the HLA-DR shared epitope, and immune recognition of this determinant has been demonstrated in RA patients [50, 52]. It has been long recognized that RA patients have increased EBV infection rates and increased titers of antibodies to various EBV antigens [157], and one antibody specific for the EBNA-1 antigen cross-reacts with denatured collagen and keratin [158]. Recently, it has been demonstrated that joint-infiltrating $CD8^+$ T cells were enriched for reactivity to EBV proteins [159]. Clones responding to autologous B lymphoblastoid cells were shown to have fine specificity for peptides derived from the BZLF1 and BMLF1 transactivator proteins of EBV [160]. Interestingly, these clones were representatives of clonotypes shown by TCR CDR3 length analysis to be expanded and persistent in the synovial compartment. Therefore, the combination of T cell reactivity corroborated by TCR analysis strengthens the argument that these $CD8^+$ cells may be relevant to the disease process. Interestingly, the 16 T cell clones reactive to BZLF1 were all unique clonotypes utilizing a total of four TCRBV gene segments. This shows that the T cell response to a single protein can involve a diverse TCR repertoire and perhaps partially account for the heterogeneous synovial TCR repertoire in RA patients.

A bacterial candidate antigen was realized with the finding that immunization of rats with *Mycobacterium tuberculosis* leads to adjuvant arthritis, and a T cell clone specific for mycobacterial HSP65 can transfer disease to naive recipients [161]. This HSP shares considerable homology with the human HSP60, and it has been hypothesized that mycobacterial HSP65-reactive T cells cross-reacting with the human equivalent or other synovial antigens may be important in synovial inflammation [162]. Consistent with this hypothesis, RA patients with early disease have pronounced synovial T cell responses to HSP65 [163, 164] and synovial T cells are enriched for clones specific for HSP65 [165, 166]. In addition, a small subset of mycobacterial HSP65-specific T cell clones cross-react with human HSP60 [165, 167], although responses to human HSP60 appears to be more characteristic of patients with juvenile chronic arthritis than RA patients [168].

As these studies indicate, T cell reactivity to multiple antigens can be detected in the peripheral blood and synovial compartment of RA patients, and the large number of potential antigens involved may correlate with the heterogeneity observed in the TCR repertoire. It is anticipated that future studies will be directed at determining the specificity of expanded synovial clonotypes for candidate self and foreign antigens.

Conclusions

In summary, there is considerable evidence that $CD4^+$ T cells are primary players in the immunopathogenesis of RA. The most compelling evidence is based on genetic contributions from HLA-DR and the central role for $CD4^+$ T cells in the different models for how the DR shared epitope results in disease. Genetic epidemiological studies appear to support a role for $CD4^+$ T cells in both the initiation of disease and the perpetuation of severe disease. There is also suggestive evidence that genes within the TCRA or TCRB complexes may also contribute to disease susceptibility. TCR repertoire studies also suggest that responses to particular antigens are ongoing in the RA synovium. Clearly, however, these TCR data will be most enlightening when the target antigens for expanded and selected synovial T cell clones are delineated.

References

1 Firestein GS, Zvaifler NJ (1990) How important are T cells in chronic rheumatoid synovitis? [published erratum appears in *Arthritis Rheum* 1990 Sep;33(9):1437]. *Arthritis Rheum* 33: 768–773

2 Panayi GS, Lanchbury JS, Kingsley GH (1992) The importance of the T cell in initiating and maintaining the chronic synovitis of rheumatoid arthritis. *Arthritis Rheum* 35: 729–735

3 Cush JJ, Lipsky PE (1988) Phenotypic analysis of synovial tissue and peripheral blood lymphocytes isolated from patients with rheumatoid arthritis. *Arthritis Rheum* 31: 1230–1238

4 Iannone F, Corrigall VM, Kingsley GH, Panayi GS (1994) Evidence for the continuous recruitment and activation of T cells into the joints of patients with rheumatoid arthritis. *Eur J Immunol* 24: 2706–2713
5 Yokota A, Murata N, Saiki O, Shimizu M, Springer TA, Kishimoto T (1995) High avidity state of leukocyte function-associated antigen-1 on rheumatoid synovial fluid T lymphocytes. *J Immunol* 155: 4118–4124
6 Hernández-Garcia C, Fernández-Gutiérrez B, Morado IC, Bañares AA, Jover JA (1996) The CD69 activation pathway in rheumatoid arthritis synovial fluid T cells. *Arthritis Rheum* 39: 1277–1286
7 MacDonald KPA, Nishioka Y, Lipsky PE, Thomas R (1997) Functional CD40 ligand is expressed by T cells in rheumatoid arthritis. *J Clin Invest* 100: 2404–2414
8 Keystone EC, Poplonski L, Miller RG, Gorczynski R, Gladman D, Snow K (1988) Reactivity of T-cells from patients with rheumatoid arthritis to anti-CD3 antibody. *Clin Immunol Immunopathol* 48: 325–337
9 Verwilghen J, Vertessen S, Stevens EAM, Dequeker J, Ceuppens JL (1990) Depressed T-cell reactivity to recall antigens in rheumatoid arthritis. *J Clin Immunol* 10: 90–98
10 Kotzin BL, Leung DYM, Kappler J, Marrack P (1993) Superantigens and their potential role in human disease. *Adv Immunol* 54: 99–166
11 Trentham DE, Townes AS, Kang AH (1977) Autoimmunity to type II collagen: an experimental model of arthritis. *J Exp Med* 146: 857–868
12 Courtenay JS, Dallman MJ, Dayan AD, Martin A, Mosedale B (1980) Immunisation against heterologous type II collagen induces arthritis in mice. Nature 283: 666–668
13 Verheijden GFM, Rijnders AWM, Bos E, Coenen-de Roo CJ, van Staveren CJJ, Miltenburg AMM, Meijerink JH, Elewaut D, de Keyser F, Veys E et al (1997) Human cartilage glycoprotein-39 as a candidate autoantigen in rheumatoid arthritis. *Arthritis Rheum* 40: 1115–1125
14 Glant TT, Mikecz K, Arzoumanian A, Poole AR (1987) Proteoglycan-induced arthritis in BALB/c mice. Clinical features and histopathology. *Arthritis Rheum* 30: 201–212
15 Theofilopoulos AN, Dixon FJ (1985) Murine models of systemic lupus erythematosus. *Adv Immunol* 37: 269–390
16 Cohen PL, Eisenberg RA (1991) *Lpr* and *gld*: single gene models of systemic autoimmunity and lymphoproliferative disease. *Annu Rev Immunol* 9: 243–269
17 Hang L, Theofilopoulos AN, Dixon FJ (1982) A spontaneous rheumatoid arthritis-like disease in MRL/l mice. *J Exp Med* 155: 1690–1701
18 O'Sullivan FX, Fassbender H-G, Gay S, Koopman WJ (1985) Etiopathogenesis of the rheumatoid arthritis-like disease in MRL/l mice. I. The histomorphologic basis of joint destruction. *Arthritis Rheum* 28: 529–536
19 O'Sullivan FX, Vogelweid CM, Besch-Williford CL, Walker SE (1995) Differential effects of $CD4^+$ T cell depletion on inflammatory central nervous system disease, arthritis and sialadenitis in MRL/lpr mice. *J Autoimmun* 8: 163–175
20 Nepom GT, Nepom BS (1992) Prediction of susceptibility to rheumatoid arthritis by human leukocyte antigen genotyping. *Rheum Dis Clin North Am* 18: 785–792

21 Gregersen PK, Silver J, Winchester RJ (1987) The shared epitope hypothesis. An approach to understanding the molecular genetics of susceptibility to rheumatoid arthritis. *Arthritis Rheum* 30: 1205–1213
22 Brown JH, Jardetzky TS, Gorga JC, Stern LJ, Urban RG, Strominger JL, Wiley DC (1993) Three-dimensional structure of the human class II histocompatibility antigen HLA-DR1. *Nature* 364: 33–39
23 Stern LJ, Brown JH, Jardetzky TS, Gorga JC, Urban RG, Strominger JL, Wiley DC (1994) Crystal structure of the human class II MHC protein HLA-DR1 complexed with an influenza virus peptide. *Nature* 368: 215–221
24 Dessen A, Lawrence CM, Cupo S, Zaller DM, Wiley DC (1997) X-ray crystal structure of HLA-DR4 (DRA*0101, DRB1*0401) complexed with a peptide from human collagen II. *Immunity* 7: 473–481
25 Brown JH, Jardetzky T, Saper MA, Samraoui B, Bjorkman PJ, Wiley DC (1988) A hypothetical model of the foreign antigen binding site of class II histocompatibility molecules [published erratum appears in *Nature* 1988 Jun 23;333(6175):786]. *Nature* 332: 845–850
26 O'Sullivan D, Arrhenius T, Sidney J, del Guercio M-F, Albertson M, Wall M, Oseroff C, Southwood S, Colón SM, Gaeta FCA et al (1991) On the interaction of promiscuous antigenic peptides with different DR alleles. Identification of common structural motifs. *J Immunol* 147: 2663–2669
27 Chicz RM, Urban RG, Lane WS, Gorga JC, Stern LJ, Vignali DA, Strominger JL (1992) Predominant naturally processed peptides bound to HLA-DR1 are derived from MHC-related molecules and are heterogeneous in size. *Nature* 358: 764–768
28 Hammer J, Takacs B, Sinigaglia F (1992) Identification of a motif for HLA-DR1 binding peptides using M13 display libraries. *J Exp Med* 176: 1007–1013
29 Chicz RM, Urban RG, Gorga JC, Vignali DAA, Lane WS, Strominger JL (1993) Specificity and promiscuity among naturally processed peptides bound to HLA-DR alleles. *J Exp Med* 178: 27–47
30 Hammer J, Valsasnini P, Tolba K, Bolin D, Higelin J, Takacs B, Sinigaglia F (1993) Promiscuous and allele-specific anchors in HLA-DR-binding peptides. *Cell* 74: 197–203
31 Sette A, Sidney J, Oseroff C, del Guercio M-F, Southwood S, Arrhenius T, Powell MF, Colon SM, Gaeta FCA, Grey HM (1993) HLA DR4w4-binding motifs illustrate the biochemical basis of degeneracy and specificity in peptide-DR interactions. *J Immunol* 151: 3163–3170
32 Marshall KW, Liu AF, Canales J, Perahia B, Jorgensen B, Gantzos RD, Aguilar B, Devaux B, Rothbard JB (1994) Role of the polymorphic residues in HLA-DR molecules in allele-specific binding of peptide ligands. *J Immunol* 152: 4946–4957
33 Wucherpfennig KW, Strominger JL (1995) Selective binding of self peptides to disease-associated major histocompatibility complex (MHC) molecules: a mechanism for MHC-linked susceptibility to human autoimmune diseases. *J Exp Med* 181: 1597–1601
34 Hammer J, Gallazzi F, Bono E, Karr RW, Guenot J, Valsasnini P, Nagy ZA, Sinigaglia F

(1995) Peptide binding specificity of HLA-DR4 molecules: correlation with rheumatoid arthritis association. *J Exp Med* 181: 1847–1855

35 Woulfe SL, Bono CP, Zacheis ML, Kirschmann DA, Baudino TA, Swearingen C, Karr RW, Schwartz BD (1995) Negatively charged residues interacting with the p4 pocket confer binding specificity to DRB1*0401. *Arthritis Rheum* 38: 1744–1753

36 Rosloniec EF, Brand DD, Myers LK, Whittington KB, Gumanovskaya M, Zaller DM, Woods A, Altmann DM, Stuart JM, Kang AH (1997) An HLA-DR1 transgene confers susceptibility to collagen-induced arthritis elicited with human type II collagen. *J Exp Med* 185: 1113–1122

37 Rosloniec EF, Brand DD, Myers LK, Esaki Y, Whittington KB, Zaller DM, Woods A, Stuart JM, Kang AH (1998) Induction of autoimmune arthritis in HLA-DR4 (DRB1*0401) transgenic mice by immunization with human and bovine type II collagen. *J Immunol* 160: 2573–2578

38 Fugger L, Rothbard JB, Sonderstrup-McDevitt G (1996) Specificity of an HLA-DRB1*0401-restricted T cell response to type II collagen. *Eur J Immunol* 26: 928–933

39 Goronzy JJ, Weyand CM (1993) Interplay of T lymphocytes and HLA-DR molecules in rheumatoid arthritis. *Curr Opin Rheumatol* 5: 169–177

40 Malhotra U, Spielman R, Concannon P (1992) Variability in T cell receptor Vβ gene usage in human peripheral blood lymphocytes. Studies of identical twins, siblings, and insulin-dependent diabetes mellitus patients. *J Immunol* 149: 1802–1808

41 Hawes GE, Struyk L, van den Elsen PJ (1993) Differential usage of T cell receptor V gene segments in $CD4^+$ and $CD8^+$ subsets of T lymphocytes in monozygotic twins. *J Immunol* 150: 2033–2045

42 Davey MP, Meyer MM, Bakke AC (1994) T cell receptor Vβ gene expression in monozygotic twins. Discordance in CD8 subset and in disease states. *J Immunol* 152: 315–321

43 Walser-Kuntz DR, Weyand CM, Weaver AJ, O'Fallon WM, Goronzy JJ (1995) Mechanisms underlying the formation of the T cell receptor repertoire in rheumatoid arthritis. *Immunity* 2: 597–605

44 Kohsaka H, Nanki T, Ollier WER, Miyasaka N, Carson DA (1996) Influence of the rheumatoid arthritis-associated shared epitope on T-cell receptor repertoire formation. *Proc Assoc Am Physicians* 108: 323–328

45 Penzotti JE, Nepom GT, Lybrand TP (1997) Use of T cell receptor/HLA-DRB1*04 molecular modeling to predict site-specific interactions for the DR shared epitope associated with rheumatoid arthritis. *Arthritis Rheum* 40: 1316–1326

46 Hiraiwa A, Yamanaka K, Kwok WW, Mickelson EM, Masewicz S, Hansen JA, Radka SF, Nepom GT (1990) Structural requirements for recognition of the HLA-Dw14 class II epitope: a key HLA determinant associated with rheumatoid arthritis. *Proc Natl Acad Sci USA* 87: 8051–8055

47 Penzotti JE, Doherty D, Lybrand TP, Nepom GT (1996) A structural model for TCR

recognition of the HLA class II shared epitope sequence implicated in susceptibility to rheumatoid arthritis. *J Autoimmun* 9: 287–293

48 Nepom GT, Ou D, Lybrand TP, DeWeese C, Domeier ME, Buckner JH, Mitchell LA, Tingle AJ (1996) Recognition of altered self major histocompatibility complex molecules modulated by specific peptide interactions. *Eur J Immunol* 26: 949–952

49 Roudier C, Auger I, Roudier J (1996) Molecular mimicry reflected through database screening: serendipity or survival strategy? *Immunol Today* 17: 357–358

50 Roudier J, Petersen J, Rhodes GH, Luka J, Carson DA (1989) Susceptibility to rheumatoid arthritis maps to a T-cell epitope shared by the HLA-Dw4 DR β-1 chain and the Epstein-Barr virus glycoprotein gp110. *Proc Natl Acad Sci USA* 86: 5104–5108

51 La Cava A, Nelson JL, Ollier WER, MacGregor A, Keystone EC, Thorne JC, Scavulli JF, Berry CC, Carson DA, Albani S (1997) Genetic bias in immune responses to a cassette shared by different microorganisms in patients with rheumatoid arthritis. *J Clin Invest* 100: 658–663

52 Albani S, Carson DA (1996) A multistep molecular mimicry hypothesis for the pathogenesis of rheumatoid arthritis. *Immunol Today* 17: 466–470

53 Salvat S, Auger I, Rochelle L, Begovich A, Geburher L, Sette A, Roudier J (1994) Tolerance to a self-peptide from the third hypervariable region of HLA DRB1*0401 in rheumatoid arthritis patients and normal subjects. *J Immunol* 153: 5321–5329

54 Albani S, Keystone EC, Nelson JL, Ollier WER, La Cava A, Montemayor AC, Weber DA, Montecucco C, Martini A, Carson DA (1995) Positive selection in autoimmunity: abnormal immune responses to a bacterial dnaJ antigenic determinant in patients with early rheumatoid arthritis. *Nat Med* 1: 448–452

55 Auger I, Escola JM, Gorvel JP, Roudier J (1996) HLA-DR4 and HLA-DR10 motifs that carry susceptibility to rheumatoid arthritis bind 70-kD heat shock proteins. *Nat Med* 2: 306–310

56 Auger I, Roudier J (1997) A function for the QKRAA amino acid motif: mediating binding of DnaJ to DnaK. Implications for the association of rheumatoid arthritis with HLA-DR4. *J Clin Invest* 99: 1818–1822

57 Zanelli E, Gonzalez-Gay MA, David CS (1995) Could HLA-DRB1 be the protective locus in rheumatoid arthritis? *Immunol Today* 16: 274–278

58 Nepom GT, Erlich H (1991) MHC class-II molecules and autoimmunity. *Annu Rev Immunol* 9: 493–525

59 Gonzalez-Gay MA, Nabozny GH, Bull MJ, Zanelli E, Douhan J, Griffiths MM, Glimcher LH, Luthra HS, David CS (1994) Protective role of major histocompatibility complex class II Eb^d transgene on collagen-induced arthritis. *J Exp Med* 180: 1559–1564

60 Nabozny GH, Baisch JM, Cheng S, Cosgrove D, Griffiths MM, Luthra HS, Davis CS (1996) HLA-DQ8 transgenic mice are highly susceptible to collagen-induced arthritis: a novel model for human polyarthritis. *J Exp Med* 183: 27–37

61 Bradley DS, Nabozny GH, Cheng S, Zhou P, Griffiths MM, Luthra HS, David CS (1997) HLA-DQB1 polymorphism determines incidence, onset, and severity of collagen-

induced arthritis in transgenic mice. Implications in human rheumatoid arthritis. *J Clin Invest* 100: 2227–2234

62 Zanelli E, Krco CJ, Baisch JM, Cheng S, David CS (1996) Immune response of HLA-DQ8 transgenic mice to peptides from the third hypervariable region of HLA-DRB1 correlates with predisposition to rheumatoid arthritis. *Proc Natl Acad Sci USA* 93: 1814–1819

63 Zanelli E, Krco CJ, David CS (1997) Critical residues on HLA-DRB1*0402 HV3 peptide for HLA-DQ8-restricted immunogenicity: implications for rheumatoid arthritis predisposition. *J Immunol* 158: 3545–3551

64 Jawaheer D, Thomson W, MacGregor AJ, Carthy D, Davidson J, Dyer PA, Silman AJ, Ollier WER (1994) "Homozygosity" for the HLA-DR shared epitope contributes the highest risk for rheumatoid arthritis concordance in identical twins. *Arthritis Rheum* 37: 681–686

65 Weyand CM, Xie C, Goronzy JJ (1992) Homozygosity for the HLA-DRB1 allele selects for extraarticular manifestations in rheumatoid arthritis. *J Clin Invest* 89: 2033–2039

66 Weyand CM, Hicok KC, Conn DL, Goronzy JJ (1992) The influence of HLA-DRB1 genes on disease severity in rheumatoid arthritis. *Ann Intern Med* 117: 801–806

67 Evans TI, Han J, Singh R, Moxley G (1995) The genotypic distribution of shared-epitope DRB1 alleles suggests a recessive mode of inheritance of the rheumatoid arthritis disease-susceptibility gene. *Arthritis Rheum* 38: 1754–1761

68 Moreno I, Valenzuela A, García A, Yélamos J, Sánchez B, Hernánz W (1996) Association of the shared epitope with radiological severity of rheumatoid arthritis. *J Rheumatol* 23: 6–9

69 Weyand CM, McCarthy TG, Goronzy JJ (1995) Correlation between disease phenotype and genetic heterogeneity in rheumatoid arthritis. *J Clin Invest* 95: 2120–2126

70 Berg LJ, Frank GD, Davis MM (1990) The effects of MHC gene dosage and allelic variation on T cell receptor selection. *Cell* 60: 1043–1053

71 Ashton-Rickardt PG, Bandeira A, Delaney JR, Van Kaer L, Pircher H-P, Zinkernagal RM, Tonegawa S (1994) Evidence for a differential avidity model of T cell selection in the thymus. *Cell* 76: 651–663

72 Hogquist KA, Jameson SC, Heath WR, Howard JL, Bevan MJ, Carbone FR (1994) T cell receptor antagonist peptides induce positive selection. *Cell* 76: 17–27

73 Ricalton NS, Paliard X, Kappler J, Marrack P, Kotzin BL (1996) Analysis of TcRBV expression in human populations for evidence of superantigen exposure. *The Immunologist* 4: 106–108

74 McDermott M, Kastner DL, Holloman JD, Schmidt-Wolf G, Lundberg AS, Sinha AA, Hsu C, Cashin P, Molloy MG, Mulcahy B et al (1995) The role of T cell receptor β chain genes in susceptibility to rheumatoid arthritis. *Arthritis Rheum* 38: 91–95

75 Mu H, Charmley P, King M-C, Criswell LA (1996) Synergy between T cell receptor β gene polymorphism and HLA-DR4 in susceptibility to rheumatoid arthritis. *Arthritis Rheum* 39: 931–937

76 Cornélis F, Hardwick L, Flipo RM, Martinez M, Lasbleiz S, Prud'Homme JF, Tran TH, Walsh S, Delaye A, Nicod A et al (1997) Association of rheumatoid arthritis with an amino acid allelic variation of the T cell receptor. *Arthritis Rheum* 40: 1387–1390

77 Hall FC, Brown MA, Weeks DE, Walsh S, Nicod A, Butcher S, Andrews LJ, Wordsworth BP (1997) A linkage study across the T cell receptor A and T cell receptor B loci in families with rheumatoid arthritis. *Arthritis Rheum* 40: 1798–1802

78 Charmley P, Nepom BS, Concannon P (1994) HLA and T cell receptor β-chain DNA polymorphisms identify a distinct subset of patients with pauciarticular-onset juvenile rheumatoid arthritis. *Arthritis Rheum* 37: 695–701

79 Maksymowych WP, Gabriel CA, Luyrink L, Melin-Aldana H, Elma M, Giannini EH, Lovell DJ, Van Kerckhove C, Leiden J, Choi E et al (1992) Polymorphism in a T-cell receptor variable gene is associated with susceptibility to a juvenile rheumatoid arthritis subset. *Immunogenetics* 35: 257–262

80 Luyrink L, Gabriel CA, Thompson SD, Grom AA, Maksymowych WP, Choi E, Glass DN (1993) Reduced expression of a human $V_{\beta}6.1$ T-cell receptor allele. *Proc Natl Acad Sci USA* 90: 4369–4373

81 Acha-Orbea H, Mitchell DJ, Timmermann L, Wraith DC, Tausch GS, Waldor MK, Zamvil SS, McDevitt HO, Steinman L (1988) Limited heterogeneity of T cell receptors from lymphocytes mediating autoimmune encephalomyelitis allows specific immune intervention. *Cell* 54: 263–273

82 Urban JL, Kumar V, Kono DH, Gomez C, Horvath SJ, Clayton J, Ando DG, Sercarz EE, Hood L (1988) Restricted use of T cell receptor V genes in murine autoimmune encephalomyelitis raises possibilities for antibody therapy. *Cell* 54: 577–592

83 Offner H, Buenafe AC, Vainiene M, Celnik B, Weinberg AD, Gold DP, Hashim G, Vandenbark AA (1993) Where, when, and how to detect biased expression of disease-relevant Vβ genes in rats with experimental autoimmune encephalomyelitis. *J Immunol* 151: 506–517

84 Keystone EC, Minden M, Klock R, Poplonski L, Zalcberg J, Takadera T, Mak TW (1988) Structure of T cell antigen receptor β chain in synovial fluid cells from patients with rheumatoid arthritis. *Arthritis Rheum* 31: 1555–1557

85 Stamenkovic I, Stegagno M, Wright KA, Krane SM, Amento EP, Colvin RB, Kurnick JT (1988) Clonal dominance among T-lymphocyte infiltrates in arthritis. *Proc Natl Acad Sci USA* 85: 1179–1183

86 Duby AD, Sinclair AK, Osborne-Lawrence SL, Zeldes W, Kan L, Fox DA (1989) Clonal heterogeneity of synovial fluid T lymphocytes from patients with rheumatoid arthritis. *Proc Natl Acad Sci USA* 86: 6206–6210

87 Miltenburg AMM, van Laar JM, Daha MR, de Vries RRP, van den Elsen PJ, Breedveld FC (1990) Dominant T-cell receptor β-chain gene rearrangements indicate clonal expansion in the rheumatoid joint. *Scand J Immunol* 31: 121–126

88 Cooper SM, Dier DL, Roessner KD, Budd RC, Nicklas JA (1991) Diversity of rheumatoid synovial tissue T cells by T cell receptor analysis. Oligoclonal expansion in interleukin-2-responsive cells. *Arthritis Rheum* 34: 537–546

89 van Laar JM, Miltenburg AMM, Verdonk MJA, Daha MR, de Vries RRP, van den Elsen PJ, Breedveld FC (1991) Lack of T cell oligoclonality in enzyme-digested synovial tissue and in synovial fluid in most patients with rheumatoid arthritis. *Clin Exp Immunol* 83: 352–358

90 van Laar JM, Miltenburg AMM, Verdonk MJA, Daha MR, de Vries RRP, van den Elsen PJ, Breedveld FC (1992) T-cell receptor β-chain gene rearrangements of T-cell populations expanded from multiple sites of synovial tissue obtained from a patient with rheumatoid arthritis. *Scand J Immunol* 35: 187–194

91 Bucht A, Oksenberg JR, Lindblad S, Grönberg A, Steinman L, Klareskog L (1992) Characterization of T-cell receptor αβ repertoire in synovial tissue from different temporal phases of rheumatoid arthritis. *Scand J Immunol* 35: 159–165

92 Fischer D-C, Opalka B, Hoffmann A, Mayr W, Haubeck H-D (1996) Limited heterogeneity of rearranged T cell receptor V_{α} and V_{β} transcripts in synovial fluid T cells in early stages of rheumatoid arthritis. *Arthritis Rheum* 39: 454–462

93 Williams WV, Fang Q, Demarco D, VonFeldt J, Zurier RB, Weiner DB (1992) Restricted heterogeneity of T cell receptor transcripts in rheumatoid synovium. *J Clin Invest* 90: 326–333

94 Bröker BM, Korthäuer U, Heppt P, Weseloh G, de la Camp R, Kroczek RAE, Emmrich F (1993) Biased T cell receptor V gene usage in rheumatoid arthritis. Oligoclonal expansion of T cells expressing Vα2 genes in synovial fluid but not in peripheral blood. *Arthritis Rheum* 36: 1234–1243

95 Lunardi C, Marguerie C, So AK (1992) An altered repertoire of T cell receptor V gene expression by rheumatoid synovial fluid T lymphocytes. *Clin Exp Immunol* 90: 440– 446

96 Maruyama T, Saito I, Miyake S, Hashimoto H, Sato K, Yagita H, Okumura K, Miyasaka N (1993) A possible role of two hydrophobic amino acids in antigen recognition by synovial T cells in rheumatoid arthritis. *Eur J Immunol* 23: 2059–2065

97 Pluschke G, Ricken G, Taube H, Kroninger S, Melchers I, Peter HH, Eichmann K, Krawinkel U (1991) Biased T cell receptor Vα region repertoire in the synovial fluid of rheumatoid arthritis patients. *Eur J Immunol* 21: 2749–2754

98 Uematsu Y, Wege H, Straus A, Ott M, Bannwarth W, Lanchbury J, Panayi G, Steinmetz M (1991) The T-cell-receptor repertoire in the synovial fluid of a patient with rheumatoid arthritis is polyclonal. *Proc Natl Acad Sci USA* 88: 8534–8538

99 Sottini A, Imberti L, Gorla R, Cattaneo R, Primi D (1991) Restricted expression of T cell receptor Vβ but not Vα genes in rheumatoid arthritis. *Eur J Immunol* 21: 461–466

100 Struyk L, Kurnick JT, Hawes GE, van Laar JM, Schipper R, Oksenberg JR, Steinman L, de Vries RRP, Breedveld FC, van den Elsen P (1993) T-cell receptor V-gene usage in synovial fluid lymphocytes of patients with chronic arthritis. *Hum Immunol* 37: 237–251

101 Davey MP, Munkirs DD (1993) Patterns of T-cell receptor variable β gene expression by synovial fluid and peripheral blood T-cells in rheumatoid arthritis. *Clin Immunol Immunopathol* 68: 79–87

102 Jenkins RN, Nikaein A, Zimmermann A, Meek K, Lipsky PE (1993) T cell receptor Vβ gene bias in rheumatoid arthritis. *J Clin Invest* 92: 2688–2701

103 Pluschke G, Ginter A, Taube H, Melchers I, Peter HH, Krawinkel U (1993) Analysis of T cell receptor Vβ regions expressed by rheumatoid synovial T lymphocytes. *Immunobiol* 188: 330–339
104 Cooper SM, Roessner KD, Naito-Hoopes M, Howard DB, Gaur LK, Budd RC (1994) Increased usage of $V_{\beta}2$ and $V_{\beta}6$ in rheumatoid synovial fluid T cells. *Arthritis Rheum* 37: 1627–1636
105 Howell MD, Diveley JP, Lundeen KA, Esty A, Winters ST, Carlo DJ, Brostoff SW (1991) Limited T-cell receptor β-chain heterogeneity among interleukin 2 receptor-positive synovial T cells suggests a role for superantigen in rheumatoid arthritis. *Proc Natl Acad Sci USA* 88: 10921–10925
106 Paliard X, West SG, Lafferty JA, Clements JR, Kappler JW, Marrack P, Kotzin BL (1991) Evidence for the effects of a superantigen in rheumatoid arthritis. *Science* 253: 325–329
107 Sioud M, Kjeldsen-Kragh J, Quayle AJ, Wiker HG, Sorskaar D, Natvig JB, Forre O (1991) Immune responses to 18.6 and 30-kDa mycobacterial antigens in rheumatoid patients, and Vβ usage by specific synovial T-cell lines and fresh T cells. *Scand J Immunol* 34: 803–812
108 Zagon G, Tumang JR, Li Y, Friedman SM, Crow MK (1994) Increased frequency of Vβ17-positive T cells in patients with rheumatoid arthritis. *Arthritis Rheum* 37: 1431–1440
109 Li Y, Sun G-R, Tumang JR, Crow MK, Friedman SM (1994) CDR3 sequence motifs shared by oligoclonal rheumatoid arthritis synovial T cells. Evidence for an antigen-driven response. *J Clin Invest* 94: 2525–2531
110 Pannetier C, Even J, Kourilsky P (1995) T-cell repertoire diversity and clonal expansions in normal and clinical samples. *Immunol Today* 16: 176–181
111 Hingorani R, Monteiro J, Furie R, Chartash E, Navarrete C, Pergolizzi R, Gregersen PK (1996) Oligoclonality of Vβ3 TCR chains in the $CD8^+$ T cell population of rheumatoid arthritis patients. *J Immunol* 156: 852–858
112 Lim A, Toubert A, Pannetier C, Dougados M, Charron D, Kourilsky P, Even J (1996) Spread of clonal T-cell expansions in rheumatoid arthritis patients. *Hum Immunol* 48: 77–83
113 Ikeda Y, Masuko K, Nakai Y, Kato T, Hasanuma T, Yoshino S-I, Mizushima Y, Nishioka K, Yamamoto K (1996) High frequencies of identical T cell clonotypes in synovial tissues of rheumatoid arthritis patients suggest the occurrence of common antigen-driven immune responses. *Arthritis Rheum* 39: 446–453
114 Alam A, Lambert N, Lulé J, Coppin H, Mazières B, de Préval C, Cantagrel A (1996) Persistence of dominant T cell clones in synovial tissues during rheumatoid arthritis. *J Immunol* 156: 3480–3485
115 Kato T, Kurokawa M, Masuko-Hongo K, Sasakawa H, Sekine T, Ueda S, Yamamoto K, Nishioka K (1997) T cell clonality in synovial fluid of a patient with rheumatoid arthritis: persistent but fluctuant oligoclonal T cell expansions. *J Immunol* 159: 5143–5149
116 Masuko-Hongo K, Sekine T, Ueda S, Kobata T, Yamamoto K, Nishioka K, Kato T

(1997) Long term persistent accumulation of CD8+ T cells in synovial fluid of rheumatoid arthritis. *Ann Rheum Dis* 56: 613–621

117 Goronzy JJ, Bartz-Bazzanella P, Hu W, Jendro MC, Walser-Kuntz DR, Weyand CM (1994) Dominant clonotypes in the repertoire of peripheral CD4+ T cells in rheumatoid arthritis. *J Clin Invest* 94: 2068–2076

118 Schmidt D, Goronzy JJ, Weyand CM (1996) CD4+ CD7− CD28− T cells are expanded in rheumatoid arthritis and are characterized by autoreactivity. *J Clin Invest* 97: 2027–2037

119 Waase I, Kayser C, Carlson PJ, Goronzy JJ, Weyand CM (1996) Oligoclonal T cell proliferation in patients with rheumatoid arthritis and their unaffected siblings. *Arthritis Rheum* 39: 904–913

120 Struyk L, Hawes GE, Dolhain RJEM, van Scherpenzeel A, Godthelp B, Breedveld FC, van den Elsen PJ (1994) Evidence for selective in vivo expansion of synovial tissue-infiltrating CD4+ CD45RO+ T lymphocytes on the basis of CDR3 diversity. *Int Immunol* 6: 897–907

121 Struyk L, Hawes GE, Chatila MK, Breedveld FC, Kurnick JT, van den Elsen PJ (1995) T cell receptors in rheumatoid arthritis. *Arthritis Rheum* 38: 577–589

122 Rock EP, Sibbald PR, Davis MM, Chien Y-H (1994) CDR3 length in antigen-specific immune receptors. *J Exp Med* 179: 323–328

123 Chien Y-H, Davis MM (1993) How αβ T-cell receptors 'see' peptide/MHC complexes. *Immunol Today* 14: 597–602

124 Fox DA (1997) The role of T cells in the immunopathogenesis of rheumatoid arthritis: new perspectives. *Arthritis Rheum* 40: 598–609

125 Hingorani R, Choi I-H, Akolkar P, Gulwani-Akolkar B, Pergolizzi R, Silver J, Gregersen PK (1993) Clonal predominance of T cell receptors within the CD8+ CD45RO+ subset in normal human subjects. *J Immunol* 151: 5762–5769

126 Posnett DN, Sinha R, Kabak S, Russo C (1994) Clonal populations of T cells in normal elderly humans: the T cell equivalent to "benign monoclonal gammapathy" [published erratum appears in *J Exp Med* 1994 Mar 1; 179(3): 1077]. *J Exp Med* 179: 609–618

127 Fitzgerald JE, Ricalton NS, Meyer A-C, West SG, Kaplan H, Behrendt C, Kotzin BL (1995) Analysis of clonal CD8+ T cell expansions in normal individuals and patients with rheumatoid arthritis. *J Immunol* 154: 3538–3547

128 DerSimonian H, Sugita M, Glass DN, Maier AL, Weinblatt ME, Rème T, Brenner MB (1993) Clonal Vα12.1+ T cell expansions in the peripheral blood of rheumatoid arthritis patients. *J Exp Med* 177: 1623–1631

129 Wang ECY, Lawson TM, Vedhara K, Moss PAH, Lehner PJ, Borysiewicz LK (1997) CD8high+ (CD57+) T cells in patients with rheumatoid arthritis. *Arthritis Rheum* 40: 237–248

130 Sercarz EE, Lehmann PV, Ametani A, Benichou G, Miller A, Moudgil K (1993) Dominance and crypticity of T cell antigenic determinants. *Annu Rev Immunol* 11: 729–766

131 Elson CJ, Barker RN, Thompson SJ, Williams NA (1995) Immunologically ignorant

autoreactive T cells, epitope spreading and repertoire limitation. *Immunol Today* 16: 71–76

132 Lanzavecchia A (1995) How can cryptic epitopes trigger autoimmunity? *J Exp Med* 181: 1945–1948

133 Martens PB, Goronzy JJ, Schaid D, Weyand CM (1997) Expansion of unusual CD4+ T cells in severe rheumatoid arthritis. *Arthritis Rheum* 40: 1106–1114

134 Ohashi PS, Oehen S, Buerki K, Pircher H, Ohashi CT, Odermatt B, Malissen B, Zinkernagel RM, Hengartner H (1991) Ablation of "tolerance" and induction of diabetes by virus infection in viral antigen transgenic mice. *Cell* 65: 305–317

135 Röcken M, Urban JF, Shevach EM (1992) Infection breaks T-cell tolerance. *Nature* 359: 79–82

136 Oldstone MBA (1997) Viruses and autoimmune diseases. *Scand J Immunol* 46: 320–325

137 Barnaba V, Sinigaglia F (1997) Molecular mimicry and T cell-mediated autoimmune disease. *J Exp Med* 185: 1529–1531

138 Garboczi DN, Ghosh P, Utz U, Fan QR, Biddison WE, Wiley DC (1996) Structure of the complex between human T-cell receptor, viral peptide and HLA-A2. *Nature* 384: 134–141

139 Wucherpfennig KW, Strominger JL (1995) Molecular mimicry in T cell-mediated autoimmunity: viral peptides activate human T cell clones specific for myelin basic protein. *Cell* 80: 695–705

140 Hemmer B, Fleckenstein BT, Vergelli M, Jung G, McFarland H, Martin R, Wiesmüller KH (1997) Identification of high potency microbial and self ligands for a human autoreactive class II-restricted T cell clone. *J Exp Med* 185: 1651–1659

141 Londei M, Savill CM, Verhoef A, Brennan F, Leech ZA, Duance V, Maini RN, Feldmann M (1989) Persistence of collagen type II-specific T-cell clones in the synovial membrane of a patient with rheumatoid arthritis. *Proc Natl Acad Sci USA* 86: 636–640

142 Melchers I, Jooss-Rüdiger J, Peter HH (1997) Reactivity patterns of synovial T-cell lines derived from a patient with rheumatoid arthritis. I. Reactions with defined antigens and auto-antigens suggest the existence of multireactive T-cell clones. *Scand J Immunol* 46: 187–194

143 Solinger AM, Bhatnagar R, Stobo JD (1981) Cellular, molecular, and genetic characteristics of T cell reactivity to collagen in man. *Proc Natl Acad Sci USA* 78: 3877–3881

144 Klareskog L, Forsum U, Scheynius A, Kabelitz D, Wigzell H (1982) Evidence in support of a self-perpetuating HLA-DR-dependent delayed-type cell reaction in rheumatoid arthritis. *Proc Natl Acad Sci USA* 79: 3632–3636

145 Cuesta IA, Sud S, Song Z, Affholter JA, Karvonen RL, Fernández-Madrid F, Wooley PH (1997) T cell receptor (Vβ) bias in the response of rheumatoid arthritis synovial fluid T cells to connective tissue antigens. *Scand J Rheumatol* 26: 166–173

146 Snowden N, Reynolds I, Morgan K, Holt L (1997) T cell responses to human type II collagen in patients with rheumatoid arthritis and healthy controls. *Arthritis Rheum* 40: 1210–1218

147 van Schooten WCA, Devereux D, Ho CH, Quan J, Aguilar BA, Rust CJJ (1994) Joint-

derived T cells in rheumatoid arthritis react with self-immunoglobulin heavy chains or immunoglobulin-binding proteins that copurify with immunoglobulin. *Eur J Immunol* 24: 93–98
148 Leroux J-Y, Guerassimov A, Cartman A, Delaunay N, Webber C, Rosenberg LC, Banerjee S, Poole AR (1996) Immunity to the G1 globular domain of the cartilage proteoglycan aggrecan can induce inflammatory erosive polyarthritis and spondylitis in BALB/c mice but immunity to G1 is inhibited by covalently bound keratan sulfate *in vitro* and *in vivo*. *J Clin Invest* 97: 621–632
149 Singer II, Kawka DW, Bayne EK, Donatelli SA, Weidner JR, Williams HR, Ayala JM, Mumford RA, Lark MW, Glant TT et al (1995) VDIPEN, a metalloproteinase-generated neoepitope, is induced and immunolocalized in articular cartilage during inflammatory arthritis. *J Clin Invest* 95: 2178–2186
150 Mikecz K, Glant TT, Buzás E, Poole AR (1990) Proteoglycan-induced polyarthritis and spondylitis adoptively transferred to naive (nonimmunized) BALB/c mice. *Arthritis Rheum* 33: 866–876
151 Guerassimov A, Duffy C, Zhang Y, Banerjee S, Leroux J-Y, Reimann A, Webber C, Delaunay N, Vipparti V, Ronbeck L et al (1997) Immunity to cartilage link protein in patients with juvenile rheumatoid arthritis. *J Rheumatol* 24: 959–964
152 Blass S, Haferkamp C, Specker Ch, Schwochau M, Schneider M, Schneider EM (1997) Rheumatoid arthritis: autoreactive T cells recognising a novel 68k autoantigen. *Ann Rheum Dis* 56: 317–322
153 Nyirkos P, Golds EE (1990) Human synovial cells secrete a 39 kDa protein similar to a bovine mammary protein expressed during the non-lactating period. *Biochem J* 269: 265–268
154 Hakala BE, White C, Recklies AD (1993) Human cartilage gp-39, a major secretory product of articular chondrocytes and synovial cells, is a mammalian member of a chitinase protein family. *J Biol Chem* 268: 25803–25810
155 Johansen JS, Jensen HS, Price PA (1993) A new biochemical marker for joint injury. Analysis of YKL-40 in serum and synovial fluid. *Br J Rheumatol* 32: 949–955
156 Toyosaki T, Tsuruta Y, Yoshioka T, Takemota H, Suzuki R, Tomita T, Ochi T (1998) Recognition of rheumatoid arthritis synovial antigen by $CD4^+$, $CD8^-$ T cell clones established from rheumatoid arthritis joints. *Arthritis Rheum* 41: 92–100
157 Vaughn JH (1995) The Epstein-Barr virus in autoimmunity. *Springer Sem Immunopathol* 17: 203–230
158 Birkenfeld P, Haratz N, Klein G, Sulitzeanu D (1990) Cross-reactivity between the EBNA-1 p107 peptide, collagen, and keratin: implications for the pathogenesis of rheumatoid arthritis. *Clin Immunol Immunopathol* 54: 14–25
159 David-Ameline J, Lim A, Davodeau F, Peyrat MA, Berthelot JM, Semana G, Pannetier C, Gaschet J, Vie H, Even J et al (1996) Selection of T cells reactive against autologous B lymphoblastoid cells during chronic rheumatoid arthritis. *J Immunol* 157: 4697–4706
160 Scotet E, David-Ameline J, Peyrat MA, Moreau-Aubry A, Pinczon D, Lim A, Even J,

Semana G, Berthelot JM, Breathnach R et al (1996) T cell response to Epstein-Barr virus transactivators in chronic rheumatoid arthritis. *J Exp Med* 184: 1791–1800

161 van Eden W, Thole JER, van der Zee R, Noordzij A, van Embden JDA, Hensen EJ, Cohen IR (1988) Cloning of the mycobacterial epitope recognized by T lymphocytes in adjuvant arthritis. *Nature* 331: 171–173

162 Jones DB, Coulson AFW, Duff GW (1993) Sequence homologies between hsp60 and autoantigens. *Immunol Today* 14: 115–118

163 Holoshitz J, Klajman A, Drucker I, Lapidot Z, Yaretzky A, Frenkel A, van Eden W, Cohen IR (1986) T lymphocytes of rheumatoid arthritis patients show augmented reactivity to a fraction of mycobacteria cross-reactive with cartilage. *Lancet* 2: 305–309

164 Res PCM, Schaar CG, Breedveld FC, van Eden W, van Embden JDA, Cohen IR, de Vries RRP (1988) Synovial fluid T cell reactivity against 65 kD heat shock protein of mycobacteria in early chronic arthritis. *Lancet* 2: 478–480

165 Quayle AJ, Wilson KB, Li SG, Kjeldsen-Kragh J, Oftung F, Shinnick T, Forre O, Capra JD, Natvig JB (1992) Peptide recognition, T cell receptor usage and HLA restriction elements of human heat-shock protein (hsp) 60 and mycobacterial 65-kDa hsp-reactive T cell clones from rheumatoid synovial fluid. *Eur J Immunol* 22: 1315–1322

166 Celis L, Vandevyver C, Geusens P, Dequeker J, Raus J, Zhang J (1997) Clonal expansion of mycobacterial heat-shock protein-reactive T lymphocytes in the synovial fluid and blood of rheumatoid arthritis patients. *Arthritis Rheum* 40: 510–519

167 Pope RM, Lovis RM, Gupta RS (1992) Activation of synovial fluid T lymphocytes by 60-kd heat-shock proteins in patients with inflammatory synovitis. *Arthritis Rheum* 35: 43–48

168 De Graeff-Meeder ER, van der Zee R, Rijkers GT, Schuurman H-J, Kuis W, Bijlsma JWJ, Zegers BJ, van Eden W (1991) Recognition of human 60 kD heat shock protein by mononuclear cells from patients with juvenile chronic arthritis. *Lancet* 337: 1368–1372

Index

adhesion receptor 132
adjuvant arthritis (AA) 77
adjuvant property 79
AIDS, and rheumatoid arthritis (RA) 60
allergy 103
animal model 75
animal model, of reactive arthritis 176
animal, germ-free 78
ankylosing spondylitis (AS) 155
anti-Epstein-Barr virus (EBV) response 160
anti-Epstein-Barr virus (EBV) T cell response 157
antigen-induced arthritis (AIA) 76
antigen, retroviral 81
apoptosis 10
arthritis 81
arthritis, chronic 155
arthritis, juvenile chronic 20
arthritis, psoriatic 20
arthritis, reactive 162
asthma 103
autoantibody 103

B7-1 98
B7-2 98
BMLF1 155
bone resorption 101
Borrelia burgdorferi (Bb) 176
bystander suppression 86
BZLF1 155

cartilage glycoprotein gp39 216, 218
cathepsin 65
CD3 20
CD4 monoclonal antibody 190
$CD4^+$ clonal expansion 213
$CD4^+$ T cell 131, 201, 202, 204, 207
CD11 119, 120, 121
CD27 98
CD40 ligand 38
CD45 98
CD45RO 38
CD60 38
CD69 119, 120, 121
cell, dendritic 37
cell-cell contact 112, 117, 118
chemokine 138
chemokine-chemoattractant 62
chemokine receptor 112
Chlamydia trachomatis, target antigen 170
chlodronate 84
class II molecule, rheumatoid arthritis (RA)-associated 206
collagen-induced arthritis (CIA) 209
collagen type II (CII), reactive T cell clone 217
complementarity determining region 3 (CDR3) motif, homologous 214
complementarity determining region 3 (CDR3), in T cell receptor (TCR) 214
cross reactivity 79
cytokine balance 93
cytokine pattern, in Lyme arthritis 178

cytokine pattern, in reactive arthritis 172
cytokine synovium 62

DNA fragmentation 10, 11
DQ molecule, mouse transgenic for 217
DR4 (DRB1*0401) molecule 206
DR4 molecule, mouse transgenic for 217
DRB1*0404 molecule 207

endothelial cell 120, 131
Epstein-Barr virus (EBV) 149
Epstein-Barr virus (EBV) antigen 155, 218
Epstein-Barr virus (EBV) glycoprotein (gp) 110 208, 218
Epstein-Barr virus (EBV)-reactive T cell 155
extravasation 135

Felty's syndrome 31
fibroblast, synovial 36
Fisher rat, germ-free 82
flare interleukin-1 (IL-1) 83

GATA-3 99

heat shock protein (hsp) 36, 95, 208, 218
heat shock protein (hsp) 60, *Chlamydia trachomatis* 171
heat shock protein (hsp) 60, human 175
heat shock protein (hsp) 60, Yersinia 171, 172, 175
histopathology 1
human histocompatibility leukocyte antigen (HLA) class II association, in Lyme arthritis 179
human histocompatibility leukocyte antigen (HLA)-DR 3, 22, 201
human histocompatibility leukocyte antigen (HLA)-DR allele, associated with rheumatoid arthritis (RA) 202
human histocompatibility leukocyte antigen (HLA)-DR1 (DRB1*0101) molecule 206
human histocompatibility leukocyte antigen (HLA)-DR1 molecule, mouse transgenic for 217
human histocompatibility leukocyte antigen (HLA)-DRB1 4
- shared epitope 202
- shared epitope in rheumatoid arthritis (RA) 205
human type II collagen (CII) 206
HTLV-1 100

inflammation, chronic 134
inflammatory cytokine 134
interferon (IFN)-γ 173
interleukin-1 (IL-1) 117, 118
interleukin-4 (IL-4) 86, 93
interleukin-4 (IL-4), in reactive arthritis 173
interleukin-5 (IL-5) 93, 94
interleukin-6 (IL-6) 93
interleukin-10 (IL-10) 93
interleukin-12 (IL-12) 78, 96
interleukin-13 (IL-13) 93
interleukin-15 (IL-15) 64, 83
interleukin-16 (IL-16) 64
interleukin-17 (IL-17) 97
interleukin-1Ra (IL-1Ra) 118

joint destruction 55

large granular lymphocyte (LGL) leukemia 31
linkage disequilibrium 4
Lyme arthritis 100

major histocompatibility complex (MHC) 19
major histocompatibility complex (MHC) class II allele 201, 202
major histocompatibility complex (MHC) class II molecule, interaction with T cell in rheumatoid arthritis (RA) 204
matrix metalloproteinase (MMP) 65, 111, 113, 115, 117

membrane-associated cytokine 118
microbial component 77
molecular mimicry 206, 217
monoclonal antibody, against the CD7 protein 192
monoclonal antibody, against the CDw52 (Campath-1H) protein 192
monocyte-marcophage activation 117, 118
motif, peptide binding 205
mouse, transgenic 81, 209
MRL/lpr mouse model 57, 65
MRL-lpr/lpr mouse 80

OspA molecule 177
osteopontin 63, 65

p53 gene, somatic mutation of 11
p53 mutation 11, 57
p53 tumor suppressor gene 10
paracine cytokine network 8
pathogenesis, of reactive arthritis 174
peptide binding 205
peptide binding motif 206, 207
peripheral CD4+ T cell, clonal expansion of 216
polymerase chain reaction (PCR) 25
proto-oncogene 66
proto-oncogene expression 59
psoriatic arthritis (PA) 155

retroviral particle, in synovial fluid 61
retrovirus 100
rheumatoid arthritis (RA) 19, 129, 149
rheumatoid arthritis (RA), gene transfer 68
rheumatoid arthritis (RA), novel therapeutic strategy 68
rheumatoid arthritis (RA) pathogenesis 149, 160
rheumatoid arthritis (RA), severe combined immunodeficiency (SCID)-mouse model 60
Sag, autoimmunity in 161
sentrin 57
severe combined immunodeficiency (SCID) 10, 80
severe combined immunodeficiency (SCID)-mouse model 60
shared epitope 3, 4, 22, 205, 208
shared epitope, in disease susceptibility 209
single strand conformational polymorphism 25
Southern blotting 24
STAT 98
streptococcal cell wall (SCW) arthritis 76
superantigen 36, 213
synovial attachment 64
synovial cell 81
synovial hyperplasia 55, 56
synovial macrophage 84
synovial proliferation 56
synoviocyte 115, 120
synoviocyte, transformation of 9
synovium apoptosis 56

T cell 149, 151, 189
T cell, antigen specificity 151
T cell, autoreactive 161
T cell, in Lyme arthritis 176, 177
T cell, infiltration of 134
T cell, mycobacterial heat shock protein (hsp)65-reactive 219
T cell, oligoclonal expansion of 33
T cell, product of 5
T cell, synovial 30
T cell clonal expansion, frequency of 214
T cell clone 26
T cell frequency, antigen-specific 170
T cell hyporesponsiveness 7
T cell product 6
T cell receptor (TCR) 19, 150, 202
αβ T cell receptor (TCR) 21
γδ T cell receptor (TCR) 21
T cell receptor (TCR) diversity 154
T cell receptor (TCR) gene complex 202, 210
T cell receptor (TCR) gene polymorphism 21

T cell receptor (TCR) gene rearrangement 211
T cell receptor (TCR) gene usage 5
T cell receptor (TCR) gene utilization 5
T cell receptor (TCR), interaction with major histocompatibility complex (MHC) 207
T cell receptor (TCR) peptide vaccination 194
T cell receptor (TCR) A repertoire 213
T cell receptor (TCR) B repertoire 213
T cell receptor (TCR) repertoire 157, 207, 212
T cell receptor (TCR) repertoire formation 207
T cell receptor (TCR) repertoire in rheumatoid arthritis (RA) 211
T cell receptor (TCR) Vβ 150, 151
T cell recognition 205
T cell repertoire 149, 151, 153, 215
T cell response CD8, in reactive arthritis 171
T cell response, bacterium-specific 169
T cell response, CD4 reactive arthritis 170
T cell specificity 158
T cell vaccination 194
T helper type (Th) 1/Th2 subset, in reactive arthritis 172
T lymphocyte activation 117, 118
target antigen in rheumatoid arthritis (RA) 216
Th1 93
Th1/Th2 cell 112
Th2 93
Th3 96
thymus 20
tolerance 78, 82
tolerance, oral 195
transendothelial migration 137
trimolecular complex 204
tumor growth factor (TGF) β 86, 96
tumor necrosis factor (TNF) 79
tumor necrosis factor (TNF) α 117
tumor necrosis factor (TNF) α, in reactive arthritis 173
type II collagen (CII) 216

Vβ clonality 27
Vβ family 27
vasculature 131

Yersinia, target antigen 170

Zeitfracht Medien GmbH
Ferdinand-Jühlke-Straße 7
99095 Erfurt, Deutschland
produktsicherheit@kolibri360.de